Clinical Dilemmas in

Primary Liver Cancer

Clinical Dilemmas in

Primary Liver Cancer

EDITED BY

Roger Williams CBE, MD, FRCP, FRCS, FMedSci
Professor of Hepatology and Director
The Institute of Hepatology
The Foundation for Liver Research
London, UK

Simon D. Taylor-Robinson MD, DA, EUMS, FRCP
Professor of Translational Medicine
Clinical Dean of the Faculty of Medicine
Department of Medicine
Imperial College
London, UK

WILEY-BLACKWELL
A John Wiley & Sons, Ltd., Publication

Wiley-Blackwell is an imprint of John Wiley & Sons, formed by the merger of Wiley's global Scientific, Technical and Medical business with Blackwell Publishing.

Registered office: John Wiley & Sons, Ltd, The Atrium, Southern Gate, Chichester, West Sussex, PO19 8SQ, UK

Editorial offices: 9600 Garsington Road, Oxford, OX4 2DQ, UK
The Atrium, Southern Gate, Chichester, West Sussex, PO19 8SQ, UK
111 River Street, Hoboken, NJ 07030-5774, USA

For details of our global editorial offices, for customer services and for information about how to apply for permission to reuse the copyright material in this book please see our website at www.wiley.com/wiley-blackwell

Library of Congress Cataloging-in-Publication Data

Clinical dilemmas in primary liver cancer / edited by Roger Williams, Simon D. Taylor-Robinson.
p. ; cm.
Includes bibliographical references and index.
ISBN-13: 978-0-470-65797-3 (pbk. : alk. paper)
ISBN-10: 0-470-65797-9 (pbk. : alk. paper)
1. Liver–Cancer. 2. Liver–Cancer–Diagnosis. 3. Liver–Cancer–Treatment. I. Williams, Roger, 1931- II. Taylor-Robinson, Simon D.
[DNLM: 1. Carcinoma, Hepatocellular–diagnosis. 2. Carcinoma, Hepatocellular–therapy. 3. Hepatitis, Viral, Human. 4. Risk Factors. WI 735]
RC280.L5C57 2012
616.99′436–dc23

2011024816

A catalogue record for this book is available from the British Library.

This book is published in the following electronic formats: ePDF [9781119962175]; Wiley Online Library [9781119962205]; ePub [9781119962182]; Mobi [9781119962199]

Set in 8.75/12pt Minion by Aptara® Inc., New Delhi, India
Printed in Singapore by Ho Printing Singapore Pte Ltd

1 2012

Contents

List of contributors

Mehtan Ahmed, BSc, MBBS
Department of Medicine
Imperial College London
London, UK

Adil Al-Nahhas, MB ChB, MSc, FRCP
Professor of Nuclear Medicine
Chief of Service of Nuclear Medicine, Imperial College Health Care Trust
London, UK

Quentin M. Anstee, BSc, MBBS, PhD, MRCP(UK)
Senior Lecturer & Honorary Consultant Hepatologist
Institute of Cellular Medicine
Newcastle University & Liver Unit
Newcastle-Upon-Tyne, UK

Tara D. Barwick, MSc, FRCR, MRCP
Consultant Radiology and Nuclear Medicine
Imperial College Health Care NHS Trust
London, UK

Michel Beaugrand, MD
Service d'hépatologie
Hôpital Jean Verdier
Bondy, France
Université Paris XIII
France

Christopher Binny, PhD
Department of Haematology
UCL Cancer Institute
London, UK

Pierre-Alain Clavien, MD, PhD, FACS, FRCS(Eng), FRCS (Ed)
Professor and Chairman, Department of Visceral and Transplantation Surgery
University Hospital Zurich
Zurich, Switzerland

Massimo Colombo
Professor and Chairman, Department of Medicine, 1st Division of Gastroenterology
Fondazione IRCCS Ca' Granda Ospedale Maggiore Policlinico and University of Milan
Milan, Italy

Matthew E. Cramp, FRCP
Consultant Hepatologist and Honorary Reader
Plymouth Hospitals NHS Trust
Plymouth, UK

Marco Della Peruta, PhD
The Institute of Hepatology London
The Foundation for Liver Research
London, UK

Hashem B. El-Serag, MD, MPH
Chief, Gastroenterology and Hepatology
Michael E. DeBakey VA Medical Center
Baylor College of Medicine
Houston, TX, USA

Wladyslaw Gedroyc, MBBS, MRCP, FRCR
Professor of Radiology
MRI Unit
St. Mary's Hospital
Imperial College Health Care Trust
London, UK

Tim F. Greten, MD
Head, Gastrointestinal Cancer Section, National Cancer Institute, NIH
Bethesda, MD, USA

Christopher N. Hacking, BSc, MBBS, FRCP, FRCR
Consultant Radiologist
Southampton University Hospitals NHS Trust
Southampton, UK

Saeed Hamid, FRCP
The Ibn-e-Sina Chair and Professor
Department of Medicine
Aga Khan University
Karachi, Pakistan

Philip J. Johnson, MD, FRCP
Professor of Oncology and Translational Research
Director of the Cancer Research UK Clinical Trials Unit
University of Birmingham
Birmingham, UK

Jia-Horng Kao, MD, PhD
Distinguished Professor and Director
Graduate Institute of Clinical Medicine
National Taiwan University College of Medicine and Hospital
Taipei, Taiwan

John Karani
Consultant Radiologist and Clinical Director of Radiology
King's College Hospital
London, UK

Shahid A. Khan, BSc, MB, BS, PhD, FRCP
Clinical Senior Lecturer and Consultant Physician
Department of Medicine
Imperial College London
London, UK

Firouzeh Korangy, PhD
National Cancer Institute, Center for Cancer Research
Medical Oncology Branch
Bethesda, MD, USA

Pradesh Kumar, MB ChB, MRCS, FRCR
Interventional Radiology Fellow
Southampton General Hospital
Southampton, UK

Nimzing G. Ladep, MBBS, FWACP
Imperial College London
Hepatology Section
Department of Medicine
St. Mary's Hospital Campus
Imperial College London
London, UK;
Formerly: Senior Lecturer, University of Jos, Nigeria

Riccardo Lencioni, MD
Associate Professor of Radiology
Director, Division of Diagnostic Imaging and Intervention
University of Pisa School of Medicine
Pisa, Italy

Mickaël Lesurtel, MD, PhD
Senior Surgeon, Department of Visceral and Transplantation Surgery
University Hospital Zurich
Zurich, Switzerland

Adrian Lim, MD, FRCR
Consultant Radiologist and Reader in Radiology
Imperial College Health Care NHS Trust
Charing Cross Hospital
London, UK

Janice Main, MB ChB, FRCP
Reader & Honorary Consultant in Infectious Diseases and General Medicine
Department of Medicine
St. Mary's Hospital Campus
Imperial College London
London, UK

Hitoshi Maruyama, MD
Department of Medicine and Clinical Oncology
Graduate School of Medicine
Chiba University
Chiba, Japan

Ryota Masuzaki, MD, PhD
Research Fellow
Department of Gastroenterology
Graduate School of Medicine
University of Tokyo
Tokyo, Japan

Emmanuel Melloul, MD
Department of Visceral and Transplantation Surgery
University Hospital Zurich
Zurich, Switzerland

Tariq Moatter, PhD
Associate Professor
Head of Molecular Pathology
Department of Pathology and Microbiology
Aga Khan University
Karachi, Pakistan

Amit C. Nathwani, MD, PhD
Department of Haematology
UCL Cancer Institute
London, UK;
NHS Blood and Transplant, UK

Gisèle N'Kontchou, MD
Service d'hépatologie
Hôpital Jean Verdier
Bondy, France

Masao Omata, MD
President/Honorary Professor
Department of Gastroenterology
Yamanashi-Ken Hospital Organization, Yamanashi, Japan/University of Tokyo, Japan

Peter Ott, MD, Dr. Sc
Head of Medical Department V
Hepatology and Gastroenterology
Aarhus University Hospital
Aarhus, Denmark

Daniel H. Palmer, FRCP, PhD
Professor of Medical Oncology
University of Liverpool
Liverpool, UK

Timothy M. Pawlik, MD, MPH
Associate Professor of Surgery and Oncology
Hepatobiliary Surgery Program Director
Director, Johns Hopkins Medicine Liver Tumor Center Multi-Disciplinary Clinic
Johns Hopkins Hospital
Baltimore, MD, USA

Peter D. Peng, MD
Surgical Oncology Fellow
Johns Hopkins Hospital
Baltimore, MD, USA

Bernard C. Portmann, MD, FRCPath
Professor Emeritus
King's College Medical School
University of London, London, UK;
Former Consultant Histopathologist and Service-lead, Liver Pathology
King's College Hospital NHS Foundation Trust, London, UK

Tania Roskams, MD
Professor, Department of Morphology and Molecular Pathology
University Hospitals Leuven
Leuven, Belgium

Angelo Sangiovanni, MD
A.M. & A. Migliavacca Center for Liver Disease
1st Division of Gastroenterology
Fondazione IRCCS Ca' Granda Ospedale Maggiore Policlinico and University of Milan
Milan, Italy

Arun J. Sanyal, MBBS, MD
Charles Caravati Professor of Medicine
Division of Gastroenterology and Hepatology
Virginia Commonwealth University
Richmond, VA, USA

Myron Schwartz, MD
The Mount Sinai Medical Center
New York, NY, USA

Olivier Seror, MD, PhD
Service de radiologie
Hôpital Jean Verdier
Bondy, France
Université Paris XIII
France

Mohamed I.F. Shariff, MA (Oxon), BM BCh, MRCP
Specialist Registrar and Clinical Research Fellow
Department of Medicine
Imperial College London
London, UK

Simon D. Taylor-Robinson, MD, DA, EUMS, FRCP
Professor of Translational Medicine
Clinical Dean of the Faculty of Medicine
Department of Medicine
Imperial College London
London, UK

Mireille B. Toledano, BA (Hons), MSc, PhD, FHEA
Senior Lecturer in Epidemiology
School of Public Health
Imperial College London
London, UK

Roger Williams, CBE, MD, FRCP, FRCS, FMedSci
Professor of Hepatology and Director
The Institute of Hepatology London
The Foundation for Liver Research
London, UK

Abigail Zabron, BSc, PhD, MBBS, MRCP
Academic Clinical Fellow
Department of Medicine
Imperial College London
London, UK

Imene Zerizer, MSc, MRCP, FRCR
Specialist Registrar Radiology/Nuclear Medicine
Imperial College Health Care NHS Trust,
London, UK

Preface

In this book, *Clinical Dilemmas in Primary Liver Cancer*, we have attempted to provide an input into difficult issues of present-day clinical practice and management of patients with end-stage liver disease and primary hepatocellular cancer. Areas of uncertainly and lack of knowledge are highlighted wherever possible. The volume complements the first in the Clinical Dilemmas series on viral liver disease and is similar in style and layout. Similarly, it is not intended to be an exhaustive and comprehensive account of the subject as is found in standard textbooks. Assembled over a few months, the material is as up to date as it can be in such a rapidly changing field, and we are grateful to the contributors worldwide, who have made it possible, for their expertise and commitment. Our personal thanks to Elisabeth Dodds, Assistant Production Manager, and Oliver Walter, the Commissioning Editor at Wiley-Blackwell, and also to Enda O'Sullivan, Editorial Assistant in the Institute of Hepatology London.

There can be no doubt about the importance of primary hepatocellular cancer. The tumour is now the fifth most common cancer worldwide and third most frequent cause of death from cancer. Most encouragingly, with the high sensitivity of imaging techniques and the institution of surveillance programmes for those at most risk, the diagnosis can be made at an early stage when treatment by liver resection or radiofrequency ablation as well as liver transplantation prolongs survival and can even be curative. The proven effectiveness of the recently introduced oral agent sorafenib with its anti-angiogenesis and antiproliferation effects is widening horizons for future improvements in outcome. This volume, we hope, will help in encouraging the necessary investment in diagnostic and treatment facilities worldwide to reduce the scourge of this currently all-too-frequent cancer.

Professor Roger Williams, CBE
Professor Simon D. Taylor-Robinson

PART 1
Learning from a Worldwide Perspective

1 Are patterns and prevalence changing?

Hashem B. El-Serag
Michael E. DeBakey VA Medical Center, Baylor College of Medicine, Houston, TX, USA

LEARNING POINTS

- Hepatocellular carcinoma (HCC) is the most common primary liver malignancy, and in the absence of early detection through tumour surveillance, it is usually fatal with almost equal incidence and mortality rates in most parts of the world
- Most cases of HCC arise in those with established cirrhosis (annual rate of HCC in cirrhosis is 1–7%)
- Most cases of HCC are reported from hepatitis B virus (HBV) endemic areas in Southeast Asia and sub-Saharan Africa; many risk factors for HCC have been identified among those with chronic hepatitis C virus (HCV) or HBV
- There is a partly unexplained 2–4-fold increase in HCC risk in men, compared with women
- Viral hepatitis (HBV and HCV) is responsible for most cases of HCC worldwide
- The HCV epidemic in many regions, including the United States, has resulted in a recent dramatic increase in HCC incidence
- New risk factors for HCC include insulin resistance syndrome, manifesting as diabetes-related liver disease or obesity-related liver disease; given the high prevalence of these risk factors, even small increases in HCC risk may result in a considerable number of future HCC cases
- Apart from alcohol (which increases HCC risk) and coffee (which decreases HCC risk), the role of dietary factors is unclear

Liver cancer is the fifth most common cancer in men (522,000 cases, 7.9% of the total) and the seventh in women (225,000 cases, 6.5% of the total). Most of the burden is in developing countries, where almost 85% of the cases occur. Owing to its high fatality (overall ratio of mortality to incidence of 0.93), liver cancer is the third most common cause of death from cancer worldwide [1]. Hepatocellular carcinoma (HCC) accounts for 85–90% of all primary liver cancer (PLC) [2]. The aetiology of HCC, with more than 80% arising in patients infected by hepatitis B virus (HBV) or hepatitis C virus (HCV) [3], explains several features of the distinct geographic variations and temporal trends of liver cancer.

Figure 1.1 shows the considerable regional heterogeneity in the incidence of PLC worldwide. The highest age-standardised rates (ASRs) (more than 20 per 100,000 underlying population) are reported from countries in Southeast Asia (North and South Korea, China, Vietnam). These regions are endemic for HBV infection, with most PLC in these regions constituted by HCC. Exceptions to this generalisation include Thailand, where cholangiocarcinoma due to high exposure to liver flukes is the predominant form of PLC. Another exception is Japan, where HCV is the predominant risk factor for HCC in this high incidence area.

Owing to its very large population and high ASRs, China alone sees more than 55% of all PLC worldwide, with rates of 38–40 per 100,000 in males and 14–15 per 100,000 in females. Other high-incidence areas outside Southeast Asia include sub-Saharan African countries such as Cameroon and Mozambique. In general, countries in southern Europe have medium–high incidence rates (ASR in males: 10–15 per 100,000), with Italy on the high end with an ASR of 15.9 in men and 5.1 in women. Intermediate incidence areas (ASR: 5–10 per 100,000) include the United

Clinical Dilemmas in Primary Liver Cancer, First Edition. Edited by Roger Williams and Simon D. Taylor-Robinson.

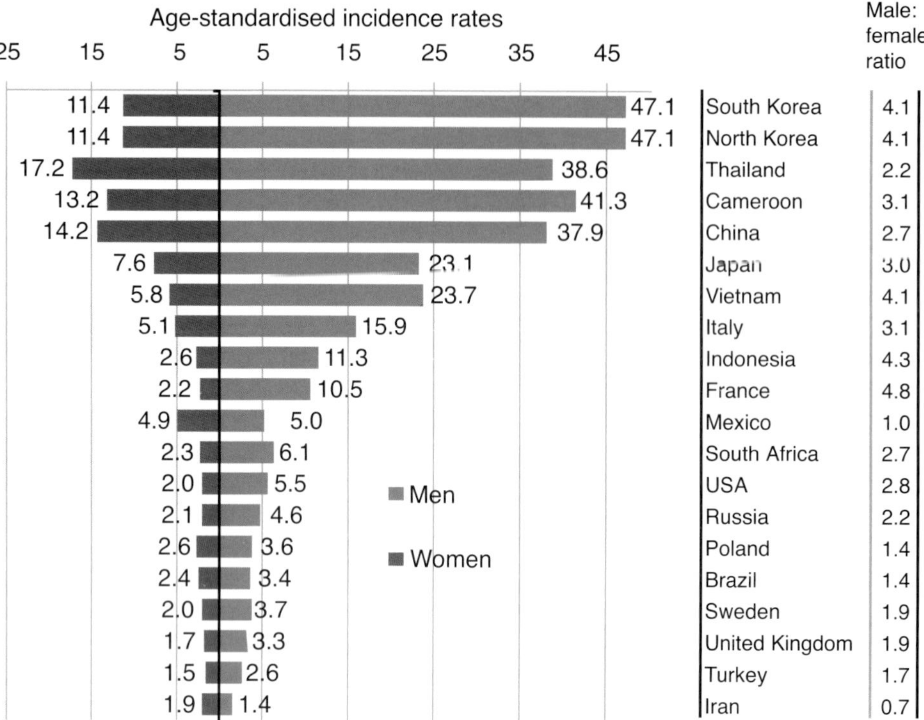

FIG 1.1 Age-standardised incidence rates of primary liver cancer per 100,000 population at risk. (GLOBOCAN 2002. The age-standardised rate is calculated using the 1960 world standard population.)

Kingdom (where cholangiocarcinoma is the commonest PLC), the United States, France and Germany. Low-incidence areas include South and Central America, Europe excluding the Mediterranean countries and North America (ASRs in males: less than 6 per 100,000).

There have been encouraging trends in liver cancer incidence in some high-rate areas [4], such as China, Japan and part of Europe, where HCC has been declining [5,6]. On the other hand, substantial increases in HCC incidence and mortality rates have been observed in areas previously considered low incidence in North America, Europe and Oceania. In these regions, HCV is the most frequent aetiologic risk factor, accounting for 30–50% of HCC cases. For example, incidence of HCC has tripled in the United States during the past two decades [7] and has become the most rapidly increasing cause of cancer-related deaths [8].

The median survival of PLC patients is estimated at less than 1 year [9]. There is considerable regional variation in mortality that tends to mirror those reported for incidence rates. In addition, there are also significant differences in the proportion of total cancer mortality attributable to PLC in different regions. For example, in Cameroon and Thailand, about one third of all cancer deaths are due to PLC, compared with less than 5% in most Western countries in Europe and North America.

Demographic features of HCC

Age

HCC is rare before age 40 and reaches a peak at around age 70. In low-risk populations (e.g. US, Canada, UK), the highest age-specific rates occur among persons 75 years and older. However, in Qidong, China, where HCC rates are among the world's highest, age-specific incidence rates among males rise until age 45 and then plateau. In all regions, female rates peak in the age group 5 years older than the peak age group for males. The variable age-specific patterns in different geographic regions are likely related to differences in the dominant hepatitis virus in the population, the age at viral infection and the existence of other risk factors.

Sex

There is a striking male predominance in HCC, with the highest male to female ratios seen in high and medium HCC incidence areas. HCC is more equally distributed among men and women in low-incidence countries in South and Central America. The prevalence of HBV, HCV, alcohol consumption and cigarette smoking is higher in men than in women. Some of the male predominance seen in HCC can be explained by higher cancer rates in males in general. A possible role of sex hormones in the development of HCC has also been suggested [10]. High serum testosterone levels have been associated with risk of HCC in nested case-control studies among HBV carriers in Taiwan and Shanghai [11].

Race/ethnicity

HCC incidence rates also vary substantially among different populations living in the same region. For example, ethnic Chinese populations of Singapore have considerably higher age-adjusted rates than Indians in the same region [12]. Another example, the age-adjusted HCC incidence rates in individuals of Asian/Pacific Islander ethnicity were almost three times higher than that in whites (ASRs 11.7 and 3.9, respectively), with Hispanics and blacks in between these two extremes (ASRs 8.0 and 7.0, respectively) [13]. Differences in the prevalence of the main risk factors may explain some of these differences; for example first generation immigrants from Southeast Asia have high HBV infection rates.

Risk factors for HCC

The main HCC risk factors are HBV, HCV, alcohol, aflatoxin and possible obesity and diabetes. Together HBV and HCV account for 80–90% of all HCC worldwide [3] (Table 1.1). Mendelian disorders (e.g. Wilson's disease, alpha-1 antitrypsin deficiency and hemochromatosis) account for a very small proportion of HCC. Cryptogenic or unknown aetiology HCC accounts for 15–30% of cases. Most HCC risk factors promote formation of cirrhosis, which is present in about 80–90% of HCC patients [14,15]. The risk of developing HCC in cirrhosis patients varies considerably with the underlying condition and severity of cirrhosis [16]. The highest 5-year cumulative risks are seen in HCV cirrhosis (30% in Japan and 17% in the West), hemochromatosis (21%), HBV cirrhosis (15% in Asia and 10% in the West), alcoholic cirrhosis (8%) and biliary cirrhosis (4%) [17].

TABLE 1.1 Estimated cases of primary liver cancer in 2002 attributable to HBV and HCV

	Primary liver cancer cases	HCV Attributable fraction (%)	HBV Attributable fraction (%)
Developed countries	110,800	23.3	19.9
Developing countries	515,300	58.8	33.4
Total	626,100	54.4	31.1

Source: Adapted from Parkin DM. The global health burden of infection-associated cancers in the year 2002. *Int J Cancer* 2006; 118(12):3030–3044.

HBV

Approximately 350 million people around the world are estimated to be chronically infected by HBV [18]. Worldwide, chronic HBV infection accounts for approximately 50% of HCC cases [19] with considerable regional variation (70% in South Korea, 10–15% in Japan [20], 3% in Sweden, 9% in the United States and 55% in Greece [21]). The lifetime risk of HCC for a person with a chronic HBV infection is between 10% and 25% [22], which is 15–20-fold higher than non-infected controls [23,24]. HBV is a notorious cause for HCC in the absence of cirrhosis; however, the great majority (70–90%) of HBV-related HCC develops in livers already afflicted by cirrhosis [2].

The increased HCC risk associated with HBV infection particularly applies to areas where HBV infection is endemic. In these areas, HBV is usually transmitted from mother to newborn (vertical transmission), and up to 90% of infected persons follow a chronic course. This pattern is different in areas with low HCC incidence rates, where HBV is acquired in adulthood through sexual and parenteral routes (horizontal transmission) with more than 90% of acute infections resolving spontaneously. The annual HCC incidence in chronic HBV carriers in Asia ranges between 0.4% and 0.6%, but is considerably lower in Caucasian HBV carriers [25].

Several additional factors increase HCC risk among HBV carriers, including male sex, older age, longer duration of infection, family history of HCC, exposure to aflatoxin, alcohol or tobacco or co-infection with HCV or delta hepatitis. HCC risk is also increased in patients with high levels of HBV hepatocellular replication, as indicated by high HBV DNA levels, presence of HBeAg [26] or HBV genotype C [27]. HBV DNA can also be detected in hepatitis B surface antigen (HBsAg)-negative individuals, but it has an unclear association with HCC risk There is moderately strong evidence that effective antiviral therapy that controls HBV infection in HBsAg-positive patients in viremic patients substantially reduces, but does not eliminate, HCC risk. One high-quality Taiwanese randomised controlled trial in patients with chronic HBV who had cirrhosis reported a significant reduction of HCC in patients treated with lamivudine for several years compared with placebo (3.9% vs. 7.4%; hazard ratio 0.49; $p = 0.047$) [28].

The risk of HCC is substantially lower in persons who are immune to HBV. For example, in the seminal study by Beasley et al. [29], the incidence of HCC was significantly lower in immune persons compared with carriers (5 vs. 495 per 100,000 per year) [29]. By using sensitive amplification assays, many studies have shown that HBV DNA persists as 'occult HBV infection' for decades among persons with serological recovery (HBsAg negative) from acute infection [30]. Although some studies have linked development of HCC in individuals with chronic HCV infection to occult HBV, others have not found an association. Frequently cited reports from Taiwan have described a reduction of HCC incidence rates in children 1–2 decades after the introduction of a universal vaccination programme against HBV [31].

Dietary aflatoxin

Aflatoxins are naturally occurring, potent hepatocarcinogenic mycotoxins produced by some *Aspergillus* species. They are moulds that grow on grains, corn, cassava, peanuts and fermented soy beans particularly under high moisture conditions in parts of sub-Saharan Africa and eastern Asia. Animal experiments demonstrated that AFB_1 is a powerful hepatocarcinogen, leading the International Agency for Research on Cancer to classify it as carcinogenic [32]. Once ingested, AFB_1 is metabolised to an active intermediate, AFB_1-*exo*-8,9-epoxide, which can bind to DNA and produce a characteristic mutation in the *p53* tumour suppressor gene (*p53 249*^{ser}) [33]. This mutation has been observed in 30–60% of HCC tumours in aflatoxin endemic areas [34,35]. Individuals infected by HBV and exposed to aflatoxin have an even higher risk of liver cancer, suggesting a synergistic effect between HBV and aflatoxin [36]. Though HBV vaccination in these areas should be the major preventive tactic, persons already chronically infected will not benefit from vaccination. However, HBV carriers could benefit by eliminating AFB_1 exposure. Efforts have been launched to accomplish this goal in China [37] and Africa [35].

HCV

The global HCV prevalence is estimated to be 2% and as high as 10% in Egypt [38]. It has been estimated that HCV began to infect large numbers of young adults in Japan in the 1920s and in southern Europe in the 1940s and in North America in the 1960s and 1970s as a result of contaminated needles and/or injection drug use [39]. The virus then migrated into national blood supplies and circulated until a screening test was developed in 1990, after which the rates of new infection dropped dramatically.

The association between HCV infection and increased HCC risk is well established and has been shown in case-control as well as cohort studies. Markers of HCV infection are found in a variable proportion of HCC cases, for example 45–65% in Italy [40,41] and 80–90% in Japan [42]. HCC risk increased 17–20-fold in HCV-infected patients compared with HCV-negative controls [43].

The rate of HCC development in HCV-infected persons ranges from 1% to 3% after 30 years of chronic infection [44]. HCV increases HCC risk by promoting fibrosis and eventually cirrhosis. Once cirrhosis is established, the annual incidence of HCC is 1–4% [16]. In HCV-infected patients, factors related to host and environment or lifestyle appear to be more important than viral factors in determining progression to cirrhosis. These factors include: older age overall as well as older age at the time of HCV acquisition, male sex, heavy alcohol intake (more than 50 g/day), diabetes, obesity and co-infection with HIV or HBV [45]. On the other hand, HCV viral load and HCV genotype have not been associated with HCC risk.

Alcohol

Heavy alcohol intake, defined as ingestion of more than 50–70 g/day for several years, is a well-established HCC risk factor. It is unclear whether the risk of HCC is significantly altered in those with low or moderate alcohol intake. There is evidence for a synergistic effect of heavy alcohol ingestion with HCV or HBV, with these factors presumably operating together to increase HCC risk by more actively promoting cirrhosis [43].

Fatty liver disease. Many studies conducted in Western countries fail to identify a major risk factor (HBV, HCV, alcohol) for chronic liver disease or HCC in a large proportion of patients (30–40%). Non-alcoholic fatty liver disease (NAFLD), including its more advanced form non-alcoholic steatohepatitis (NASH), has been proposed as the aetiologic factor for many cases of cryptogenic HCC. Insulin resistance has been proposed as the major pathogenic mechanism for this disorder as well as its progression to NASH. Obesity and diabetes are the major clinical manifestations of the insulin resistance syndrome.

There is epidemiologic evidence in support of a potential association between NAFLD/NASH and a modest increase in HCC risk. The few available population-based cohort studies of patients with NAFLD/NASH provide a modest support for this association [46,47]. Cross-sectional and case-control studies are limited due to the requisite histopathological features for confirmed NAFLD/NASH diagnosis being less evident, or even absent, once cirrhosis is established. Indirect evidence to the NAFLD–HCC association is provided by multiple cross-sectional and case-control studies showing significantly higher prevalence of obesity and diabetes among patients with cryptogenic cirrhosis compared with controls with other causes of liver disease [48–51]. It is clear that development of cirrhosis related to NASH signals a considerable increase in HCC risk. Most studies that evaluated cryptogenic cirrhosis or documented NASH-related cirrhosis reported high HCC incidence. While the progression of NAFLD/NASH to cirrhosis and NAFLD/NASH-related HCC may very well be infrequent, given vast and increasing prevalence, obesity and diabetes could still contribute a large HCC.

Obesity

It has been estimated that up to 90% of all obese individuals (BMI >30 kg/m^2) and up to 70% of all people with diabetes have some type of fatty liver disease [52]. The effect of obesity on HCC risk has been examined in several cohort studies. In a large prospective cohort study of more than 900,000 individuals from around the United States followed for a 16-year period, liver cancer mortality rates were 4.5 higher in men with a BMI >35 kg/m^2 and 1.7 higher in women with a BMI >35 kg/m^2, compared with normal-weight individuals [53]. Two other population-based cohort studies from Sweden and Denmark found a 2–3-fold increased HCC risk in obese men and women compared with those with normal BMI [54,55]. Diabetes, particularly type 2, has been proposed to be a risk factor for both chronic liver disease and HCC. Several case-control studies have examined the association between diabetes and HCC. The majority found a statistically significant association with 50–100% increased HCC risk in the presence of diabetes. However, reverse causality is a concern in all these studies because in some cases diabetes might itself be a result of cirrhosis. A few cohort studies, better suited to evaluate temporality, have been conducted, showing that individuals with type 2 diabetes had on average a doubled risk to develop HCC, with one showing an association between longer duration of diabetes and increased HCC risk [41,56]. Additional research is needed to examine how any excess risk conveyed by diabetes is mediated by the duration and treatment of diabetes, a family history of diabetes, by obesity and by physical activity.

Tobacco smoking

The relationship between cigarette smoking and HCC has been examined in more than 50 studies in both low- and high-rate areas. In almost all countries, both positive association and lack of association findings have been reported. Taken together, available evidence suggests that any effect of smoking on HCC is likely to be weak and limited to a subset of the general population.

Diet

The role of diet, except for alcohol and coffee drinking, in the aetiology of HCC in human populations is largely unknown. Coffee drinking has been studied extensively in relation to HCC. Several epidemiological studies have previously reported coffee drinking reduces risk of elevated liver enzymes and of cirrhosis, while animal studies suggest that coffee reduces liver carcinogenesis. Further, coffee drinking has also been associated with reduced insulin levels as well as reduced risk of type 2 diabetes, in itself considered to be a risk factor for HCC [57].

Both case-control and cohort studies conducted in Japan and Southern Europe specifically evaluated the relationship between coffee consumption and HCC risk, most reporting a significantly reduced risk of HCC with increased consumption [58–60].

Future trends

HBV continues to be the major HCC risk factor worldwide, although its importance will most likely decrease during the coming decades because of the widespread use of the HBV vaccine in the newborns in HBV endemic and HCC high-incidence areas. This effect may become more tangible as the first individuals to get immunised grow older. HCV has been the dominant viral cause in HCC in North America, some Western countries and Japan. Obesity and diabetes are increasing at a fast pace throughout the world, and if they are established as HCC risk factors, whether independently or in the presence of viral hepatitis or alcohol abuse, these conditions would plausibly account for more HCC cases in the future.

References

1. Ferlay J, Bray F, Pisani P, Parkin DM. GLOBOCAN 2000: Cancer Incidence, Mortality and Prevalence Worldwide, Version 1.0. IARC Cancer Base No. 5. IARC Press, Lyon; 2001. Available from: http://globocan.iarc.fr .
2. El-Serag HB, Rudolph KL. Hepatocellular carcinoma: epidemiology and molecular carcinogenesis. *Gastroenterology* 2007; 132(7):2557–2576.
3. Bosch FX, Ribes J, Cleries R, et al. Epidemiology of hepatocellular carcinoma. *Clin Liver Dis* 2005; 9(2):191–211, v.
4. McGlynn KA, Tsao L, Hsing AW, et al. International trends and patterns of primary liver cancer. *Int J Cancer* 2001; 94(2):290–296.
5. Bosetti C, Bianchi C, Negri E, et al. Estimates of the incidence and prevalence of hepatocellular carcinoma in Italy in 2002 and projections for the years 2007 and 2012. *Tumori* 2009; 95(1):23–27.
6. Jepsen P, Vilstrup H, Tarone RE, et al. Incidence rates of hepatocellular carcinoma in the US and Denmark: recent trends. *Int J Cancer* 2007; 121(7):1624–1626.
7. El-Serag HB. Hepatocellular carcinoma: recent trends in the United States. *Gastroenterology* 2004; 127(5 suppl 1):S27–S34.
8. Ries L, Melbert D, Krapcho M, et al. *SEER Cancer Statistics Review, 1975–2004.* National Cancer Institute, Bethesda, MD; 2007.
9. Nguyen VT, Law MG, Dore GJ. Hepatitis B-related hepatocellular carcinoma: epidemiological characteristics and disease burden. *J Viral Hepat* 2009; 16(7):453–463.
10. Yu MW, Chang HC, Chang SC, et al. Role of reproductive factors in hepatocellular carcinoma: Impact on hepatitis B- and C-related risk. *Hepatology* 2003; 38(6):1393–1400.
11. Yuan JM, Ross RK, Stanczyk FZ, et al. A cohort study of serum testosterone and hepatocellular carcinoma in Shanghai, China. *Int J Cancer* 1995; 63(4):491–493.
12. Parkin DM, Whelan SL, Ferlay J, Teppo L, Thomas DB. *Cancer Incidence in Five Continents,* Vol. VIII. IARC Scientific Publications No. 155. IARC Press, Lyon; 2002.
13. Altekruse SF, McGlynn KA, Reichman ME. Hepatocellular carcinoma incidence, mortality, and survival trends in the United States from 1975 to 2005. *J Clin Oncol* 2009; 27(9):1485–1491.
14. Colombo M, de FR, Del NE, et al. Hepatocellular carcinoma in Italian patients with cirrhosis. *N Engl J Med* 1991; 325(10):675–680.
15. Tiribelli C, Melato M, Croce LS, et al. Prevalence of hepatocellular carcinoma and relation to cirrhosis: comparison of two different cities of the world – Trieste, Italy, and Chiba, Japan. *Hepatology* 1989; 10(6):998–1002.
16. Fattovich G, Giustina G, Degos F, et al. Morbidity and mortality in compensated cirrhosis type C: a retrospective follow-up study of 384 patients. *Gastroenterology* 1997; 112(2): 463–472.
17. Fattovich G, Stroffolini T, Zagni I, et al. Hepatocellular carcinoma in cirrhosis: incidence and risk factors. *Gastroenterology* 2004; 127(5 suppl 1):S35–S50.
18. WHO. Hepatitis B. 2008 (Fact Sheet No. 204). 2010. 11-10-2009.
19. Parkin DM. The global health burden of infection-associated cancers in the year 2002. *Int J Cancer* 2006; 118(12): 3030–3044.
20. Kim SR, Kudo M, Hino O, et al. Epidemiology of hepatocellular carcinoma in Japan and Korea. A review. *Oncology* 2008; 75(suppl 1):13–16.
21. Raza SA, Clifford GM, Franceschi S. Worldwide variation in the relative importance of hepatitis B and hepatitis C viruses in hepatocellular carcinoma: a systematic review. *Br J Cancer* 2007; 96(7):1127–1134.
22. Seeger C, Mason WS. Hepatitis B virus biology. *Microbiol Mol Biol Rev* 2000; 64(1):51–68.
23. Donato F, Boffetta P, Puoti M. A meta-analysis of epidemiological studies on the combined effect of hepatitis B and C virus infections in causing hepatocellular carcinoma. *Int J Cancer* 1998; 75(3):347–354.
24. Shi J, Zhu L, Liu S, et al. A meta-analysis of case-control studies on the combined effect of hepatitis B and C virus infections in causing hepatocellular carcinoma in China. *Br J Cancer* 2005; 92(3):607–612.
25. McMahon BJ, Alberts SR, Wainwright RB, et al. Hepatitis B-related sequelae. Prospective study in 1400 hepatitis B surface antigen-positive Alaska native carriers. *Arch Intern Med* 1990; 150(5):1051–1054.

26. Chen CJ, Yang HI, Iloeje UH, REVEAL-HBV Study Group. Hepatitis B virus DNA levels and outcomes in chronic hepatitis B. *Hepatology* 2009; 49(5 suppl):S72–S84.
27. Yang HI, Yeh SH, Chen PJ, et al. Associations between hepatitis B virus genotype and mutants and the risk of hepatocellular carcinoma. *J Natl Cancer Inst* 2008; 100(16):1134–1143.
28. Liaw YF, Sung JJ, Chow WC, et al. Lamivudine for patients with chronic hepatitis B and advanced liver disease. *N Engl J Med* 2004; 351(15):1521–1531.
29. Beasley RP. Hepatitis B virus. The major etiology of hepatocellular carcinoma. *Cancer* 1988; 61(10):1942–1956.
30. Torbenson M, Thomas DL. Occult hepatitis B. *Lancet Infect Dis* 2002; 2(8):479–486.
31. Chang MH, Chen CJ, Lai MS, et al. Universal hepatitis B vaccination in Taiwan and the incidence of hepatocellular carcinoma in children. Taiwan Childhood Hepatoma Study Group. *N Engl J Med* 1997; 336(26):1855–1859.
32. IARC Monographs. *Overall evaluations of carcinogenicity: An updating of IARC monographs volumes 1–42.* Suppl. 7. Lyon: IARC Press 1987; 83–87.
33. Garner RC, Miller EC, Miller JA. Liver microsomal metabolism of aflatoxin B 1 to a reactive derivative toxic to Salmonella typhimurium TA 1530. *Cancer Res* 1972; 32(10):2058–2066.
34. Bressac B, Kew M, Wands J, et al. Selective G to T mutations of p53 gene in hepatocellular carcinoma from southern Africa. *Nature* 1991; 350(6317):429–431.
35. Turner PC, Sylla A, Diallo MS, Castegnaro JJ, Hall AJ, Wild CP. The role of aflatoxins and hepatitis viruses in the etiopathogenesis of hepatocellular carcinoma: a basis for primary prevention in Guinea-Conakry, West Africa. *J Gastroenterol Hepatol* 2002; 17(suppl):S441–S448.
36. Qian GS, Ross RK, Yu MC, et al. A follow-up study of urinary markers of aflatoxin exposure and liver cancer risk in Shanghai, People's Republic of China. *Cancer Epidemiol Biomarkers Prev* 1994; 3(1):3–10.
37. Yu S. Primary prevention of hepatocellular carcinoma. *J Gastoenterol Hepatol* 1995; 10:674–682.
38. Shepard CW, Finelli L, Alter MJ. Global epidemiology of hepatitis C virus infection. *Lancet Infect Dis* 2005; 5(9):558–567.
39. Armstrong GL, Alter MJ, McQuillan GM, et al. The past incidence of hepatitis C virus infection: implications for the future burden of chronic liver disease in the United States. *Hepatology* 2000; 31(3):777–782.
40. Fasani P, Sangiovanni A, De FC, et al. High prevalence of multinodular hepatocellular carcinoma in patients with cirrhosis attributable to multiple risk factors. *Hepatology* 1999; 29(6):1704–1707.
41. Stroffolini T, Andreone P, Andriulli A, et al. Gross pathologic types of hepatocellular carcinoma in Italy. *Oncology* 1999; 56(3):189–192.
42. Yoshizawa H. Hepatocellular carcinoma associated with hepatitis C virus infection in Japan: projection to other countries in the foreseeable future. *Oncology* 2002; 62(suppl 1): 8–17.
43. Donato F, Tagger A, Gelatti U, et al. Alcohol and hepatocellular carcinoma: the effect of lifetime intake and hepatitis virus infections in men and women. *Am J Epidemiol* 2002; 155(4):323–331.
44. Hassan MM, Frome A, Patt YZ, et al. Rising prevalence of hepatitis C virus infection among patients recently diagnosed with hepatocellular carcinoma in the United States. *J Clin Gastroenterol* 2002; 35(3):266–269.
45. Cramp ME. HBV + HCV = HCC? *Gut* 1999; 45(2):168–169.
46. Ong JP, Pitts A, Younossi ZM. Increased overall mortality and liver-related mortality in non-alcoholic fatty liver disease. *J Hepatol* 2008; 49(4):608–612.
47. Younossi ZM, Stepanova M. Hepatitis C virus infection, age, and Hispanic ethnicity increase mortality from liver cancer in the United States. *Clin Gastroenterol Hepatol* 2010; 8(8):718–723.
48. Abe H, Yoshizawa K, Kitahara T, et al. Etiology of non-B non-C hepatocellular carcinoma in the eastern district of Tokyo. *J Gastroenterol* 2008; 43(12):967–974.
49. Bugianesi E, Leone N, Vanni E, et al. Expanding the natural history of nonalcoholic steatohepatitis: from cryptogenic cirrhosis to hepatocellular carcinoma. *Gastroenterology* 2002; 123(1):134–140.
50. Marrero JA, Fontana RJ, Su GL, et al. NAFLD may be a common underlying liver disease in patients with hepatocellular carcinoma in the United States. *Hepatology* 2002; 36(6):1349–1354.
51. Regimbeau JM, Colombat M, Mognol P, et al. Obesity and diabetes as a risk factor for hepatocellular carcinoma. *Liver Transpl* 2004; 10(2 suppl 1):S69–S73.
52. Neuschwander-Tetri BA, Caldwell SH. Nonalcoholic steatohepatitis: summary of an AASLD Single Topic Conference. *Hepatology* 2003; 37(5):1202–1219.
53. Calle EE, Rodriguez C, Walker-Thurmond K, et al. Overweight, obesity, and mortality from cancer in a prospectively studied cohort of U.S. adults. *N Engl J Med* 2003; 348(17):1625–1638.
54. Moller H, Mellemgaard A, Lindvig K, et al. Obesity and cancer risk: a Danish record-linkage study. *Eur J Cancer* 1994; 30A(3):344–350.
55. Wolk A, Gridley G, Svensson M, et al. A prospective study of obesity and cancer risk (Sweden). *Cancer Causes Control* 2001; 12(1):13–21.
56. El-Serag HB, Tran T, Everhart JE. Diabetes increases the risk of chronic liver disease and hepatocellular carcinoma. *Gastroenterology* 2004; 126(2):460–468.

57. El-Serag HB, Hampel H, Javadi F. The association between diabetes and hepatocellular carcinoma: a systematic review of epidemiologic evidence. *Clin Gastroenterol Hepatol* 2006; 4(3):369–380.
58. Bravi F, Bosetti C, Tavani A, et al. Coffee drinking and hepatocellular carcinoma risk: a meta-analysis. *Hepatology* 2007; 46(2):430–435.
59. Montella M, Polesel J, La VC, et al. Coffee and tea consumption and risk of hepatocellular carcinoma in Italy. *Int J Cancer* 2007; 120(7):1555–1559.
60. Shimazu T, Tsubono Y, Kuriyama S, et al. Coffee consumption and the risk of primary liver cancer: pooled analysis of two prospective studies in Japan. *Int J Cancer* 2005; 116(1):150–154.

2 Why is the tumour different in Africa?

Nimzing G. Ladep
Hepatology Section, Department of Medicine, St. Mary's Hospital Campus, Imperial College London, London, UK

LEARNING POINTS

- Sub-Saharan Africa ranks second after Asia in the incidence and mortality of liver cancer
- Hepatitis B virus (HBV) is most frequently encountered risk factor, modified by aflatoxin, produced by contamination of food substrates by *Aspergillus spp.*
- Suboptimal management of liver diseases due to inadequate health financing, poor HBV vaccination coverage and iron overload syndromes associated with locally brewed alcohol drinks is contributory
- Whereas most sites have peak incidence of this cancer in the elderly, most African countries record high incidence during the middle age
- With a high HIV co-infection of hepatitis B and C in this region, and more people living with the virus, information about the contribution of HIV to the known risk factors might soon become available
- There is a dire need for cheap and socially acceptable screening systems for the detection of early liver cancer if the picture of 'enlarged painful liver', characterising a typical patient from this region, is to change
- Collaborations are encouraged with scientists working in Africa to work in the area of prevention, treatment and control of risk factors for hepatocellular carcinoma (HCC)
- Screening for early carcinoma using conventional as well as investigational methods (metabonomics and proteomics) and treatment of early tumour will be beneficial contribution to this region

Introduction

Hepatocellular carcinoma (HCC) is a commonly occurring tumour worldwide, with at least half of the 600,000 associated global deaths occurring in China alone and majority of the other 300,000 deaths occurring in the sub-Saharan African region. There are many factors responsible for the distinct epidemiological patterns seen in Africa with vertical or horizontal transmission at an early age, environmental interplay with food contaminants such as aflatoxins, suboptimal management of predisposing disease conditions such as chronic hepatitis B and cirrhosis and poorly managed strategies for health delivery, including absent neonatal vaccination for hepatitis B in many countries.

The global high case fatality associated with HCC is most significant in Africa. The countries in the sub-Saharan African region present with HCC incidence mortality ratio close to unity owing to very late patient presentation, when very little can be offered to them. Some reasons that are discussed for this dismal picture are: (i) high prevalence of risk factors, such as viral hepatitis with HIV co-infection; (ii) failure to recognise those at risk; (iii) absence of effective management of the risk factors as a result of inadequate medical expertise; and (iv) inadequate facilities for early diagnosis. Additionally, lack of surveillance systems, as well as absence of treatment for those diagnosed with early HCC, has also contributed in no small measure to the overall burden of the disease. As a result of these, the dictum 'An adult African who presents with upper abdominal

Clinical Dilemmas in Primary Liver Cancer, First Edition. Edited by Roger Williams and Simon D. Taylor-Robinson.

pain and an enlarged, hard, nodular liver should be considered a case of hepatocellular carcinoma' has since become adopted as the most frequent presentation for HCC. This is contrasted to the Western society that has enough capacity to detect some cases early enough for curative management. Moreover, sorafenib, a recently licensed drug shown to have potent activity in the management of advanced HCC, is too expensive for sufferers in this region of the world.

The burden of liver cancer in sub-Saharan Africa

The distribution of HCC in Africa is very diverse. Areas of high incidence include the Gambia, Guinea and Senegal in West Africa. In these countries, the incidence in men has been documented to range between 30/100,000 and 50/100,000 and in women, 12/100,000–20/100,000 [1]. In Rwanda and the Democratic Republic of Congo (countries in Central Africa), the estimated rate is 15.4/100,000 men and 8.9/100,000 women. Mozambique, a Southern African country, has always led the league table in the incidence of this disorder. Early reports date back as far as 1965 [2] and latter data have shown only slight decline in HCC incidence in Mozambique [3]. There is stable rate in the incidence among men in Uganda and about 50% increase in females over 30-year period [4]. A tertiary hospital-based cancer centre in Nigeria did not demonstrate any trend over time in this highly populated country [5].

The poor survival of these patients leading to premature death, rather than long-term illness, is most illustrated in the African context. Most of the affected people are at the most productive age of their lives, suggesting that HCC contributes in no small measure in reducing the economic productivity of this region of the world. Whereas the incidence of HCC in more developed countries of the world, as well as East Asia peaks in people above 75 years of age, younger age of highest incidence is the case in most African countries. The male rates in countries like the Gambia and Mali tend to peak between 60 and 65, while that of females peak at 65 and 75. Younger age peaks of 40 years have been described in some countries in this region [6]. Data from the International Agency for Research on Cancer demonstrate that although the age-specific mortality rate of this cancer in 2007 is highest in Japan, a further look at the lower age range, 20–44, featured South Africa leading in the mortality figures. Some of the reasons for the distinct characteristics of HCC in Africa are discussed in the following sections.

High prevalence of risk factors

The most common risk factors for HCC are the infectious viral agents hepatitis B virus (HBV) and hepatitis C virus (HCV). HBV is endemic in Africa, and the prevalence of HBV in different parts of Africa, documented using hepatitis B surface antigen (HBsAg), highlights this (Plate 2.1). Although there are different rates of this virus in the sub-Saharan region, with some up to 20% [7], all countries in this region are in the endemic zone. Of the worldwide 1.5 million deaths attributable to HBV-related illnesses, about 20% occur in sub-Saharan Africa.

More Africans have longer durations of HBV infections than individuals in the developed world who acquire the infection much later in life. Eighty per cent of persons in Africa acquire HBV by age 10 years [8] with consistently high carrier rates up to 20% leading to proportional proneness to HCC. Inadequate data representation might actually be downplaying the true burden of HBV and its sequel (liver cancer) in many African countries.

HCV infection is also prevalent in Africa, though most significantly associated with HCC in the developed world. Though the transmission route in this region is not well established and most cases are thought to be due to use of unsterile sharps during injections at drugstores, traditional practices such as tattoos and reception of unscreened blood products are widespread; sexual transmission is thought to be rare [9]. Until early 2000, blood products were not being screened for HCV because of an incorrect assumption that it was not cost-effective to screen for it as the prevalence of this virus was thought to be insignificant in most African countries. However, some of the highest prevalence of HCV is in Africa, with Egypt badly affected [10]. The central African region (Cameroon, Gabon, Congo-Brazzaville and Central African Republic) has the highest prevalence in sub-Saharan Africa, estimated at 6% (twice the world average), with West Africa at 2.5–9.9%, while Southern and East Africa coming in at 1.6% [9]. The overall import of this is the fact that HCV is contributing in no small way to the whole burden of HCC in Africa.

Multiracial studies of HCC have demonstrated that the prevalence of this tumour is higher among blacks than Caucasians. A study from the United States showed that of a population of HBV-associated HCC, 6% were whites compared with 16% blacks and 50% Asians [1,11]. A genetic polymorphism distinct to the black races of Africa might be playing a role in the aggressive nature of this disease. Studies of the cirrhosis-engendering potential of HBV have been postulated to be distinct for each viral genotype in different populations. The distribution of HBV differs from one region to another. For example, genotype E is restricted to Africa, genotypes B and C more prevalent in Southeast Asia, China and Japan, and genotype F is found in Central and South America [12]. There is evolving evidence to suggest that these genotypes may influence the clinical outcomes of patients with chronic HBV infection. Studies from Asia have demonstrated an increase in the development of HCC among patients with HBV genotype C compared with genotype B [13–16]. However, this association is controversial and remains a subject of further studies. These studies may demonstrate that the carcinogenic potential of the genotype subsisting in Africa produces characteristically aggressive tumour found in this region. Kew and co-workers in South Africa recently showed that HBV genotype A had a greater hepatocarcinogenic potential than non-A genotypes [17]. Collaborative studies between centres in Africa and the developed world would be helpful to investigate this hypothesis. The roles of iron overload and aflatoxin are discussed in Section 'Contribution of other factors'.

Failure to recognise those at risk

Many patients in this region of the world get to know their HBV status only at diagnosis of the tumour. This late diagnosis, as it applies to many other diseases in Africa, is worse for HCC and is not explained by health-seeking behaviour only. A less than satisfactory health care system leading to many HBsAg-positive patients resorting to herbal and alternative medications that potentially worsen liver function, complicating the whole picture might be plausible. Many cases of liver failure might have resulted from this malady. Few individuals who want to get quality care for their HBV hardly receive adequate management; hence, an unabated tendency to progress to cirrhosis. It is a known fact that more than 80% of HCCs in HBV patients among the Africans arise in a background of cirrhosis, in contrast to a lower proportion in developed regions [18]. Malignancy on a poor hepatic reserve with superimposed toxic substances (as these remedies have unknown compositions) in most instances tips the patients to develop liver failure sooner than later.

Poor HBV vaccine coverage

Countries that introduced HBV vaccine have recorded significant declines in childhood HCCs. The Gambia Hepatitis Intervention Study (GHIS), a study within the region, has shown that the vaccine is capable of decreasing chronic HBsAg carrier status by more than 83% [19]. Similar results have been obtained in South Africa and Senegal [20,21]. Despite these observations, only a handful of African countries have ensured adequate coverage in their national immunisation programmes as of 2008. The high cost of this vaccine on one hand and the technical difficulty on another might be the mitigating factors towards ensuring the massive implementation of HBV vaccination programmes in this part of the world. Moreover, the Global Alliance for Vaccines and Immunisation (GAVI) funding supporting HBV vaccination programmes has led to a little change in the coverage in sub-Saharan Africa, suggesting a significant logistic difficulty interplaying more than poor health budgets. As at 2007, the HBV vaccine coverage for Africa was dwindling at 69%.

Contribution of other factors

Aflatoxin, a mycotoxin produced by *Aspergillus spp.*, grows on a large number of substrates, including corn, peanuts and cassava, under high-moisture conditions in parts of Africa and eastern Asia. These foods are staples in Africa, some of which are consumed unprocessed (ground nuts). Subsistence farming, poor farm produce storage and suboptimal processing systems facilitate the dissemination of this organism; thus exposing the populace to its carcinogenic toxin. Studies to establish the role of aflatoxin in the carcinogenesis of the liver are being carried out. Chronic HBV and aflatoxin can act synergistically to increase the risk of HCC, but the underlying cellular and molecular mechanisms of interaction are still being studied. A possibility suggested by studies in HBV transgenic mice is that chronic liver damage alters the expression of carcinogen-metabolising proteins, modulating the level of binding of aflatoxin to DNA [22]. The ultimate result is the inhibition of cytochrome p53, leading to the prevention of apoptosis of damaged hepatocytes. Moreover, researchers in the Gambia have shown that exposure to aflatoxin, assessed both by high lifetime groundnut (peanut) intake and by the presence of the 249 (ser) TP53 mutations in plasma, is associated with a significant increase in the risk of cirrhosis [23].

The contribution of alcohol to HCC in Africa is quite intriguing. Although anecdotally more quantity of alcohol is consumed in the developed world, early reports have indicated a link between the locally brewed fermented drinks in Africa and HCC. These studies postulated that the containers within which these beverages are brewed release iron in vivo, leading to an 'iron overload syndrome' akin to primary haemochromatosis. Severe iron overload is prevalent in more than 10% in some populations in sub-Saharan Africa [24,25]. Iron absorption is enhanced in the presence of alcohol. A synergistic role by these two factors is suggested to raise HCC risk by more actively promoting cirrhosis in chronically infected HBV or HCV patients. In 1998, iron levels were demonstrated to be higher among Africans with liver cancer than controls by an odds ratio of up to 10.6 [26]. Although excess iron is excreted by normal individuals, this becomes altered in the face of a genetic mutation. Polymorphism in the ferroportin 1 (protein for iron excretion) gene has been demonstrated in samples of subjects from Southern Africa [27]. The risk of primary haemochromatosis to develop HCC increases 200-folds in those who are above 55 years of age, seropositive for HBsAg and who drink excess alcohol [28,29]. More widespread studies in the countries of this region are required to establish the role of iron overload versus ferroportin 1 polymorphism in the enhanced carcinogenic potential of HBV in chronically infected Africans.

HBV/HCV co-infection of HIV

Although both HBV and HIV are highly prevalent in Africa, reports on the impact of HIV and how it may alter the natural history of HBV have been lacking from this region. Africa stands to yield substantial data in the wake of HIV/AIDS pandemic. Several cohort studies in the developed world have established a definite link between HIV/HBV and HIV/HCV co-infections and higher mortality rates associated with HCC than either infections alone [30,31]. Before the provision of antiretrovirals and international funding for highly active antiretroviral treatment (HAART) to Africa, most of these patients died earlier because of opportunistic infections than they could survive long enough for complications of HBV or HCV (cirrhosis and HCC) to be noted. With successes recorded in well-monitored HAART centres [32], most co-infected patients are expected to survive longer and may probably contribute to the burden of HCC in the future. Also, the impact of HIV infection on the long-term efficacy of the HBV vaccine in this part of the world is yet to be determined and might pose grave consequences for the gains already made in places that have attained a wide coverage [33].

Inadequate management of liver diseases

The management of patients with liver diseases predisposing to HCC is suboptimal in many countries of Africa. Lack of trained medical personnel, poor training curricula, 'brain-draining' of medical professionals and absence of guidelines locally adaptable to these countries are contributory. Poor funding of the health sectors, besides low performance, are in no small measure significant towards this. In a recently published review, an example of this was highlighted in a highly populated country in West Africa [34]. The public expenditure on health is four times less than the $34 per capita internationally recommended for this country [34]. Because of poor or non-functional referral systems, many of the primary health care facilities serve only about 10% of their potential patient load. These inefficient referral systems in some parts of Africa contribute in no small way to the poor outcome of patients with liver diseases. In a few cases, some persons get referred when discovered at blood donation campaigns.

There is insufficient public health action and a flourishing of self-acclaimed 'curers' of hepatitis. The contribution of this alternative medication to the burden of HCC is enormous, yet remains undocumented and treated with levity by health authorities. The situation is worse in one country as those who should be making policies claim to possess cure and treat patients without firm scientific proof of the potency of their concoctions and methods. With general lack of confidence in the health system, many patients seek care from these set-ups.

There is paucity of sound epidemiological programmes that could provide advice to governments in this region such that what is being reported in literature is only a 'tip of the iceberg' as research data emerge from pockets of investigations within the continent. With HBsAg and anti-HCV prevalence of 15–20% and 2.9–10.3% respectively in Nigeria, it was only in 2009 that a guideline for the management of HBV was produced. With the prohibitive cost of antivirals and a non-insured system of health care where the patient pays for services, only those who can afford get treated. The ultimate result of this is that a large pool of those who could have been 'cured' of their disease goes on to develop HCC.

Lack of surveillance systems

Early HCC is often asymptomatic. The majority of HCC are detected at advanced stages, particularly profound in Africa where patients seek medical advice late in the disease [35]. This precludes curative treatment. The advantage of surveillance of at-risk populations with attempts to decrease mortality from HCC has been documented by Zhang and colleagues, who observed that a 6-monthly alpha-fetoprotein and ultrasound surveillance significantly reduced HCC mortality by 37% compared with a non-surveyed disease population [36]. The absence of surveillance programmes in most parts of this region could account for the dismal prognosis of this tumour in Africa. In a bold attempt to mitigate this gap in the screening for HCC in developing countries, The World Gastroenterology Organisation has proposed simplified modalities for intervening based on the resources of each region. The governments of Africa are essential partners in the implementation of this guideline.

Conclusions

Regional efforts and future work

HCC is a major cause of cancer-related death in sub-Saharan Africa, approaching 200,000 deaths each year [37]. The fact that this tumour presents in an aggressively rapid manner and in a younger population than occurs elsewhere gives room for postulation of the interplay of multiple factors in African. Poor health service provision, insufficient personnel and specialists, lack of adherence to or absence of guidelines for the treatment of at-risk populations as well as lackadaisical governmental commitment to health delivery are among these factors. Demonstrated intervention programmes using HBV vaccine administration, such as the Gambia Hepatitis Intervention Study, has encouraged some governments to include the vaccine in their national immunisation schedules. Implementation teething problems continue to tone down the coverage of this programme in many countries. Reduction to aflatoxin exposure after harvest of crops in Guinea has led to less contamination of staple foods and individual exposures [38]. This effort is feasible and requires a multisocial approach in terms of the provision of long-term education, adequate storage facilities and mechanised farming systems among others. No doubt, a sturdy governmental commitment is a desirable in this regard. Systems to attract and retain specialists in public health response, upgraded annual health budgets, funding of national cancer registries with supportive histopathology laboratories and aggressive HBV vaccination campaigns should be in place.

For these interventions to begin to yield results, there is a pool of at-risk population that will go on to develop HCC in Africa. It has been suggested that the burden of HCC in this region is likely to get higher than currently observed in the next 40–50 years [39]. Novel programmes aimed at comprehensive care for patients with HBV are underway. Large data is expected from this endeavour that will inform further care to the best epidemiological approaches to this problem. More energetic systems are invited to help combat HCC in Africa, including prevention and treatment of risk factors for HCC as well as screening for early carcinoma, using conventional and investigational methods (metabonomics and proteomics) as well as treatment of incident cases.

References

1. Nordenstedt H, White DL, El-Serag HB. The changing pattern of epidemiology in hepatocellular carcinoma. *Dig Liver Dis* 2010; 42(suppl 3):S206–S214.
2. Oettle AG. Cancer in Africa, especially in regions south of the Sahara. *J Natl Cancer Inst* 1964; 33:383–439.
3. Prates MD, Torres FO. A cancer survey in Lourenco Marques, Portuguese East Africa. *J Natl Cancer Inst* 1965; 35(5): 729–757.
4. Harington JS, Bradshaw EM, McGlashan ND. Changes in primary liver and esophageal cancer rates among black goldminers, 1964–1981. *S Afr Med J* 1983; 64(17):650.
5. Ocama P, Nambooze S, Opio CK, Shiels MS, Wabinga HR, Kirk GD. Trends in the incidence of primary liver cancer in Central Uganda, 1960–1980 and 1991–2005. *Br J Cancer* 2009; 100(5):799–802.
6. Echejoh GO, Tanko MN, Manasseh AN, Ogala-Echejoh S, Ugoya SO, Mandong BM. Hepatocellular carcinoma in Jos, Nigeria. *Niger J Med* 2008; 17(2):210–213.
7. Seleye-Fubara D, Jebbin NJ. Hepatocellular carcinoma in Port Harcourt, Nigeria: clinicopathologic study of 75 cases. *Ann Afr Med* 2007; 6(2):54–57.
8. Barin F, Perrin J, Chotard J, et al. Cross-sectional and longitudinal epidemiology of hepatitis B in Senegal. *Prog Med Virol* 1981; 27:148–162.

9. Kew MC, Rossouw E, Hodkinson J, Paterson A, Dusheiko GM, Whitcutt JM. Hepatitis B virus status of southern African Blacks with hepatocellular carcinoma: comparison between rural and urban patients. *Hepatology* 1983; 3(1): 65–68.
10. Madhava V, Burgess C, Drucker E. Epidemiology of chronic hepatitis C virus infection in sub-Saharan Africa. *Lancet Infect Dis* 2002; 2(5):293–302.
11. Hassan MM, Zaghloul AS, El-Serag HB, et al. The role of hepatitis C in hepatocellular carcinoma: a case control study among Egyptian patients. *J Clin Gastroenterol* 2001; 33(2): 123–126.
12. Di Bisceglie AM, Lyra AC, Schwartz M, et al. Hepatitis C-related hepatocellular carcinoma in the United States: influence of ethnic status. *Am J Gastroenterol* 2003; 98(9): 2060–2063.
13. Tangkijvanich P, Mahachai V, Komolmit P, Fongsarun J, Theamboonlers A, Poovorawan Y. Hepatitis B virus genotypes and hepatocellular carcinoma in Thailand. *World J Gastroenterol* 2005; 11(15):2238–2243.
14. Kao JH, Chen PJ, Lai MY, Chen DS. Hepatitis B genotypes correlate with clinical outcomes in patients with chronic hepatitis B. *Gastroenterology* 2000 ; 118(3):554–559.
15. Fujie H, Moriya K, Shintani Y, Yotsuyanagi H, Iino S, Koike K. Hepatitis B virus genotypes and hepatocellular carcinoma in Japan. *Gastroenterology* 2001 ; 120(6):1564–1565.
16. Fung SK, Lok AS. Hepatitis B virus genotypes: do they play a role in the outcome of HBV infection? *Hepatology* 2004; 40(4):790–792.
17. Kew MC, Kramvis A, Yu MC, Arakawa K, Hodkinson J. Increased hepatocarcinogenic potential of hepatitis B virus genotype A in Bantu-speaking sub-saharan Africans. *J Med Virol* 2005; 75(4):513–521.
18. El-Serag HB, Rudolph KL. Hepatocellular carcinoma: epidemiology and molecular carcinogenesis. *Gastroenterology* 2007; 132(7):2557–2576.
19. van der Sande MA, Waight P, Mendy M, et al. Long-term protection against carriage of hepatitis B virus after infant vaccination. *J Infect Dis* 2006; 193(11):1528–1535.
20. Hino K, Katoh Y, Vardas E, Sim J, Okita K, Carman WF. The effect of introduction of universal childhood hepatitis B immunization in South Africa on the prevalence of serologically negative hepatitis B virus infection and the selection of immune escape variants. *Vaccine* 2001; 19(28–29): 3912–3918.
21. Coursaget P, Leboulleux D, Soumare M, et al. Twelve-year follow-up study of hepatitis B immunization of Senegalese infants. *J Hepatol* 1994; 21(2):250–254.
22. Turner PC, Sylla A, Diallo MS, Castegnaro JJ, Hall AJ, Wild CP. The role of aflatoxins and hepatitis viruses in the etiopathogenesis of hepatocellular carcinoma: A basis for primary prevention in Guinea-Conakry, West Africa. *J Gastroenterol Hepatol* 2002; 17(suppl): S441–S448.
23. Kuniholm MH, Lesi OA, Mendy M, et al. Aflatoxin exposure and viral hepatitis in the etiology of liver cirrhosis in the Gambia, West Africa. *Environ Health Perspect* 2008; 116(11): 1553–1557.
24. Gordeuk VR, Boyd RD, Brittenham GM. Dietary iron overload persists in rural sub-Saharan Africa. *Lancet* 1986; 1(8493):1310–1313.
25. Gordeuk VR. Hereditary and nutritional iron overload. *Baillieres Clin Haematol* 1992; 5(1):169–186.
26. Mandishona E, MacPhail AP, Gordeuk VR, et al. Dietary iron overload as a risk factor for hepatocellular carcinoma in Black Africans. *Hepatology* 1998; 27(6):1563–1566.
27. Gordeuk VR, Caleffi A, Corradini E, et al. Iron overload in Africans and African-Americans and a common mutation in the SCL40A1 (ferroportin 1) gene. *Blood Cells Mol Dis* 2003; 31(3):299–304.
28. Fargion S, Piperno A, Fracanzani AL, Cappellini MD, Romano R, Fiorelli G. Iron in the pathogenesis of hepatocellular carcinoma. *Ital J Gastroenterol* 1991 ; 23(9):584–588.
29. Colombo M, de FR, Del NE, et al. Hepatocellular carcinoma in Italian patients with cirrhosis. *N Engl J Med* 1991; 325(10):675–680.
30. Thio CL, Seaberg EC, Skolasky R, Jr., et al. HIV-1, hepatitis B virus, and risk of liver-related mortality in the Multicenter Cohort Study (MACS). *Lancet* 2002; 360(9349):1921–1926.
31. Hoffmann CJ, Charalambous S, Thio CL, et al. Hepatotoxicity in an African antiretroviral therapy cohort: the effect of tuberculosis and hepatitis B. *AIDS* 2007; 21(10):1301–1308.
32. Idoko JA, Agbaji O, Agaba P, et al. Direct observation therapy-highly active antiretroviral therapy in a resource-limited setting: the use of community treatment support can be effective. *Int J STD AIDS* 2007; 18(11):760–763.
33. Burnett RJ, Francois G, Kew MC, et al. Hepatitis B virus and human immunodeficiency virus co-infection in sub-Saharan Africa: a call for further investigation. *Liver Int* 2005; 25(2):201–213.
34. Ladep NG, Taylor-Robinson SD. Management of liver disease in Nigeria. *Clin Med* 2007; 7(5):439–441.
35. Shariff MI, Cox IJ, Gomaa AI, Khan SA, Gedroyc W, Taylor-Robinson SD. Hepatocellular carcinoma: current trends in worldwide epidemiology, risk factors, diagnosis and therapeutics. *Expert Rev Gastroenterol Hepatol* 2009; 3(4): 353–367.

36. Zhang BH, Yang BH, Tang ZY. Randomized controlled trial of screening for hepatocellular carcinoma. *J Cancer Res Clin Oncol* 2004; 130(7):417–422.
37. Parkin DM. The global health burden of infection-associated cancers in the year 2002. *Int J Cancer.* 2006; 118(12): 3030–3044.
38. Turner PC, Sylla A, Gong YY, et al. Reduction in exposure to carcinogenic aflatoxins by postharvest intervention measures in west Africa: a community-based intervention study. *Lancet* 2005; 365(9475):1950–1956.
39. Hainaut P, Boyle P. Curbing the liver cancer epidemic in Africa. *Lancet* 2008; 371(9610):367–368.

3 Control by vaccination: Asian and Taiwan experience

Jia-Horng Kao

Graduate Institute of Clinical Medicine, National Taiwan University College of Medicine and Hospital, Taipei, Taiwan

LEARNING POINTS

- Hepatocellular carcinoma (HCC) is one of the most common cancers and causes of cancer-related death worldwide
- More than half of HCC patients have tumours that are attributable to persistent hepatitis B virus (HBV) infections worldwide, and nearly 75% of HBV-related HCC patients reside in Asia
- Vaccines against HBV infection have been available since early 1980s, and reduction of hepatitis B surface antigen (HBsAg) carriage has been clearly demonstrated in vaccinated subjects
- Nationwide surveys documented that the best and cheapest measure to prevent HBV-related HCC is the implementation of universal hepatitis B vaccination programmes, by which the incidence rates of HCC in children and young adults are reduced in several Asian countries, including Taiwan

Introduction

Hepatocellular carcinoma (HCC) is the major primary cancer of the liver, and it has become the fifth most common cancer in men and the seventh in women in the world. There is an estimated 0.5–1 million new cases per year, and 80% of these occur in developing countries [1]. HCC is also the third leading cause of cancer-related death worldwide, suggesting that current therapy for HCC is far from satisfactory. Remarkable geographic and ethnic variations have been found in the incidence of HCC, from the low rate of 3.8 per 100,000 among white men in the United States to the high rate of 18–35 per 100,000 among Asian men in the Far East and Southeast Asia [2]. Most of the new cases occur in East or Southeast Asia. In contrast, the prevalence of HCC in Western countries has traditionally been low; however, increasing incidence has been reported in the United States and in some European countries [3].

The risk factors associated with the development of HCC include chronic infection with either hepatitis B virus (HBV) or hepatitis C virus (HCV) [1], the presence of cirrhosis, carcinogen exposure, especially aflatoxin B1 (AFB1), alcohol abuse, genetic factors, male gender, cigarette smoking and advanced age [4]. Overall, at least 50% of HCC are attributable to persistent HBV infections. Several lines of evidence have strongly indicated an aetiological association between persistent HBV infection and HCC, including the geographical correlation between prevalence of chronic HBV infection and the incidence of HCC, high prevalence of hepatitis B surface antigen (HBsAg) in HCC patients, increased relative risk of HCC in HBsAg carriers, the presence of integrated HBV DNA in HCC, reduced incidence of childhood HCC after HBV vaccination and association of chronic hepadnavirus infection with HCC in animal models [4]. In this chapter, the successful control of HBV-related HCC by universal hepatitis B vaccination in Asian countries including Taiwan will be reviewed and discussed.

Control of hepatitis B virus infection

Similar to other infectious agents, successful HBV infection is composed of three major components: an infection source, a susceptible host and established transmission routes [5]. Thus, the most cost-effective measure to control

Clinical Dilemmas in Primary Liver Cancer, First Edition. Edited by Roger Williams and Simon D. Taylor-Robinson.

HBV infection is to prevent any susceptible individual from contracting the virus infection, rather than treating those who are already infected.

There are two approaches to prevent susceptible people from infection of virus. The first is to interrupt the route of infection and the second is to immunise the susceptible host. Public health measures should at least include these two approaches, which demand considerable input from society, the government and health professionals, both locally and internationally.

Hepatitis B vaccination

The development of highly effective vaccines against HBV since 1982 represents a major advancement in preventive medicine and public health. The first commercially available HBV vaccines were plasma-derived HBsAg subunit vaccines. At present, the plasma-derived vaccines have largely been replaced by recombinant vaccines [6]. All these vaccines are safe and have a protective efficacy of 90–95% [7]. On the basis of the disease burden of hepatitis B and the availability of a safe and effective vaccine, the Global Advisory Group of the Expanded Programme on Immunization of the World Health Organization (WHO) recommended that hepatitis B vaccine be incorporated into routine infant and childhood immunisation programmes for countries with HBV carrier rates greater than 8% by 1995 and for all countries by 1997 [6]. As of 2007, according to WHO, 171 (89%) of the 193 member states had initiated a hepatitis B vaccination programme. The global coverage of completing three doses of hepatitis B vaccine was 65% on average, ranging from 89% in the American region to 28% in the Southeast Asian region [8].

Although the current vaccines are highly effective with a rate of 94–98% in protecting from chronic HBV infection for at least 20 years [9], they are far from perfect. For example, a small yet significant proportion of individuals do not respond adequately to the vaccine. A third-generation recombinant hepatitis B vaccine containing pre-S1, pre-S2 and S antigenic components of viral surface antigen subtypes *adw* and *ayw* has been developed. Pre-S1 and pre-S2 domains of the virus are thought to increase antibody to HBsAg (anti-HBs) responses [10]. Also, these domains stimulate cellular immune responses and can help bypass genetic non-responsiveness to the S antigen. This novel vaccine was developed to produce a superior immune response to that of the currently approved vaccines. Clinical trials have confirmed that the vaccine is well tolerated in human beings and that a 20-μg dose is adequate and effective for vaccination of naive subjects [11].

Effectiveness of hepatitis B vaccination

Hepatitis B vaccination is highly effective in both pre-exposure and post-exposure prophylaxis. Anti-HBs is neutralising and serum levels of more than 10 mIU/mL are protective. The efficacy of a hepatitis B vaccination programme can be assessed at various stages. The effect of routine infant and childhood hepatitis B vaccination programmes is usually not apparent because almost all HBV infections in infants and young children are symptomless, and HBV-related sequelae as a result of the long-term consequences of chronic infection usually manifest after middle age. Nevertheless, the immediate effect of vaccination programmes can be investigated firstly by comparing the prevalence of HBsAg carriage rate between vaccinated and unvaccinated populations. The serological surveys are important evaluation tools and indeed provide a means of predicting the eventual effect of vaccination on HBV-related diseases. More directly, the effectiveness of vaccination programmes can be measured by studying their influence on HBV-related morbidity and mortality rates.

In Taiwan, the carrier rate of HBsAg in the general population has been as high as 15–20% – one of the highest in the world. This has resulted in chronic hepatitis, cirrhosis and HCC in patients with chronic HBV infection. In about half of the Taiwanese chronic HBsAg carriers, the infection is attributed to perinatal transmission of the virus from mothers to infants. To control this serious public health problem in Taiwan, a mass vaccination programme against HBV infection was launched on July 1, 1984 – one of the earliest national programmes in the world [12]. This programme provided the scientific community with an excellent opportunity to observe the effectiveness of universal hepatitis B mass vaccination.

Control of HBV-related HCC by vaccination: a success story in Taiwan

Ample evidence has documented that vaccination of infants against HBV infection in Taiwan has effectively reduced persistent HBV infections in children and teenagers [13]. In brief, all infants received three to four doses of plasma or recombinant HBV vaccines. Meanwhile, newborns of HBeAg-positive mothers also received 0.5 mL of hepatitis B immunoglobulin (HBIg) within 24 hours after

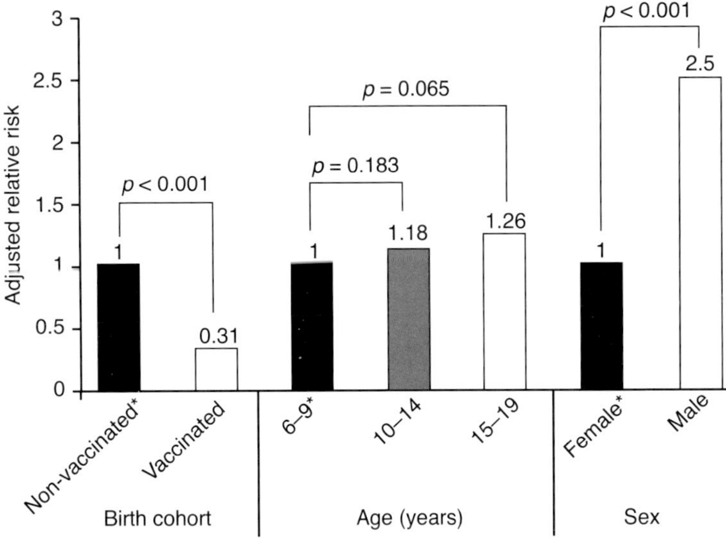

FIG 3.1 Multivariable-adjusted relative risk of developing HCC between July 1983 and June 2004 in birth cohorts born before vs. after the national HBV vaccination programme. (Adapted from Chang MH, You SL, Chen CJ, et al. Decreased incidence of hepatocellular carcinoma in hepatitis B vaccinees: a 20-year follow-up study. *J Natl Cancer Inst* 2009; 101:1348–1355.)

birth. The vaccination coverage rate was more than 97% countrywide. Subsequent surveys in Taipei City showed that the seroprevalence rate of HBsAg declined from 9.8% (pre-vaccination period) to 0.6% in children after 20 years of mass vaccination. The seropositive rates for HBsAg, anti-HBs and antibody to hepatitis B core antigen (anti-HBc) were 1.2%, 50.5% and 3.7%, respectively, in those born after the era of vaccination programme (<20 years old) in 2004 [5,14].

With the decline of chronic HBV infection, the incidence rate of HCC also decreased in children in Taiwan. From 1981 to 1994, the incidence of HCC in 6–9-year-olds declined from 0.52 per 100,000 for those born between 1974 and 1984 to 0.13 for those born between 1984 and 1986 ($p < 0.001$) [15]. In addition, a recent population-based study in Taiwan further documented that the control of HBV-related HCC by vaccination has extended from childhood to early adulthood [16]. The study included 1958 individuals aged 6–29 diagnosed with HCC between July 1, 1983 and June 30, 2004. Of these, 508 were aged 6–19 at diagnosis (444 unvaccinated, 64 vaccinated) and 1450 were aged 20–29 at diagnosis (all unvaccinated). In the unvaccinated cohorts, there was a trend for higher incidence of HCC with increasing age; this was significant for those aged 20 years or older ($p < 0.001$), but not for those below age 20. For children aged 6–19, vaccination was associated with a significant reduction in the age-specific incidence of HCC ($p < 0.001$ for each age group [6–9,10–14 and 15–19 years old at diagnosis]). In each age group and in both vaccinated and unvaccinated cohorts, HCC was more common in boys than in girls. Multivariate analysis adjusted for birth cohort, age and sex showed an adjusted relative risk of HCC of 0.31 for vaccinated birth cohorts compared with unvaccinated birth cohorts ($p < 0.001$) and an adjusted relative risk of 2.50 for boys compared with girls ($p < 0.001$) (Figure 3.1). With the longer term follow-up, the efficacy of universal HBV vaccination in preventing adulthood HCC is anticipated.

Several reasons have been implicated for a successful hepatitis B control programme in Taiwan [17]. These include (1) the government has shown determination in controlling hepatitis B in the Taiwanese people, and the actions have involved many different sections, including the Department of Health, the Ministry of Education, the office of information services, the academic institutions and the local governments; (2) the well-designed infrastructure of the public health system, which has close links with private hospitals and clinics and can provide convenient locations for vaccination; and (3) the control programme was designed carefully and implemented step by step. The research, evaluations and educational activities were started first, followed by stepwise vaccination.

TABLE 3.1 Rates of HBsAg carriage before and after hepatitis B vaccination in Asian countries

	HBsAg (%)		
Country	Before	After	Efficacy (%)
China, rural	14.6	1.4	90.4
China (Shanghai)	11	0.63	94.3
Indonesia (Lombok)	6.2	1.4	61.1
Japan (Iwate)	0.9	0.03	96.7
(Shizuoka)	0.3	0.03	90.0
Korea	7.5	0.38	94.9
Malaysia	2.5	0.4	84.0
Singapore	4.1	0	100
Taiwan (Taipei)	10	0.7	93.0
(Hualien)	9.3	1.9	79.6
(Taichung)	14	1.2	91.4
Thailand	4.3	0.7	83.7

Source: Adapted from Chen DS. Toward elimination and eradication of hepatitis B. *J Gastroenterol Hepatol* 2010; 25:19–25.

Asian experience of hepatitis B vaccination

Since the availability of hepatitis B vaccination in 1982, there has been a dramatic impact on the outcome of liver disease in Asian countries [18]. Studies from Malaysia and Singapore indicated a noticeable reduction in the prevalence rate of HBsAg in selected populations after the implementation of hepatitis B vaccination programme [19,20]. Table 3.1 shows the rates of HBsAg carriage before and after hepatitis B vaccination in some Asian countries [21]. Although the WHO Western Pacific Region has committed to reduce chronic HBV infection in children aged <5 years to <2% by 2012 [22], the wide variation (40–100%) of infant hepatitis B vaccination coverage rate among different Asian countries is an urgent issue needed to be tackled.

Like Taiwan, a similar trend in the decrease of HCC after hepatitis B vaccination has been observed in China, Singapore, Saudi Arabia and more recently in the Khon Kaen region of northeast Thailand [23–25]. For example, a universal hepatitis B vaccination programme was implemented in Singapore on September 1, 1987. The age-standardised incidence rate of HCC in males had dropped from 27.8 per 100,000 per year between 1978 and 1982 to 19.0 per 100,000 per year between 1988 and 1992 [26].

Given estimates that approximately 75% of HCC in Asian Pacific countries are attributable to persistent HBV infection, universal hepatitis B vaccination could prevent more than 500,000 HCC cases per year in this region [27]. These facts clearly highlight the importance of a global perspective for the prevention of chronic HBV infection and HBV-related HCC.

Challenges ahead to control HBV infection and HBV-related HCC

Although hepatitis B vaccines have been available for nearly three decades, and at least 1 billion people have received the vaccine, many susceptible people have not been immunised. According to the statement of WHO, 35% of infants worldwide had not received a complete course of hepatitis B vaccine in 2007. The coverage rate was especially low in Southeast Asia. The reasons of failing to offer mass hepatitis B vaccination in each country are complex. In brief, the infrastructure of public health delivery system needs to be improved and education should be strengthened for the general public, medical personnel, as well as the opinion of political leaders [8]. Economical burdens of hepatitis B vaccination are always a major obstacle. Constant endeavours from governments and the WHO are required, and continued support from non-government organisations are also essential. The effort from the Global Alliance on Vaccines and Immunization (GAVI) is particularly notable. Millions of children have received hepatitis B vaccine with the assistance of GAVI since 2000. It has been estimated that 2.5 million deaths will be averted through the GAVI vaccination project against HBV infection.

Despite the success of hepatitis B vaccination in Taiwan, childhood chronic HBV infection and HCC are not totally eliminated by the universal vaccination programme [14]. Among child HBsAg carriers born after the vaccination programme, 89% of their mothers were found to be HBsAg-positive, indicating the importance of maternal or vertical transmission. This fact also holds true for mothers of children with HCC, 96% of which were positive for HBsAg. In other words, approximately 10% of infants born to HBsAg-positive and e antigen (HBeAg)-positive mothers are still infected by HBV and suffer from chronic hepatitis B [28]. Our recent study also demonstrated that in the post-immunisation era, most HBV breakthrough infections are from maternal transmission, and immunised children born to HBV genotype C mothers may have a higher rate of breakthrough infection than those born to HBV genotype B mothers [29]. These HBV carrier children still carry an increased risk of HCC development later in life, especially those with HBV genotype C infection [30]. Therefore,

HBV breakthrough infection through maternal transmission remains a challenge to the global control of HBV infection. Further studies are urgently required to identify risk factors associated with perinatal infection despite complete immunisation. They also need to implement better prevention strategies, including the use of pregnancy category B anti-HBV agents in the late trimester of highly viremic carrier mothers to reduce HBV breakthrough infection in these high-risk infants.

On the basis of existing evidence, the vaccination failure caused by the emergence of escape mutant does not impose an increased risk of chronic HBV infection at present. Nevertheless, development of new hepatitis B vaccines may overcome the issue of vaccine failure [14].

Conclusions

HCC is one of the most common cancers worldwide, and more than half of the patients have tumours that are attributable to persistent HBV infection. The most important strategy to reduce HBV-related HCC is hepatitis B vaccination, and this programme has already had major impact since its implementation in the 1980s, not only with a reduction in burden of hepatitis B disease, but also a significant reduction in childhood and early adulthood HCC in several Asian countries, including Taiwan. However, there are still hundreds of millions of HBV carriers that remain a global health challenge. In the past decade, several hepatitis B viral factors, such as serum HBV DNA level, genotype and naturally occurring mutants that influence liver disease progression and HCC development in HBV carriers, have been identified [31]. In addition, the role of non-viral factors in HBV-related HCC has also been increasingly recognised. In the start of a new decade, the focus should be on screening and identifying high-risk individuals for antiviral therapy before the development of HCC. With all these measures, the eradication of HBV infection and HBV-related HCC is plausible. However, every endeavour should be pursued to make it become a reality. Even if the goal cannot be reached in a short period of time, all these efforts will result in a marked decrease of HBV infection, leading to the reduction of huge disease burden caused by HBV infection worldwide.

References

1. Kao JH, Chen DS. Changing disease burden of hepatocellular carcinoma in the Far East and Southeast Asia. *Liver Int* 2005; 25:696–703.
2. Gomaa AI, Khan SA, Toledano MB, Waked I, Taylor-Robinson SD. Hepatocellular carcinoma: epidemiology, risk factors and pathogenesis. *World J Gastroenterol* 2008; 14: 4300–4308.
3. Jemal A, Siegel R, Ward E, Hao Y, Xu J, Thun MJ. Cancer statistics, 2009. *CA Cancer J Clin* 2009; 59:225–249.
4. Lok AS. Prevention of hepatitis B virus-related hepatocellular carcinoma. *Gastroenterology* 2004; 127(5 suppl 1):S303–S309.
5. Kao JH, Chen DS. Global control of hepatitis B virus infection. *Lancet Infect Dis* 2002; 2:395–403.
6. Kane M. Global programme for control of hepatitis B infection. *Vaccine* 1995; 13(suppl 1):47–49.
7. Margolis HS, Coleman PJ, Brown RE, Mast EE, Sheingold SH, Arevalo JA. Prevention of hepatitis B virus transmission by immunisation: an economic analysis of current recommendations. *JAMA* 1995; 264:1201–1208.
8. Chen DS. Hepatitis B vaccination: the key towards elimination and eradication of hepatitis B. *J Hepatol* 2009; 50:805–816.
9. Ni YH, Huang LM, Chang MH, et al. Two decades of universal hepatitis B vaccination in Taiwan: impact and implication for future strategies. *Gastroenterology* 2007; 132:1287–1293.
10. Milich DR, McLachlan A, Chisari FV, Kent SB, Thornton GB. Immune response to the pre-S(1) region of hepatitis B surface antigen (HBsAg): a pre-S(1)-specific T cell response can bypass nonresponsiveness to the pre-S(2) and S regions of the HBsAg. *J Immunol* 1986; 137:315–322.
11. Young MD, Schneider DL, Zuckerman AJ, Du W, Dickson B, Maddrey WC. Adult hepatitis B vaccination using a novel triple antigen recombinant vaccine. *Hepatology* 2001; 34:372–376.
12. Chen DS, Hsu HM, Sung JL, et al. A mass vaccination programme in Taiwan against hepatitis B virus infection in infants of hepatitis B surface antigen carrier mothers. *JAMA* 1987; 257:2597–2603.
13. Kao JH, Chen DS. Universal hepatitis B vaccination: killing 2 birds with 1 stone. *Am J Med* 2008; 121:1029–1031.
14. Ni YH, Chen DS. Hepatitis B vaccination in children: the Taiwan experience. *Pathol Biol (Paris)* 2010; 58:296–300.
15. Chang MH, Chen CJ, Lai MS, et al. Universal hepatitis B vaccination in Taiwan and the incidence of hepatocellular carcinoma in children. Taiwan Childhood Hepatoma Study Group. *N Engl J Med* 1997; 336:1855–1859.
16. Chang MH, You SL, Chen CJ, et al. Decreased incidence of hepatocellular carcinoma in hepatitis B vaccinees: a 20-year follow-up study. *J Natl Cancer Inst* 2009; 101:1348–1355.

17. Huang K, Lin S. Nationwide vaccination: a success story in Taiwan. *Vaccine* 2000; 18:S35–S38.
18. Lim SG, Mohammed R, Yuen MF, Kao JH. Prevention of hepatocellular carcinoma in hepatitis B virus infection. *J Gastroenterol Hepatol* 2009; 24:1352–1357.
19. Ng KP, Saw TL, Baki A, Rozainah K, Pang KW, Ramanathan M. Impact of the Expanded Program of Immunization against hepatitis B infection in school children in Malaysia. *Med Microbiol Immunol* 2005; 194:163–168.
20. Goh KT. Prevention and control of hepatitis B virus infection in Singapore. *Ann Acad Med Singapore* 1997; 26:671–681.
21. Chen DS. Toward elimination and eradication of hepatitis B. *J Gastroenterol Hepatol* 2010; 25:19–25.
22. Clements CJ, Baoping Y, Crouch A, et al. Progress in the control of hepatitis B infection in the Western Pacific Region. *Vaccine* 2006; 24:1975–1982.
23. Wichajarn K, Kosalaraska P, Wiangnon S. Incidence of hepatocellular carcinoma in children in Khon Kaen before and after national hepatitis B vaccine program. *Asian Pac J Cancer Prev* 2008; 9:507–510.
24. Jia JD, Zhuang H. A winning war against hepatitis B virus infection in China. *Chin Med J (Engl)* 2007; 120:2157–2158.
25. Poovorawan Y, Theamboonlers A, Vimolket T, et al. Impact of hepatitis B immunisation as part of the EPI. *Vaccine* 2000; 19:943–949.
26. Goh KT. Prevention and control of hepatitis B virus infection in Singapore. *Ann Acad Med Singapore* 1997; 26:671–681.
27. Kao JH, Chen DS. Recent updates in hepatitis vaccination and the prevention of hepatocellular carcinoma. *Int J Cancer* 2002; 97:269–271.
28. Hsu HM, Lee SC, Wang MC, Lin SF, Chen DS. Efficacy of a mass hepatitis B immunization program after switching to recombinant hepatitis B vaccine: a population-based study in Taiwan. *Vaccine* 2001; 19:2825–2829.
29. Wen WH, Chen HL, Ni YH, et al. Secular trend of the viral genotype distribution in children with chronic hepatitis B virus infection after universal infant immunization. *Hepatology* 2011; 53:429–436.
30. Kao JH, Chen PJ, Lai MY, Chen DS. Hepatitis B genotypes correlate with clinical outcomes in patients with chronic hepatitis B. *Gastroenterology* 2000; 118:554–559.
31. Kao JH, Chen PJ, Chen DS. Recent advances in the research of hepatitis B virus-related hepatocellular carcinoma: epidemiologic and molecular biological aspects. *Adv Cancer Res* 2010; 108:21–72.

4 The view from the United Kingdom

Shahid A. Khan[1], Mireille B. Toledano[2], Abigail Zabron[1], Mehtan Ahmed[1], Simon D. Taylor-Robinson[1]

[1]Department of Medicine, Imperial College London, London, UK
[2]School of Public Health, Imperial College London, London, UK

LEARNING POINTS

- Incidence and mortality rates for both chronic liver disease (CLD) and liver cancer are increasing steadily in the United Kingdom
- This is related to an increase in known risk factors
- Alcohol consumption and non-alcoholic fatty liver disease (NAFLD) have increased over recent decades
- Chronic viral hepatitis has also increased because of increased immigration from hepatitis C virus (HBV)-endemic regions of the world and because of patients infected with hepatitis C virus (HCV) 20–30 years ago now presenting with clinical disease
- There is currently a need for organised, formal hepatocellular carcinoma (HCC) surveillance, while increased incidence presents challenges for allocation of resources for treatment of HCC
- Political help will be required, as the increasing health burden of liver disease raises public health issues in relation to health funding and addressing the underlying causes

Epidemiology

Worldwide, primary liver cancer (PLC) accounts for approximately 5% of all new cancer diagnoses, is the third commonest cause of cancer death in men and the sixth commonest in women [1,2]. The global annual incidence of PLC is almost 600,000 and an estimated 500,000 people die from PLC yearly, emphasising the overall poor prognosis of this disease. Over 80% of all PLC worldwide are HCCs, and the terms PLC and HCC are often used interchangeably [2].

The United Kingdom

Incidence rates for liver disease are important when discussing PLC because over 80% of all HCCs occur on the background of CLD. In the United Kingdom, the incidence and consequent mortality from liver disease are increasing at an alarming pace. Liver disease is the fifth commonest cause of death in those under 65 years of age, and of all top five causes, it is the only one that is increasing (Plate 4.1) [3]. Data from the UK Office of National Statistics showed that from 1979 to 2005, age-standardised incidence rates for PLC had increased in men from around 2.0 to 2.80 per 100,000 population and remained relatively static in women (Plate 4.2) [4]. Age-standardised mortality rates have risen to 2.32 per 100,000, the highest since records began [4]. HCC kills over 900 people per year in the United Kingdom, with most deaths in men, as is found in most of the world. Most of these deaths occur in older men, particularly those over 65 [4]. The rising incidence and mortality from HCC in the United Kingdom – despite greater awareness for the need of surveillance in patients with cirrhosis, plus improvements in diagnostic imaging and access to therapy – are likely to be a result of the increasing burden of CLD in general. Various factors have been postulated for this.

Alcohol

Alcohol excess is the single commonest cause of clinically significant liver disease in the United Kingdom and most Western industrialised countries. The proportion of HCC cases attributable to HCC to alcohol in Europe has been estimated at around 40–50% [5]. Overall alcohol consumption has increased in the United Kingdom over recent

Clinical Dilemmas in Primary Liver Cancer, First Edition. Edited by Roger Williams and Simon D. Taylor-Robinson.

decades, driven by fiscal, cultural and marketing factors [5]. An increase in wine consumption is thought to have been influenced by increasing foreign holidays, globalisation and European Union membership requiring harmonisation of tax duty on wine [5]. A significant increase in the number of financially important national supermarket chains in the United Kingdom changed the way alcohol was advertised and also reduced its overall cost, as stores wanted to attract customers with low prices. Successful industry lobbying on alcohol taxation led to duty on spirits being reduced during the 1990s [5]. Since 1980, spirits have become 350% more affordable, wine 270% and beer 170% [6]. Alcohol advertising expenditure increased by over 50% and the marketing focus shifted towards younger people, for example with the introduction of 'alco-pops' (alcohol-containing sweet-flavoured drinks aimed at the teenage market) and alcohol industry sponsorship of music festivals. The average alcohol consumption of 11–15-year-old children has increased by two-thirds since 1980 in the United Kingdom. These changes have been associated with a concomitant increase in liver-related deaths. Unless this trend is reversed, as some European countries have seen, rates of liver disease and HCC are unlikely to abate [5].

Non-alcoholic fatty liver disease

NAFLD has become the commonest cause of abnormal LFTs in the Western world, with an annual incidence estimated to be as high as 10% [7]. It is also emerging as a cause of HCC [7]. NAFLD is believed to be the hepatic manifestation of the metabolic syndrome, with insulin resistance deemed the common pathophysiological mechanism. Although visceral adipose tissue (VAT) is thought to be the important risk factor for obesity and its related metabolic disturbances, recent studies suggest that *intrahepatic* fat content, rather than VAT, is a better marker of metabolic derangements [8,9]. The prevalence of NAFLD, including its more aggressive form of non-alcoholic steatohepatitis (NASH), is increasing alongside the rising epidemics of diabetes and obesity. Around 30% of patients with NASH demonstrate progression of fibrosis over time with up to 10% progressing to cirrhosis [10]. Growing evidence suggests NASH accounts for many cases of what was previously labelled 'cryptogenic' cirrhosis. In the United Kingdom, as elsewhere in the Western industrialised nations, NAFLD is principally a disease of middle and old age. Previous studies suggested it was benign in older people; however, more recent studies suggest an increased mortality in over 60-year-olds. A retrospective, cohort study in the United Kingdom found that older patients had significantly greater fibrosis on biopsy with less percentage fat; patients with cirrhosis being significantly older than those without cirrhosis [11]. Insulin resistance and the subsequent inflammatory cascade that is associated with NASH are believed to play a significant role in the HCC carcinogenesis [7]. In addition to NAFLD, diabetes and obesity have been established as independent risk factors for the development of HCC [7]. At present, there are no large-scale studies that delineate the specific risk of HCC in NAFLD and the risk of cardiovascular-related death in patients with NAFLD currently outweighs the risk of liver-related death. Nonetheless, there are also reports of HCC developing in NAFLD patients who do not have cirrhosis. Given the high prevalence of NAFLD in the United Kingdom and Western industrialised nations, it may well eventually become a major cause of end-stage liver disease and HCC [5].

Of course, fatty liver disease can also develop in patients with other risk factors for CLD, such as alcohol and viral hepatitis. Multiple aetiologies can cause a supra-additive risk of developing cirrhosis and HCC. For example, obesity can lead to steatohepatitis via its effects on insulin sensitivity, and the lipid solubility of alcohol makes adipose tissue a target for its toxic effects [12]. Furthermore, alcohol itself leads to fatty liver that promotes peripheral insulin resistance, this promoting obesity [12]. A recent analysis of prospective cohort studies in the United Kingdom, with decades of follow-up and involving almost 10,000 men, found that moderate to heavy alcohol drinkers had adjusted relative rates (RR) for liver disease mortality of 3.16 for normal or underweight men, 7.01 for overweight and 18.9 for obese men. The excess RR due to interaction between high BMI and alcohol consumption was 5.58 [12]. Perhaps worryingly, most of the men in the study were from working populations and thus likely to be healthier on average than the general population – the results may, therefore, be underestimating the absolute risks of liver disease.

Hepatitis B and immigration

Chronic HBV infection is the most prevalent cause of HCC worldwide, accounting for over 50% of global cases and approximately 80% of HCCs occur in countries where HBV is endemic [13]. Although the incidence of HBV in the native UK population is very low, the British Liver Trust estimates 1 in a 1000 (0.1%) is infected. [13,14]. Like many other Western European countries, the United Kingdom has seen a rise in immigration from HBV-endemic countries over the past few decades. Immigrants to Western industrialised countries tend to have higher HCC incidence rates compared with the indigenous population [15]. Of note, however, the second generation of immigrants appears to have a lower incidence of HCC than their parents according to data from the United States [16]. However, these data are over a decade old, and the risks of HBV associated HCC include being male, older age, co-exposure to aflatoxin B(1), the presence of cirrhosis, co-infection with HCV and/or HIV, obesity and diabetes mellitus [13]. Obesity, diabetes and related NAFLD are increasingly common in the United Kingdom and the Western world, including both in the indigenous populations and also in immigrants who have settled in the developed world. It is as yet unclear how the incidence of HCC will develop in second and third generation immigrants in whom the incidence and severity of chronic HBV is likely to be less, but concomitantly additional risk factors for HCC may develop. Immigration from HBV-endemic parts of the world is likely to continue for the foreseeable future, for economic reasons including the impact of an ageing Western population. Although the global incidence of chronic HBV infection is beginning to decrease in high-risk areas as a result of immunisation programmes, HBV-induced HCC incidence is projected to increase for at least another two decades [13].

Changes in the proportion of immigrants from different parts of the world could also affect liver disease and HCC rates in the United Kingdom in the future. A recent study compared alcohol-related and HCC deaths by country of birth in England and Wales. Mortality from alcohol-related deaths was found to be particularly high for UK citizens born in Ireland and Scotland and men born in India, but low in women born in other countries and men born in Bangladesh, the Middle East, West Africa, Pakistan, China and the countries of the former British West Indies. However, mortality from HCC was particularly high in people born in Bangladesh, China and West Africa [17].

Hepatitis C

Chronic HCV infection is another major cause of liver disease globally, accounting for an estimated 20% of all cases of HCC, usually in the presence of cirrhosis. The major route of transmission of HCV in the United Kingdom is through infected needles and most patients have a history of intravenous drug usage. The cohort effect of ageing people with HCV infected between the Second World War and up to the 1980s is another postulated reason for the rise in liver disease in the United Kingdom and other Western countries. Indeed, it has been estimated that the emergence of HCV could account for up to half of the increase in HCC in developed countries [18,19]. The UK Health Protection Agency estimates the UK prevalence of HCV infection to be 0.4%, but the true incidence is unknown as HCV, similar to HBV, is largely asymptomatic until severe liver damage has occurred [20]. The clinical impact of CLD from this cohort, plus those infected up to the early 1990s, before HCV screening in blood products and needle exchange/public information programmes driven by the emergence of HIV was introduced in the United Kingdom, is likely to continue.

Management issues

As CLD increases in the United Kingdom, various management issues arise, including surveillance for HCC and therapy. Detecting early stage disease is likely to be the major advance in curing HCC for the foreseeable future, rather than curative drugs for extensive disease. It is generally accepted that patients with cirrhosis require HCC surveillance by ultrasound on a 6-monthly basis and a recent study confirmed that this is cost-effective in the context of the UK National Health Service (NHS), in terms of quality-adjusted life-years (QALY) gained. However, confirming the diagnosis of cirrhosis currently requires liver biopsy. Non-invasive techniques that can monitor progressive liver fibrosis and diagnose cirrhosis without the need for serial liver biopsies would be a welcome step forward. Early clinical studies suggested transient elastography, possibly in combination with serum markers of fibrosis, may take up this role, but results are conflicting and large-scale validatory trials are awaited [21,22].

HCC is a major indication in the United Kingdom for orthotopic liver transplantation (OLT), which raises another important issue. There is currently already a lack of available organs for liver transplantation in the United Kingdom and yet the demand for donor livers is increasing. This gap between supply and need is likely to further widen over the next decade or so as liver disease rises and the limits for OLT in HCC are extended further and further, beyond the original Milan criteria [23,24]. There is ongoing debate in the United Kingdom about how to increase the donor pool, for example by having an opt-out rather than opt-in policy at national level. One potential solution is the increased use of living-donor-liver-transplantation (LDLT). LDLT was pioneered in the Far East, initially to treat liver failure in children. As experience with the technique has grown and innovations have continued, the application of LDLT for HCC beyond Milan criteria seems feasible [25]. However, the cost may be a slightly compromised survival, and a higher rate of healthy donor mortality than currently seen in kidney transplantation for example [25]. At the time of writing, LDLT is in its infancy in the United Kingdom and not widely available in the NHS. It will be interesting to see how this develops in time.

A significant advance in the treatment of advanced HCC has been the multikinase inhibitor, sorafenib. This was the first chemotherapy agent to demonstrate a statistically significant improvement in survival for patients with advanced HCC [26]. The high cost of this drug, for a real, but relatively modest increase in survival, has meant that it is not currently approved for National Health Service (NHS) use in the United Kingdom. This raises another challenge: how to deal with the spiralling costs of novel drugs.

Political issues

The old adage states that prevention is better than cure. The likely causes of increasing liver disease and cancer, and the potential effects on the NHS, have clear relevance for health education, public health policies and funding. Important issues Governments need to address include licensing laws (extended by the previous Government), taxation/price on alcohol and high calorie foods, advertising and sponsorship regulation, involvement of alcohol and food companies in health policy, immigration health etc. Despite the challenges of rising liver disease and cancer in the United Kingdom, to both health care workers and politicians, we face the future with optimism. Knowledge and preparedness are key – being forewarned is forearmed.

References

1. Nordenstedt H, White DL, El-Serag HB. The changing pattern of epidemiology in hepatocellular carcinoma. *Dig Liver Dis* 2010; 42(suppl 3):S206–S214.
2. El-Serag HB, Rudolph KL. Hepatocellular carcinoma: epidemiology and molecular carcinogenesis. *Gastroenterology* 2007; 132(7):2557–2576.
3. UK Department of Health Report 2009.
4. Ahmed M et al., BSG 2009.
5. Jewell J, Sheron N. Trends in European liver death rates: implications for alcohol policy. *Clin Med* 2010; 10(3):259–263.
6. British Beer and Pub Association. *British Beer and Pub Association Handbook*. British Beer and Pub Association, London; 2008.
7. Starley BQ, Calcagno CJ, Harrison SA. Nonalcoholic fatty liver disease and hepatocellular carcinoma: a weighty connection. *Hepatology* 2010; 51(5):1820–1832.
8. Salamone F, Bugianesi E. Nonalcoholic fatty liver disease: the hepatic trigger of the metabolic syndrome. *J Hepatol* 2010; 53(6):1146–1147.
9. Fabbrini E, Magkos F, Mohammed BS, et al. Intrahepatic fat, not visceral fat, is linked with metabolic complications of obesity. *Proc Natl Acad Sci U S A* 2009; 106(36):15430–15435.
10. Adams LA, Sanderson S, Lindor KD, Angulo P. The histological course of nonalcoholic fatty liver disease: a longitudinal study of 103 patients with sequential liver biopsies. *J Hepatol* 2005; 42:132–138.
11. Frith J, Day CP, Henderson E, Burt AD, Newton JL. Nonalcoholic fatty liver disease in older people. *Gerontology* 2009; 55(6):607–613.
12. Hart CL, Morrison DS, Batty GD, Mitchell RJ, Davey Smith G. Effect of body mass index and alcohol consumption on liver disease: analysis of data from two prospective cohort studies. *BMJ* 2010; 340:c1240.
13. Kew MC. Epidemiology of chronic hepatitis B virus infection, hepatocellular carcinoma, and hepatitis B virus-induced hepatocellular carcinoma. *Pathol Biol (Paris)* 2010; 58(4):273–277.
14. British Liver Trust: fighting liver disease. 2009. Available from: http://www.britishlivertrust.org.uk/home/the-liver/liver-diseases/hepatitis-b.aspx.
15. Sherman M. Hepatocellular carcinoma: epidemiology, surveillance, and diagnosis. *Semin Liver Dis* 2010; 30(1):3–16.
16. Rosenblatt KA, Weiss NS, Schwartz SM. Liver cancer in Asian migrants to the United States and their descendants. *Cancer Causes Control* 1996; 7(3):345–350.
17. Bhala N, Bhopal R, Brock A, Griffiths C, Wild S. Alcohol-related and hepatocellular cancer deaths by country of birth in England and Wales. *J Public Health (Oxf)* 2009; 31(2):250–257.
18. Gomaa AI, Khan SA, Toledano MB, Waked I, Taylor-Robinson SD. Hepatocellular carcinoma: epidemiology, risk factors and pathogenesis. *World J Gastroenterol* 2008; 14(27):4300–4308.
19. El-Serag HB, Mason AC. Rising incidence of hepatocellular carcinoma in the United States. *N Engl J Med* 1999; 340(10):745–750

20. The Health Protection Agency (HPA). *Annual Report 2008: Hepatitis C in the UK*. Health Protection Agency Centre for Infection, London; 2008.
21. Cobbold JF, Crossey MM, Colman P, et al. Optimal combinations of ultrasound-based and serum markers of disease severity in patients with chronic hepatitis C. *J Viral Hepat* 2010; 17(8):537–545.
22. Myers RP, Elkashab M, Ma M, Crotty P, Pomier-Layrargues G. Transient elastography for the noninvasive assessment of liver fibrosis: a multicentre Canadian study. *Can J Gastroenterol* 2010; 24(11):661–670.
23. Mazzaferro V, Regalia E, Doci R, et al. Liver transplantation for the treatment of small hepatocellular carcinomas in patients with cirrhosis. *N Engl J Med* 1996; 334(11):693–699.
24. Duffy JP, Vardanian A, Benjamin E, et al. Liver transplantation criteria for hepatocellular carcinoma should be expanded: a 22-year experience with 467 patients at UCLA. *Ann Surg* 2007; 246(3):502–509; discussion 509–511.
25. Jeon H, Lee SG. Living donor liver transplantation. *Curr Opin Organ Transplant* 2010; 15(3):283–287.
26. Llovet JM, Ricci S, Mazzaferro V, et al. *N Engl J Med* 2008; 359(4):378–390.

5 The view from the United States

Hitoshi Maruyama[1], Arun J. Sanyal[2]

[1]Department of Medicine and Clinical Oncology, Graduate School of Medicine, Chiba University
[2]Division of Gastroenterology and Hepatology, Virginia Commonwealth University, Richmond, VA, USA

LEARNING POINTS

- Hepatocellular carcinoma (HCC) is increasing worldwide and is one of the most common carcinomas in the Western countries as well as in Asia
- More than 70% HCC patients are accompanied with chronic liver disease or cirrhosis, caused by chronic infection with hepatitis B virus, hepatitis C virus, alcoholic liver disease and non-alcoholic steatohepatitis
- The average annual incidence of HCC in the United States from 2001 to 2006 was 3.0 per 100,000 persons
- In the United States in 2009, an estimated 22,620 cases of liver and intrahepatic bile duct cancer were diagnosed and an estimated 18,160 HCC patients died of the disease
- Health care providers should also have thorough knowledge of the epidemiology of HCC to make the most of algorithms for early identification and treatment of HCC

Introduction

Hepatocellular carcinoma (HCC) is increasing worldwide and is one of the most common carcinomas in the Western countries as well as in Asia [1]. The development of HCC has a profound influence on the prognosis of patients with chronic liver disease. More than 70% HCC patients are accompanied with chronic liver disease or cirrhosis, caused by chronic infection with hepatitis B virus (HBV), hepatitis C virus (HCV), alcoholic liver disease and non-alcoholic steatohepatitis (NASH) [2,3]. There are additional risk factors for developing HCC, diabetes, obesity, certain hereditary conditions such as haemochromatosis, some metabolic disorders and intake of aflatoxin-contaminated food [2,4]. Various aetiologic factors as well as geographic location may influence the characteristics of HCC patients during their clinical course [5]. In this chapter, the authors review the literature to assess the current epidemiology of HCC and to identify risk factors for developing HCC in the United States.

Epidemiology of HCC in the United States

It is reported that HCC is the fifth leading cause of new cancer cases worldwide [6]. HCC is almost universally fatal within a year unless detected early. In the United States in 2009, an estimated 22,620 cases of liver and intrahepatic bile duct cancer were diagnosed and an estimated 18,160 HCC patients died of the disease [6]. HCC is one of the eight cancer types that, as a group, account for 50% of the mortality related to cancer in the United States [7]. This neoplasm is also the third leading cause of cancer death in men, and the sixth leading cause in women [6]. The incidence of HCC is highest in middle Africa (15.8%), followed by eastern Asia (14.1%) and western Africa (10.6%) [8].

The incidence of HCC is rising alarmingly in the United States, and it is projected that the total deaths from HCC will rise from 21,000 in 2010 to 34,000 in 2030 [7] (Figure 5.1). The average annual incidence of HCC in the United States from 2001 to 2006 was 3.0 per 100,000 persons [9]. In another analysis of population-based data using insurance claims based information on 18 million Americans followed from 2002 to 2008, the incidence of HCC was 0.23% (230 cases for every 100,000 individuals) [10]. The

Clinical Dilemmas in Primary Liver Cancer, First Edition. Edited by Roger Williams and Simon D. Taylor-Robinson.

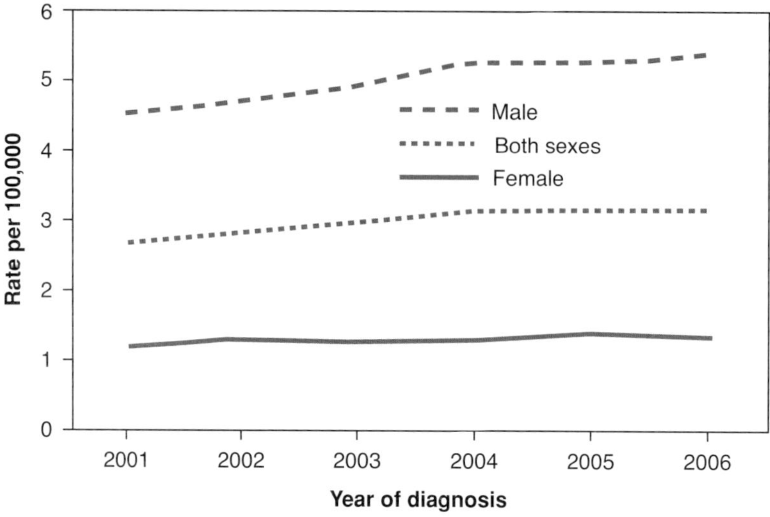

FIG 5.1 Hepatocellular carcinoma incidence rate, by sex – United States, 2001–2006. (O'Connor S, Ward JW, Watson M, Momin B, Richardson LC. Hepatocellular carcinoma – United States, 2001–2006. *Morbid Mortal Wkly Rep* 2010; 59(17):517–520.)

study also revealed that the mean annual rate of new HCC patients between 2003 and 2008 was 0.04 per 100 patients. These discrepancies may reflect the varying populations and methods used in these two studies. While the former were based on the CDC National Program of Cancer Registries and the Surveillance, Epidemiology and End Results (SEER) system, the latter was based on the MarketScan database, which includes data from a variety of third-party medical insurers and claims submitted for medical care. It is likely that the hospital and disease-specific registries, which focus on the numerator, i.e. cases of HCC, overestimate the disease, while claims-based data focus on the true denominator and are more likely to provide true population-based information.

Risk factors for developing HCC

Cirrhosis

The major risk factor for developing HCC is cirrhosis, which is a sequence of chronic liver disease. It is characterised by destruction of liver cells, altered hepatocyte proliferation and an increase in fibrous tissue. The leading cause of cirrhosis is viral infection; almost half of HCC cases worldwide are associated with HBV infection, and a further 25% cases associated with HCV infection [11]. An emergent trend in the United States is a growing number of reports of HCC in chronic liver disease without cirrhosis. A population-based study in the United States showed that mild chronic liver disease (1289/4406, 29.3% vs. 239/44,060, 0.5%; $p<0.0001$) and moderate to severe liver disease (607/4406, 13.8% vs. 113/44,060, 0.3%; $p<0.0001$) were both significantly more frequent in HCC group than control group [10]. These findings, along with recent reports of HCC in the absence of cirrhosis from other parts of the world, are of great public health concern because of their implications for liver cancer screening [12]. There are several possible mechanisms which are considered to be involved in the development of HCC in cirrhosis, such as telomere dysfunction and alterations in the micro- and macro-environment that stimulate cellular proliferation [2].

Viral infection

HBV

Acute or chronic liver disease caused by HBV infection increases the risk of developing liver cancer 100-fold in chronic carriers [13]. HBV infection accounts for approximately 340,000 cases of liver cancer (54.4% of cases globally), with the majority of these in Africa, Asia and the western Pacific region [14]. It causes hepatocyte injury and chronic necroinflammation, with subsequent hepatocyte proliferation, fibrosis and cirrhosis. The continuous regeneration leads to increased liver cell turnover and accumulation of mutations in the host genome that could result in genetic alterations, chromosomal rearrangements, activation of oncogenes and inactivation of tumour suppressor genes [15]. Furthermore, it should be noted that HCC can develop in the absence of cirrhosis in subjects with HBV infection. HBV can integrate its DNA into host cells and so may act as a mutagenic agent, causing secondary chromosomal rearrangement and increasing genomic instability [14].

HCV

Chronic inflammation, cell death, proliferation and cirrhosis caused by HCV infection increases the risk of HCC by 17-fold. The risk depends on the degree of liver fibrosis [15,16]. HCV infection accounts for approximately 195,000 cases of liver cancer (31.1% of cases globally); northern and middle Africa are the areas of highest prevalence [14]. In the United States, the prevalence of HCV is estimated at between 4.1 and 5 million as the number of infected individuals defined by anti-HCV antibody positivity; of these, 3.2–3.4 million subjects are chronically infected [17,18]. Although the number of new HCV infection cases has decreased from a peak of an estimated 262,000/year in 1986 to 17,000/year in 2007 in the United States [17], the prevalence of individuals who have been infected with HCV for over 20 years will continue to increase until 2015 [19]. In the National Health and Nutrition Examination Survey (NHANES; 1999–2002), patients aged 40–49 years accounted for 66% of HCV-infected patients in US; the prevalence of HCV infection was 2.7 times higher in this age group compared with the general population [18]. Subjects with HCV and HCC are often older males with diabetes, obesity and concomitant alcohol abuse or HBV co-infection.

HCV, an RNA-containing virus, is unable to integrate into the host genome; HCV may cause HCC by various mechanisms. HCV core protein is thought to enter the host cell and activate key signalling pathways such as the p38 mitogen-activated protein kinase and nuclear factor kappa B pathways, resulting in cytokine production and subsequent inflammation, alterations in apoptotic pathways and tumour formation [20]. The non-structural proteins of HCV, NS3 and NS5A may also act as key mediators to induce oxidative stress and inflammation [20]. Patients with both HCV infection and alcohol abuse have been shown to develop more severe fibrosis and have higher rates of cirrhosis and HCC than non-drinkers [21]. Hepatocarcinogenesis could be a more rapid and aggressive process in human immunodeficiency virus (HIV)/HCV co-infected patients [22].

Non-alcoholic fatty liver disease

Non-alcoholic fatty liver disease (NAFLD) is the most common liver disorder in Western countries, with up to 20% of individuals affected [23]. The histologic phenotype of NAFLD extends from a fatty liver alone to steatohepatitis. NASH is the most serious form of NAFLD [24,25], being associated with multiple components of the metabolic syndrome, and is thought to increase the risk of developing chronic liver disease, cirrhosis and HCC [26].

In the largest prospective study of subjects with cirrhosis due to NASH, the cumulative incidence of HCC was 6.7% at 10 years compared with 17% in those with cirrhosis due to HCV [27] (Figure 5.2). These findings were corroborated by a recent study where mild alcohol consumption was also found to be a risk factor for HCC [28] (Figure 5.3). In a population-based analysis of claims-based data, it was found that 54.6% of cases of HCC were associated with NAFLD/NASH (ICD9 codes: 571.8, 571.9, 573.4, 573.8, 573.9) [10]. In addition, of the 22% of subjects with HCC who also had HCV infection, 68% also carried a diagnosis of

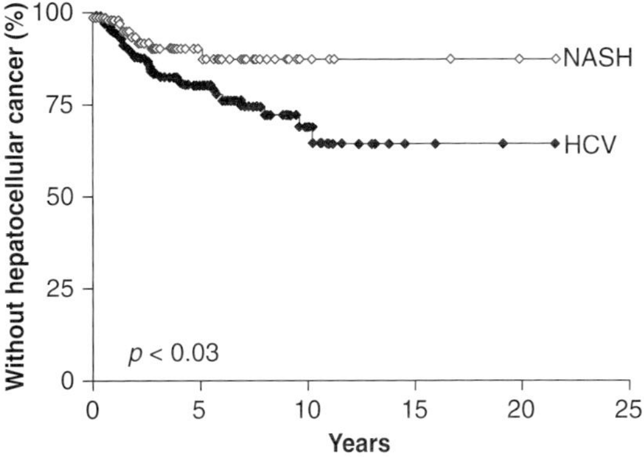

FIG 5.2 Comparison of occurrence of hepatocellular cancer between NASH-related cirrhosis and HCV-related cirrhosis. Development of hepatocellular cancer is less in cirrhosis due to NASH compared with HCV. (Sanyal AJ, Banas C, Sargeant C, et al. Similarities and differences in outcomes of cirrhosis due to non-alcoholic steatohepatitis and hepatitis C. *Hepatology* 2006; 43:682–689. Wiley publication; STM agreement.)

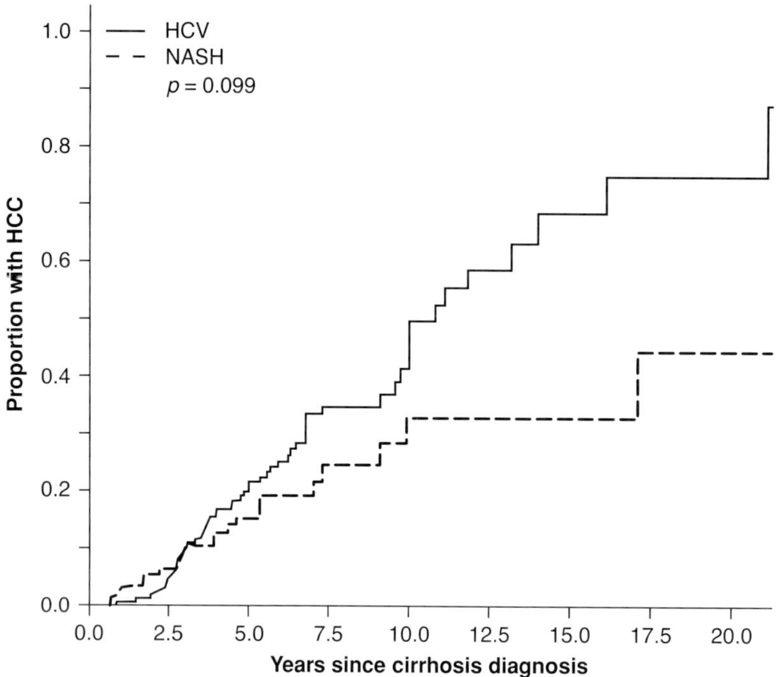

FIG 5.3 Annual cumulative incidence of hepatocellular carcinoma. (Ascha MS, Hanouneh IA, Lopez R, et al. The incidence and risk factors of hepatocellular carcinoma in patients with non-alcoholic steatohepatitis. *Hepatology* 2010; 51:1972–1978.)

hepatic steatosis. Diabetes mellitus, which is closely related to NASH and the metabolic syndrome, has also emerged as a major risk factor for HCC. Type 2 diabetes mellitus was present in 35.8% of cases of HCC [10]. The yearly cumulative incidence of HCC was 2.6% in NASH-cirrhosis and 4.0% in HCV-cirrhosis ($p = 0.09$) [28].

Alcohol

Alcoholic liver disease is also a risk factor for developing HCC, being common in Western countries. Heavy alcohol intake (50–70 g/day) is the most common cause of liver cirrhosis [29] and is a well-established risk factor for HCC [1,4]. Alcohol is often seen as a co-factor in subjects with chronic liver diseases of other causes who develop HCC. In addition, even minor amounts of alcohol consumption appears to be the most significant factor associated with risk of HCC development, as alcohol consumption ($p = 0.002$) was an independent variable associated with development of HCC in patients with NASH-cirrhosis, and patients who reported any regular alcohol consumption were at greater risk of HCC development in comparison with non-drinkers (hazard ratio: 3.6; P25: 1.5; P75: 8.3) [28].

Management dilemmas

There are still numerous problems with the implementation of existing practice guidelines for HCC. Only a minority of subjects with cirrhosis has been identified and the diagnosis is often made when the patient presents with a complication of end-stage liver disease. In addition, even after identification or suspicion of cirrhosis, only a minority of subjects undergoes routine screening for HCC [10]. It has been shown that failure to screen is associated with the higher likelihood of presentation with advanced cancer with limited options [30]. Once HCC is diagnosed, many subjects are offered no treatment, and of those who are offered treatment, systemic intravenously administered chemotherapy is still the most prevalent modality being used in the general community. Thus, despite robust screening and treatment guidelines [1], the majority of at-risk subjects and those who develop HCC receive suboptimal care. Improvement of this situation is a major public health priority in the United States.

Conclusions

Variable and complex aetiology may affect the clinical course and prognosis in HCC patients. Considering a difference of aetiology from the geographic aspect, further analysis will be necessary all over the world for the global understanding in this field. In addition, investigation of the diverse mechanisms involved in the pathogenesis of HCC in relation to different aetiologic factors may develop effective surveillance programmes, which may lead to improved long-term survival by identifying patients with early-stage disease. Health care providers should also have thorough knowledge of the epidemiology of HCC to make the most of algorithms for early identification and treatment of HCC.

References

1. Bruix J, Sherman M. Management of hepatocellular carcinoma. *Hepatology* 2005; 42:1208–1236.
2. El-Serag HB, Rudolph KL. Hepatocellular carcinoma: epidemiology and molecular carcinogenesis. *Gastroenterology* 2007; 132:2557–2576.
3. Poon D, Anderson BO, Chen LT, et al. Management of hepatocellular carcinoma in Asia: consensus statement from the Asian Oncology Summit 2009. *Lancet Oncol* 2009; 10:1111–1118.
4. Gomaa AI, Khan SA, Toledano MB, et al. Hepatocellular carcinoma: epidemiology, risk factors and pathogenesis. *World J Gastroenterol* 2008; 14:4300–4308.
5. Venook AP, Papandreou C, Furuse J, de Guevara LL. The incidence and epidemiology of hepatocellular carcinoma: a global and regional perspective. *Oncologist* 2010; 15suppl 4:5–13.
6. American Cancer Society. Cancer Facts & Figures 2009. American Cancer Society, Atlanta, GA; 2009.
7. Smith BD, Smith GL, Hurria A, Hortobagyi GN, Buchholz TA. Future of cancer incidence in the United States: burdens upon an aging, changing nation. *J Clin Oncol* 2009; 27(17):2758–2765.
8. Garcia M, Jemal A, Ward EM, et al. Global Cancer Facts & Figures 2007. American Cancer Society, Atlanta, GA; 2007.
9. O'Connor S, Ward JW, Watson M, Momin B, Richardson LC. Hepatocellular carcinoma – United States, 2001–2006. *Morbid Mortal Wkly Rep* 2010; 59(17):517–520.
10. Sanyal AJ, Poklepovic A, Moyneur E, Barghout V. Population-based risk factors and resource utilization for HCC: US perspective. *Curr Med Res Opin* 2010; 26:2183–2191.
11. Gurtsevitch VE. Human oncogenic viruses: hepatitis B and hepatitis C viruses and their role in hepatocarcinogenesis. *Biochemistry (Mosc)* 2008; 73:504–513.
12. Paradis V, Zalinski S, Chelbi E, et al. Hepatocellular carcinoma in patients with metabolic syndrome often develop without significant liver fibrosis: a pathological analysis. *Hepatology* 2009; 49:851–859.
13. Szabó E, Páska C, Kaposi Novák P, Schaff Z, Kiss A. Similarities and differences in hepatitis B and C virus induced hepatocarcinogenesis. *Pathol Oncol Res* 2004; 10: 5–11.
14. Parkin DM. The global health burden of infection-associated cancers in the year 2002. *Int J Cancer* 2006; 118:3030–3044.
15. But DYK, Lai CL, Yuen MF. Natural history of hepatitis-related hepatocellular carcinoma. *World J Gastroenterol* 2008; 14:1652–1656.
16. Donato F, Tagger A, Gelatti U, et al. Alcohol and hepatocellular carcinoma: the effect of lifetime intake and hepatitis virus infections in men and women. *Am J Epidemiol* 2002; 155:323–331.
17. Jacobson IM, Davis GL, El-Serag H, Negro F, Trepo C. Prevalence and challenges of liver diseases in patients with chronic hepatitis C virus infection. *Clin Gastroenterol Hepatol* 2010; 8:924–933.
18. Armstrong GL, Wasley A, Simard EP, et al. The prevalence of hepatitis C virus infection in the United States, 1999 through 2002. *Ann Intern Med* 2006; 144:705–714.
19. Armstrong GL, Alter MJ, McQuillan GM, et al. The past incidence of hepatitis C virus infection: implications for the future burden of chronic liver disease in the United States. *Hepatology* 2000; 31:777–782.
20. Sheikh MY, Choi J, Qadri I, et al. Hepatitis C virus infection: molecular pathways to metabolic syndrome. *Hepatology* 2008; 47:2127–2133.
21. Singal AK, Anand BS. Mechanisms of synergy between alcohol and hepatitis C virus. *J Clin Gastroenterol* 2007; 41:761–772.
22. Puoti M, Bruno R, Soriano V, et al. Hepatocellular carcinoma in HIV-infected patients: epidemiological features, clinical presentation and outcome. *AIDS* 2004; 18:2285–2293.
23. Bedogni G, Miglioli L, Masutti F, et al. Prevalence of and risk factors for nonalcoholic fatty liver disease: the Dionysos nutrition and liver study. *Hepatology* 2005; 42:44–52.
24. Falck-Ytter Y, Younossi ZM, Marchesini G, et al. Clinical features and natural history of nonalcoholic steatosis syndromes. *Semin Liver Dis* 2001; 21:17–26.
25. Angulo P, Keach JC, Batts KP, et al. Independent predictors of liver fibrosis in patients with nonalcoholic steatohepatitis. *Hepatology* 1999; 30:1356–1362.

26. Bugianesi E, Vanni E, Marchesini G. NASH and the risk of cirrhosis and hepatocellular carcinoma in type 2 diabetes. *Curr Diab Rep* 2007; 7:175–180.
27. Sanyal AJ, Banas C, Sargeant C, et al. Similarities and differences in outcomes of cirrhosis due to nonalcoholic steatohepatitis and hepatitis C. *Hepatology* 2006; 43:682–689.
28. Ascha MS, Hanouneh IA, Lopez R, et al. The incidence and risk factors of hepatocellular carcinoma in patients with nonalcoholic steatohepatitis. *Hepatology* 2010; 51:1972–1978.
29. Heidelbaugh JJ, Bruderly M. Cirrhosis and chronic liver failure: Part I. Diagnosis and evaluation. *Am Fam Physician* 2006; 74:756–762.
30. Stravitz RT, Heuman DM, Chand N, et al. Surveillance for hepatocellular carcinoma in patients with cirrhosis improves outcome. *Am J Med* 2008; 121:119–126.

6 New challenges of the NAFLD and HIV epidemics

Quentin M. Anstee[1], Janice Main[2]

[1]Institute of Cellular Medicine, Newcastle University & Liver Unit, Newcastle-Upon-Tyne, UK
[2]Department of Medicine, St. Mary's Campus, Imperial College London, London, UK

LEARNING POINTS

- Non-alcoholic fatty liver disease/non-alcoholic steatohepatitis (NAFLD/NASH; often associated with obesity, insulin resistance/diabetes and other features of the metabolic syndrome) is a leading cause of liver dysfunction worldwide
- NASH may cause progressive liver fibrosis, leading to cirrhosis and hepatocellular carcinoma (HCC)
- Obesity and diabetes are associated with greater risk of malignancy and worse outcomes
- HCC may rarely develop before progression to cirrhosis in the presence of the metabolic syndrome
- Advances in antiretroviral therapy have resulted in improved life expectancy for HIV/viral hepatitis co-infected patients who are now at increased risk of cirrhosis and HCC

Introduction

Worldwide, the development of HCC has primarily been associated with the presence of hepatitis B virus (HBV) or hepatitis C virus (HCV) infection in 80–90% of cases [1]. While these remain the most common causes of HCC, other aetiological factors are becoming increasingly prevalent and are frequently encountered in clinical practice. In particular, the worldwide 'metabolic syndrome' epidemic (characterised by obesity, insulin resistance/type II diabetes mellitus and dyslipidaemia) has, through its hepatic manifestation, NAFLD, exposed an ever-greater proportion of the population to the morbidity associated with progressive liver disease. Similarly, with the advent of highly active antiretroviral (ARV) therapy, patients with HIV-HCV or HIV-HBV co-infection are enjoying significantly greater life expectancy and are, therefore, at risk of conditions with long latent periods such as liver cirrhosis and HCC. Addressing these will pose a major challenge for health care providers and consume an increasing proportion of the available resources during the next decade and beyond.

NAFLD and HCC

Epidemiology of NAFLD/NASH

NAFLD represents a spectrum of liver disease ranging from steatosis (fatty change) through NASH to cirrhosis in the absence of alcohol abuse [2]. With the advent of increasingly sedentary lifestyles and changing dietary patterns, an increase in the prevalence of obesity, insulin resistance/type 2 diabetes mellitus, dyslipidaemia and other associated features of the metabolic syndrome has been observed worldwide. NAFLD/NASH, considered to be the hepatic manifestation of the metabolic syndrome, has become the most common cause of liver dysfunction in many developed countries during the last two decades. Studies in apparently healthy living liver donors indicate a NAFLD prevalence of 12–18% in Europe and 27–38% in the United States with NASH being found in 3–16% and 6–15%, respectively [3,4]. These surprisingly high levels of fatty liver disease are broadly similar to those seen in unselected epidemiological studies where highly sensitive MR spectroscopy techniques estimate that ~34% of US adults have NAFLD [5]. NASH is recognised as the most common cause of hepatic fibrosis and cirrhosis in the non-alcoholic, viral

Clinical Dilemmas in Primary Liver Cancer, First Edition. Edited by Roger Williams and Simon D. Taylor-Robinson.

hepatitis-negative patient population. Independent risk factors for disease progression are age over 45–50 years, presence of diabetes (or severity of insulin resistance), obesity (BMI > 28–30 kg/m^2) and hypertension [5]. Although long-term prospective data are scarce, retrospective studies suggest that progression of fibrosis may occur in 38% of NASH patients [5].

The rise in the burden of NAFLD/NASH within the population of many countries coincides with a marked increase in the annual incidence of HCC. Worldwide estimates suggest that 80–90% of HCC are related to chronic viral hepatitis infection, but in developed countries more than half of all cases of HCC occur in the viral hepatitis-negative population [1]. In general, the majority of NASH-HCC patients are male and tend to be slightly older (mean 66.7, range 45–82 years) at presentation than those with other underlying liver diseases. Most patients have features consistent with the metabolic syndrome including diabetes (64%) and obesity (58%) [6]. Longitudinal studies indicate HCC prevalence to be up to 0.5% in NAFLD and up to 2.8% in NASH and so, while HCC remains a relatively rare complication of fatty liver disease, the high prevalence of NAFLD/NASH contributes significantly to the growing HCC case-load in many developed countries [6]. This was highlighted by a recent US-based population study [7]. NAFLD/NASH was found to be the most common aetiology present in 58.5% of 4406 HCC patients surveyed, followed by diabetes which was present in 35.8% [7]. While it may be argued that the health-insurance population studied was skewed towards higher socio-economic status and so viral hepatitis and alcohol-related disease may have been underrepresented, the data also suggest that the role of NAFLD/NASH in HCC pathogenesis was not simply as a co-factor accelerating progression of viral hepatitis or alcohol related liver disease, since NASH remained the most common association (38.2%) present in the subset of patients that only possessed a single risk factor for HCC [7].

NASH cirrhosis and HCC

Irrespective of underlying aetiology, cirrhosis is present in ~80% of patients with HCC [8]. Retrospective studies from tertiary centres show that 25–33% of NASH patients have at least bridging fibrosis at diagnosis, with 10–15% of these patients having already progressed to cirrhosis [9]. To date, evidence from well-designed prospective studies showing progression of NASH to HCC has been scant. However, a recent publication by Ascha and colleagues that followed patients with NASH-cirrhosis ($n = 195$) and HCV-cirrhosis ($n = 315$) from diagnosis to the development of HCC has estimated cumulative HCC incidence in NASH-cirrhosis to be 2.6% per annum (compared with 4% in HCV-cirrhosis) [10]. Given that both hepatic steatosis and steatohepatitis tend to regress as cirrhosis develops, NASH is likely to be underdiagnosed in the setting of advanced liver disease and is now thought to be the underlying aetiology in 30–75% of so called cryptogenic cirrhosis [5]. Given that varying estimates suggest that between 6.9% and 50% of HCC diagnosed in developed countries arise on a background of cryptogenic cirrhosis, this is a potentially important misclassification that may have led to an underestimation of the morbidity associated with NASH [11]. Retrospective studies that have examined the association between cryptogenic cirrhosis related HCC and NASH provide additional support for this assertion; demonstrating that HCC patients with cryptogenic cirrhosis were much more likely to have diabetes, insulin resistance, dyslipidaemia and obesity than those with HCV, HBV or alcohol-related cirrhosis and HCC [6,12].

Non-cirrhotic NASH and HCC

While (as discussed above) HCC is predominantly found in the presence of underlying cirrhosis, there are several small series and numerous case reports describing its occurrence in non-cirrhotic NASH. The extent to which this occurs remains unclear; one recent retrospective study reported that only 46% of patients with NAFLD/NASH-related HCC had underlying cirrhosis [7]. Although this may be an underestimate, evidence now suggests that many features of the metabolic syndrome associated with NAFLD/NASH such as obesity, diabetes and hepatic iron deposition are themselves independent risk factors for HCC (Table 6.1). This adds biological plausibility to the view that carcinogenesis may occur in the absence of advanced fibrosis in NAFLD [6,21]. Indeed, published data suggest that HCC occurring on a background of non-cirrhotic metabolic syndrome/NASH may have distinct histological characteristics, or may arise through malignant transformation of hepatic adenoma [22].

Beyond serving as a driver of the metabolic syndrome and initiator of NAFLD/NASH, obesity has been implicated as a risk factor for the development of a number of different cancers and also a marker of worse prognosis and higher mortality in both solid organ and haematological malignancies. Supporting this, a large prospective study

TABLE 6.1 Selected evidence for metabolic syndrome risk factors for HCC

Risk factor	Study population	Study size	Relative risk	Reference
Obesity	USA	Population: M 404,576; F 495,477	M 4.52; F 1.68	[15]
	Denmark	Population: 40,000	1.92	[14]
	Korea	Population: 19,271	1.53	[15]
Diabetes	USA	Cohort: 173,643	2.16	[16]
	Sweden	Population: 153,852	3	[17]
	Denmark	Population: 109,581	M 4; F 2.1	[18]
	Greece	Case control: 374/385	1.86	[19]
Iron deposition	Italy	Case control: 52/102	7.08	[20]

by the American Cancer Society estimated the relative risk (RR) of mortality from liver cancer to be 1.68-fold greater in women and 4.52-fold greater in men with a BMI > 35 kg/m^2 than those of normal BMI [13]. Similarly, studies in Denmark and Korea place the overall risk of HCC in obese patients at 1.53–1.92-fold greater than those of normal weight [14,15]. Insulin resistance and type 2 diabetes are strongly associated with obesity. Diabetes was initially thought to be a co-factor predisposing to more aggressive liver disease only in the presence of concomitant alcohol excess or viral hepatitis. However, studies supporting the association are mixed; three of the larger cohort studies suggest that the presence of diabetes alone can increase the risk of developing HCC 2–3-fold [16,23]. As already alluded to, many countries are experiencing a sharp increase in the prevalence of obesity and metabolic syndrome and so even small increase in HCC risk related to these factors, when applied across a large population, could translate into a significant increase in new cases.

The challenges of NASH and HCC

The mechanisms of HCC development in NAFLD/NASH remain unresolved, but many of the same pathological processes (such as increased oxidative stress, lipid peroxidation, apoptotic and necrotic cell death and hepatocellular regenerative responses driven growth factor release) that underlie the pathogenesis of steatohepatitis are pro-carcinogenic (reviewed in [23]). While, to date, it has been the developed countries that have been at the forefront of the obesity and NASH epidemic, obesity rates are climbing worldwide, and with this, the prospect of accelerated disease progression in populations where viral hepatitis is more prevalent.

HIV infection and HCC

Background

Chronic liver disease is common in patients with HIV infection. The routes of infection of HIV and hepatitis viruses are similar and thus many patients have co-existent HBV or HCV infection. Furthermore, many of the ARV agents are hepatotoxic, while patients have high levels of alcohol consumption, and NAFLD is also common in this population. Therefore, patients with HIV infection often have multiple risk factors for the development of chronic hepatitis, cirrhosis and HCC.

Early in the HIV epidemic, patients died because of immunosuppression-related opportunistic infection or malignancy. In effect, hepatitis virus co-infected patients died before they developed the life-threatening complications of chronic viral hepatitis. It is only since the mid-1990s with the availability of more effective combination ARV therapy and improved survival [24] that hepatitis co-infection and risks of hepatic decompensation or HCC development have become clinically relevant. Therefore, the co-infected patients now have a reasonable prognosis in terms of their HIV infection and may survive to face the potentially life-threatening complications of their liver disease.

A French study reviewed the cause of death in 822 HIV-positive patients in the year 2000 [25]. HCV infection was present in 29%, HBV infection in 8% and both HBV and HCV infection in 4% of patients. Of the 110 patients who died of end-stage liver disease, the risk of HCC was 15%. The rate was highest in the HBV-infected patients (50%) compared with the 10% risk in those with HCV infection and a risk of 13% in those with both HBV and HCV infection. A follow-up study in 2005 [26] described an increasing incidence of HCC (25%) and the increasing importance of HCV infection that accounted for 25% of the HCC cases. Approximately 50% of the patients who died because of HCV sequela had received antiviral treatment for HCV, but 98% of them had HCV viraemia at the time of death. This most likely reflects the lower sustained virological response (SVR) rates in co-infected patients and in those with more advanced liver disease.

The introduction of more effective ARV therapy has resulted in changes in the patterns of hospital admissions of HIV-infected patients. A New York study [27] reported a decrease in HIV-related hospital admissions from 1995 to 2001. However, the rates of hospital admission for hepatitis and cirrhosis did not fall significantly. A Spanish study of HIV-positive individuals [28] described an increase in admissions because of decompensated liver disease from 9.1% in 1996 to 26% in 2002. Interestingly, by 2004 this had decreased to 11% and the authors attribute this to improved results of antiviral therapy for HBV and HCV in this setting and also, perhaps, secondarily to the improvement in immune function which is seen with more effective ARV therapy [29].

In co-infected patients, HCC development occurs at an earlier age than in HBV or HCV mono-infected patients [30] and has a more rapidly progressive course with reduced survival [31].

HIV and hepatitis B virus infection

HBV is mainly transmitted via contaminated blood, sexually and vertically (mother to baby).

High prevalence areas include (i) regions in Southeast Asia, where, prior to vaccination programmes, 20% of the population were HBV-infected and (ii) sub-Saharan Africa, where prevalence rates are estimated to be around 10%. In the setting of a Western HIV clinic, men who have sex with men (MSM) and sub-Saharan Africans are the two main population groups at high risk of HIV/HBV co-infection. The prevalence of HBV in the northern European EuroSIDA cohort is 9.1% [32].

The risk of HBV chronicity varies according to the age of the patient with high rates seen in those infected neonatally (more than 90%), compared with a 5% risk in healthy adults. Immunocompromised individuals are more at risk of HBV chronicity and this has been noted in patients with underlying HIV infection. Early natural history studies suggested that HBV had an adverse effect on HIV outcome [33,34], but more recent European studies have not shown this [32] and this has been attributed to the use of ARV regimens that include agents that also inhibit HBV replication, such as lamivudine, emtricitabine and tenofovir. However, it is apparent that despite the availability of effective suppressive therapy, HBV must be recognised as a significant co-morbidity. For example, the EuroSIDA study of HIV-infected patients showed that liver-related mortality was higher in the HIV/HBV-infected patients [32].

In a US prospective cohort study [35], 5293 MSM underwent regular HIV and HBV checks. 326 (6%) men had HBV infection and 65% of them were also HIV positive. The liver-related mortality rate was higher in men with HIV/HBV co-infected men than in the men with HIV monoinfection. HIV/HBV co-infected men with low nadir CD4 counts had higher risks of liver-related death. A follow-up study [36] reviewed patients taking ARV therapy for a median of 7 years. AIDS-related mortality was the most common cause of death and the risk was highest in those with chronic HBV infection. These patients also had the highest rate of non-AIDS mortality – mainly liver disease. These studies highlight the need for expert hepatitis management of this patient group. It is recommended that patients with HIV and HBV infection receive an ARV regimen with two drugs active against HBV and are carefully monitored [37].

However, there are concerns that, in sub-Saharan Africa, some of the ARV regimens in widespread use have only one agent with activity against HBV, which for the most part is usually lamivudine. Patients with HIV and HBV infection generally have high levels of HBV replication and higher risks of antiviral resistance. Therefore, although the ARV regimen may be life-saving in terms of HIV infection, patients with limited access to newer and more expensive treatments will then have to face the sequela of chronic HBV, including that of HCC development [38].

It is important that patients with HIV/HBV infection are assessed from a hepatological viewpoint and encouraged to take part in HCC screening programmes if they are available. Recognition of HBV infection is important in HIV-infected patients, and HBV testing is recommended at baseline and then on an annual basis. Patients should be reminded about safer sex measures, and HBV vaccination is recommended for those partners and family members at risk. Reduced antibody responses following HBV vaccination and a more rapid decline of protective anti-HBs antibodies are seen.

HIV and hepatitis C virus infection

As is well known, HCV is mainly spread via contaminated blood and blood products. Therefore, HIV/HCV co-infection is particularly seen in intravenous drug users and in those who have received contaminated blood products. Mother-to-baby transmission can occur and the risk of this appears higher in HIV/HCV co-infection. This presumably relates to the higher levels of HCV RNA seen in this setting. It has been estimated that there are 4–5 million people with HIV/HCV co-infection worldwide [39]. Sexual transmission of HCV is rare in heterosexuals, but an outbreak of HCV infection among HIV-infected individuals [40] has raised concerns that sexual transmission may be a risk among MSM. The rate of HCV chronicity is higher in HIV-positive patients [41] and several studies have shown more rapid progression of HCV-related liver disease [42]. There may also be an effect of HCV on the outcome and treatment response of HIV infection. The Swiss cohort study [43], for example, compared the CD4 response following initiation of ARV in HIV mono-infected versus HIV/HCV co-infected patients. A reduced CD4 response was noted in the co-infected group.

Treating HCV patients with acute HCV has resulted in SVR rates of approximately 60% [40] and does not appear to be influenced by the HCV genotype.

The SVR rates for chronic hepatitis C treatment in HIV/HCV infection are generally 60% of those seen in patients with HCV mono-infection [44]. Therefore, current treatment guidelines encourage treatment with pegylated interferon and ribavirin combination therapy for HIV-infected patients with genotype 2 or 3 infection, where SVR rates are around 60%, but suggest a more cautious approach for those with harder to treat genotypes (such as genotypes 1 and 4) and reduced response rates [37]. In the APRICOT study [44], for example, the SVR in those with genotype 1 infection was only 29%. Therefore, it is suggested that, for those with harder to treat genotypes and mild disease on liver biopsy, it may be best to defer therapy until more effective agents such as HCV protease and polymerase inhibitors become available.

ARV therapy has now been shown to increase cellular immune response to HCV antigens and inhibit viral replication [45]. It is hoped that more effective antiviral therapy of HCV will reduce the risks of progression to cirrhosis [29,46] and reduce the risk of HCC development.

Sadly, current and future treatments may be outside the budgetary limits of resource-poor settings.

HIV and alcohol consumption

Several studies have reported high levels of alcohol consumption in patients with HIV infection. In one US study, the rates of heavy drinking amongst HIV-positive patients were almost twice those of the general population [47]. Those with HIV/HCV co-infection have particularly high levels of alcohol consumption, which is likely to increase their risk of liver-related death [25].

HIV and NAFLD

NAFLD is also common in patients with HIV infection. At the start of the HIV epidemic, this mainly appeared to be related to those with HIV-associated wasting or 'slim disease'. Now NAFLD is seen in several subgroups of patients with HIV infection and there are concerns that this could result in an increased incidence of HCC. It is also increasingly recognised that a subgroup of HIV patients with metabolic syndrome may be predisposed to NAFLD with risks of cirrhosis and HCC. It is unclear whether this relates to HIV infection or to antiviral agents. Thirty-one per cent of HIV-positive, HBV- and HCV-negative patients were found to have NAFLD in one ultrasound study [48]. Risk factors included dyslipidaemia and high waist measurement, but the authors found no correlation with ARV therapy. Conversely another study reported that use of nucleoside reverse transcriptase inhibitors was an independent risk factor for NAFLD [49].

Careful monitoring of these patients is required. Many of these patients have elevated transaminase values, and as with HIV-negative patients with NAFLD, it is difficult to identify which patients are at particular risk of cirrhosis and HCC. The dilemma of when to perform liver biopsy on these patients is similar to that with patient who is HIV negative. It is hoped that non-invasive methods of assessing fibrosis (such as ultrasound transient elastography) will be helpful in this setting and that the patients with HIV will also benefit from the results of controlled trials of lifestyle changes and other interventions.

Conclusion

The challenges posed by the NAFLD/NASH epidemic are multiple, but from a clinical perspective they can be distilled into one: how can existing health care infrastructures handle such an apparently large at-risk population and provide effective primary prevention (of NASH and the metabolic syndrome), as well as detection/diagnosis and therapy for the consequent increase in HCC? In order to rise to this challenge, additional research is urgently needed to identify and understand the role of genetic modifiers of disease progression to identify novel biomarkers that may be used as screening tools for early tumour detection and to ascertain the effects of insulin sensitising treatment, weight loss and duration of risk exposure on the carcinogenic potential of NASH.

Similarly, the HIV epidemic has resulted in increased risk of HCC, particularly for those with HBV or HCV co-infection. With improved survival in HIV infection, other liver diseases, such as NAFLD, have also become important risk factors for cirrhosis and HCC. It is hoped that this can be successfully countered by advances in antiviral therapy and appropriate monitoring.

References

1. Parkin DM. The global health burden of infection-associated cancers in the year 2002. *Int J Cancer* 2006; 118(12):3030–3044.
2. Day CP. From fat to inflammation. *Gastroenterology* 2006; 130(1):207–210.
3. Minervini MI, Ruppert K, Fontes P, et al. Liver biopsy findings from healthy potential living liver donors: reasons for disqualification, silent diseases and correlation with liver injury tests. *J Hepatol* 2009; 50(3):501–510.
4. Nadalin S, Malago M, Valentin-Gamazo C, et al. Preoperative donor liver biopsy for adult living donor liver transplantation: risks and benefits. *Liver Transpl* 2005; 11(8):980–986.
5. Ratziu V, Bellentani S, Cortez-Pinto H, Day C, Marchesini G. A position statement on NAFLD/NASH based on the EASL 2009 special conference. *J Hepatol* 2010; 53(2):372–384.
6. Starley BQ, Calcagno CJ, Harrison SA. Nonalcoholic fatty liver disease and hepatocellular carcinoma: a weighty connection. *Hepatology* 2010; 51(5):1820–1832.
7. Sanyal A, Poklepovic A, Moyneur E, Barghout V. Population-based risk factors and resource utilization for HCC: US perspective. *Curr Med Res Opin* 2010; 26(9):2183–2191.
8. Hashimoto E, Yatsuji S, Tobari M, et al. Hepatocellular carcinoma in patients with nonalcoholic steatohepatitis. *J Gastroenterol* 2009; 44(suppl 19):89–95.
9. Argo CK, Caldwell SH. Epidemiology and natural history of non-alcoholic steatohepatitis. *Clin Liver Dis* 2009; 13(4):511–531.
10. Ascha MS, Hanouneh IA, Lopez R, Tamimi TA, Feldstein AF, Zein NN. The incidence and risk factors of hepatocellular carcinoma in patients with nonalcoholic steatohepatitis. *Hepatology* 2010; 51(6):1972–1978.
11. Bugianesi E. Non-alcoholic steatohepatitis and cancer. *Clin Liver Dis* 2007; 11(1):191–207, x–xi.
12. Bugianesi E, Leone N, Vanni E, et al. Expanding the natural history of nonalcoholic steatohepatitis: from cryptogenic cirrhosis to hepatocellular carcinoma. *Gastroenterology* 2002; 123(1):134–140.
13. Calle EE, Rodriguez C, Walker-Thurmond K, Thun MJ. Overweight, obesity, and mortality from cancer in a prospectively studied cohort of U.S. adults. *N Engl J Med* 2003; 348(17):1625–1638.
14. Moller H, Mellemgaard A, Lindvig K, Olsen JH. Obesity and cancer risk: a Danish record-linkage study. *Eur J Cancer* 1994; 30A(3):344–350.
15. Oh SW, Yoon YS, Shin SA. Effects of excess weight on cancer incidences depending on cancer sites and histologic findings among men: Korea National Health Insurance Corporation Study. *J Clin Oncol* 2005; 23(21):4742–4754.
16. El-Serag HB, Tran T, Everhart JE. Diabetes increases the risk of chronic liver disease and hepatocellular carcinoma. *Gastroenterology* 2004; 126(2):460–468.
17. Adami HO, Chow WH, Nyren O, et al. Excess risk of primary liver cancer in patients with diabetes mellitus. *J Natl Cancer Inst* 1996; 88(20):1472–1477.
18. Wideroff L, Gridley G, Mellemkjaer L, et al. Cancer incidence in a population-based cohort of patients hospitalized with diabetes mellitus in Denmark. *J Natl Cancer Inst* 1997; 89(18):1360–1365.
19. Lagiou P, Kuper H, Stuver SO, Tzonou A, Trichopoulos D, Adami HO. Role of diabetes mellitus in the etiology of hepatocellular carcinoma. *J Natl Cancer Inst* 2000; 92(13):1096–1099.
20. Sorrentino P, D'Angelo S, Ferbo U, Micheli P, Bracigliano A, Vecchione R. Liver iron excess in patients with hepatocellular carcinoma developed on non-alcoholic steato-hepatitis. *J Hepatol* 2009; 50(2):351–357.
21. Guzman G, Brunt EM, Petrovic LM, Chejfec G, Layden TJ, Cotler SJ. Does nonalcoholic fatty liver disease predispose patients to hepatocellular carcinoma in the absence of cirrhosis? Arch Pathol Lab Med 2008; 132(11):1761–1766.
22. Paradis V, Zalinski S, Chelbi E, et al. Hepatocellular carcinomas in patients with metabolic syndrome often develop without significant liver fibrosis: a pathological analysis. *Hepatology* 2009; 49(3):851–859.
23. El-Serag HB, Rudolph KL. Hepatocellular carcinoma: epidemiology and molecular carcinogenesis. *Gastroenterology* 2007; 132(7):2557–2576.
24. Palella FJ Jr, Delaney KM, Moorman AC, et al. Declining morbidity and mortality among patients with advanced human immunodeficiency virus infection. HIV Outpatient Study Investigators. *N Engl J Med* 1998; 338:853–860.

25. Salmon-Ceron D, Lewden C, Morlat P, et al. Mortality 2000 study group. Liver disease as a major cause of death among HIV-infected patients: role of hepatitis C and B viruses and alcohol. *J Hepatol* 2005; 42:799–805.
26. Salmon-Ceron D, Rosenthal E, Lewden C, et al. ANRS EN19 Mortalite Study Group and Mortavic. Emerging role of hepatocellular carcinoma among liver-related causes of deaths in HIV-infected patients: The French national Mortalite 2005 study. *J Hepatol* 2009; 50:736–745.
27. Paul S, Gilbert HM, Lande L, et al. Impact of antiretroviral therapy on decreasing hospitalization rates of HIV-infected patients in 2001. *AIDS Res Hum Retroviruses* 2002; 18:501–506.
28. Martin-Carbonero L, Sanchez-Somolinos M, Garcia-Samaniego J, et al. Reduction in liver-related hospital admissions and deaths in HIV-infected patients since the year 2002. *J Viral Hepat* 2006; 13:851–857.
29. Qurishi N, Kreuzberg C, Luchters G, et al. Effect of antiretroviral therapy on liver-related mortality in patients with HIV and hepatitis C virus coinfection. *Lancet* 2003; 362:1708–1713.
30. Brau N, Fox RK, Xiao P, et al. North American Liver Cancer in HIV Study Group. Presentation and outcome of hepatocellular carcinoma in HIV-infected patients: a US–Canadian multicenter study. *J Hepatol* 2007; 47:527–537.
31. Puoti M, Bruno R, Soriano V, et al. HIV HCC Cooperative Italian–Spanish Group. Hepatocellular carcinoma in HIV-infected patients: epidemiological features, clinical presentation and outcome. *AIDS* 2004; 18:2285–2293.
32. Konopnicki D, Mocroft A, de Wit S, et al. EuroSIDA Group. Hepatitis B and HIV: prevalence, AIDS progression, response to highly active antiretroviral therapy and increased mortality in the EuroSIDA cohort. *AIDS* 2005; 19:593–601.
33. Eskild A, Magnus P, Petersen G, et al. Hepatitis B antibodies in HIV-infected homosexual men are associated with more rapid progression to AIDS. *AIDS* 1992; 6:571–574.
34. Ockenga J, Tillmann HL, Trautwein C, Stoll M, Manns MP, Schmidt RE. Hepatitis B and C in HIV-infected patients. Prevalence and prognostic value. *J Hepatol* 1997; 27: 18–24.
35. Thio CL, Seaberg EC, Skolasky R Jr, et al. Multicenter AIDS Cohort Study. HIV-1, hepatitis B virus, and risk of liver-related mortality in the Multicenter Cohort Study (MACS). *Lancet* 2002; 360:1921–1926.
36. Hoffmann CJ, Seaberg EC, Young S, et al. Hepatitis B and long-term HIV outcomes in coinfected HAART recipients. *AIDS* 2009; 23:1881–1889.
37. Brook G, Main J, Nelson M, et al. BHIVA Viral Hepatitis Working Group. British HIV Association guidelines for the management of coinfection with HIV-1 and hepatitis B or C virus 2010. *HIV Med* 2010; 11:1–30.
38. Lessells RJ, Cooke GS. Effect of the HIV epidemic on liver cancer in Africa. *Lancet* 2008; 371:1504.
39. Alter MJ. Epidemiology of viral hepatitis and HIV co-infection. *J Hepatol* 2006; 44(1 suppl):S6–S9.
40. Gilleece YC, Browne RE, Asboe D, et al. Transmission of hepatitis C virus among HIV-positive homosexual men and response to a 24-week course of pegylated interferon and ribavirin. *J Acquir Immune Defic Syndr* 2005; 40:41–46.
41. Thomson EC, Fleming VM, Main J, et al. Predicting spontaneous clearance of acute hepatitis C virus in a large cohort of HIV-1-infected men. *Gut* 2011; 60(6):837–845.
42. Benhamou Y, Bochet M, Di Martino V, et al. Liver fibrosis progression in human immunodeficiency virus and hepatitis C virus coinfected patients. *The Multivirc Group.* Hepatology 1999; 30(4):1054–1058.
43. Greub G, Ledergerber B, Battegay M, et al. Clinical progression, survival, and immune recovery during antiretroviral therapy in patients with HIV-1 and hepatitis C virus coinfection: the Swiss HIV Cohort Study. *Lancet* 2000; 356:1800–1805.
44. Torriani FJ, Rodriguez-Torres M, Rockstroh JK, et al. APRICOT Study Group. Peginterferon Alfa-2a plus ribavirin for chronic hepatitis C virus infection in HIV-Infected patients. *N Engl J Med* 2004; 351(5):438–450.
45. Rohrbach J, Robinson N, Harcourt G, et al. Swiss HIV Cohort Study. Cellular immune responses to HCV core increase and HCV RNA levels decrease during successful antiretroviral therapy. *Gut* 2010; 59:1252–1258.
46. Brau N, Salvatore M, Rios-Bedoya CF, et al. Slower fibrosis progression in HIV/HCV-coinfected patients with successful HIV suppression using antiretroviral therapy. *J Hepatol* 2006; 44:47–55.
47. Galvan FH, Bing EG, Fleishman JA, et al. The prevalence of alcohol consumption and heavy drinking among people with HIV in the United States: results from the HIV Cost and Services Utilization Study. *J Stud Alcohol* 2002; 63:179–186.
48. Crum-Cianflone N, Dilay A, Collins G, et al. Nonalcoholic fatty liver disease among HIV-infected persons. *J Acquir Immune Defic Syndr* 2009; 50(5):464–473.
49. Guaraldi G, Squillace N, Stentarelli C, et al. Nonalcoholic fatty liver disease in HIV-infected patients referred to a metabolic clinic: prevalence, characteristics, and predictors. *Clin Infect Dis* 2008; 47:250–257.

PART 2

Influence of Tumour Characteristics

7 Controversies in pathology

Tania Roskams

Department of Morphology and Molecular Pathology, University Hospitals Leuven, Leuven, Belgium

LEARNING POINTS

- Understand that carcinogenesis is a stepwise process, whereby early cancer does not show all classical imaging features of more advanced cancer. Biopsy can discriminate early cancer from dysplastic nodules (DNs) using immunohistochemistry for molecular markers glypican-3, heath shock protein 70 and glutamin synthetase
- Understand the heterogeneity of primary liver cancer. Next to hepatocellular and cholangiocellular carcinoma, mixed/intermediate types of primary cancer exist, which have a worse prognosis. To recognise these mixed features, K19 is recommended as the best validated marker at the moment

Introduction

The diagnosis of a malignant tumour usually requires a histological confirmation before a curative or palliative treatment is considered. Recent guidelines published by the professional associations for the study of the liver and liver disease have challenged this paradigm in patients with cirrhosis [1]. The proposed current decision tree for diagnosis of possible hepatocellular carcinoma (HCC) nodules greater than 1 cm in diameter requires liver biopsy only if there is no arterial hypervascularity and venous or delayed washout on the first and a repeated contrast-enhanced imaging study [1].

In recent years, non-invasive imaging techniques for the diagnosis of HCC before liver transplantation have been widely used in different centres. In the study by Hayashi et al. [2], 27% of 30 patients with a pre-transplantation diagnosis of HCC had no evidence of tumour in the explanted liver and this led to incorrect organ allocation in 7% of their patients [2]. Wiesner and colleagues reported that in 31% and 9% of the patients, who underwent liver transplantation for stage 1 (1 nodule ≤ 1.9 cm) and stage 2 HCC (1 nodule 2.0–5.0 cm or 2–3 nodules all ≤3), respectively, there was no evidence of tumour in the explanted liver [3]. Similar results were also reported from a recent study in France, where a false positive pre-operative diagnosis of HCC was made in 20% of the patients [4]. Results from these studies suggest that the non-invasive diagnosis of HCC is associated with a significant false positive rate. Nevertheless, a correct pre-transplant diagnosis of HCC is not only of utmost importance for the patient but it also has a major impact on organ allocation. In several countries, for example the United States, patients with stage 2 HCC are awarded extra Model for End-stage Liver Disease points to allow for transplantation in a timely manner, whereas for patients with stage 1 HCC (1 nodule ≤ 1.9 cm) no extra points are assigned.

With the current guidelines, HCC is the only clinically significant malignant tumour that is considered not to require histological examination and confirmation to establish the diagnosis. Since for HCC diagnosis, tissue analysis is not mandatory in clinical trials, this can have a deleterious effect on the interpretation of the trial results. Currently, it is impossible to determine whether certain molecularly defined tumour subgroups show a better response than other to experimental therapies. Targeted therapy with a tissue-based histopathological and molecular evaluation prior to treatment is a reality for other cancers, for example carcinoma of the breast, lung

Clinical Dilemmas in Primary Liver Cancer, First Edition. Edited by Roger Williams and Simon D. Taylor-Robinson.

and colon. If this standard diagnosis certainly is not applied soon to HCC, clinical trial reliability will lag father behind for standards expected in other branches of oncology. Individualised HCC therapy requires definition of patient subgroups that could benefit most, or should be protected from therapy failure and unwarranted side effects. The decision not to make biopsy of HCC mandatory was made in previous decades, when no customised systemic therapy seemed feasible or imminent. This decision also clearly must be revisited urgently in the light of modern therapeutic options. Ultimately, it is also an ethical necessity to design clinical trials in a way that optimises data interpretation for the sake of future generations of patients.

From the histopathological and molecular point of view, it is now clear that primary liver cancer is even more heterogeneous than we previously thought.

Pathology diagnosis should take advantage of molecular techniques, so that a diagnosis of primary liver carcinoma is not based solely on classical staining methods but also on immunohistochemistry and characterisation of molecular markers and signalling pathways. According to the current guidelines described earlier, pathologists preferentially receive biopsies from small lesions that have an atypical vascularisation pattern. In this context, differentiating between a high-grade dysplastic nodule and early HCC is the first challenge.

High-grade dysplastic nodule versus early HCC

Hepatocarcinogenesis in the human liver is a stepwise process, in which a small monoclonal focus (dysplastic focus, <1 mm) expands into a dysplastic nodule (>1 mm). Low-grade dysplastic nodules (LGDNs) evolve into high-grade dysplastic nodules (HGDNs) [5]. The evolution into true carcinoma includes induction of an arterial blood supply, stromal invasion, venous invasion and finally metastasis [5,6] (Figure 7.1). In the early stages of HCC, the typical arterial hypervascular pattern is not yet present. In 1995, the

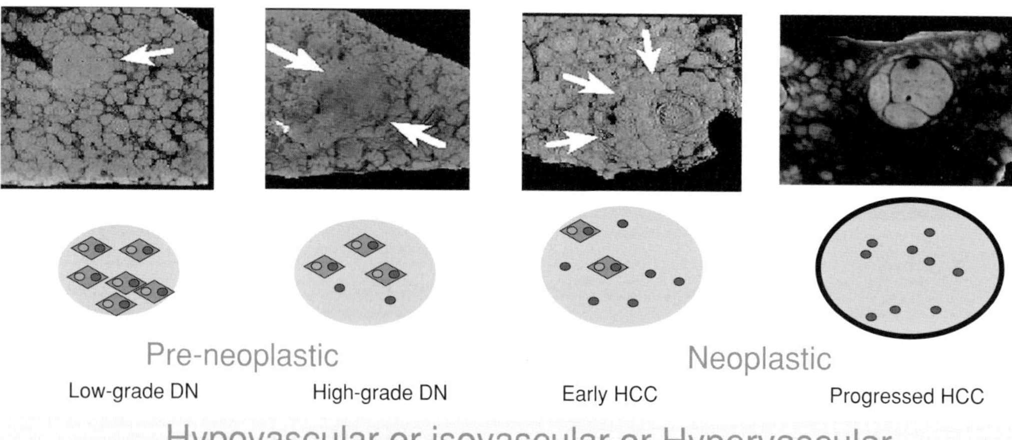

FIG 7.1 Scheme of (pre)neoplastic nodules. Grossly, many of HGDNs and most of well-differentiated HCCs of the early type (early HCC) are vaguely nodular and contain portal tracts within the nodule. Stromal invasion is not observed in either LG or HGDNs, but is present in early HCC. Unpaired arteries are sporadic in DNs, but increased in early HCC. On the other hand, moderately differentiated HCCs are distinctly nodular even when they are small and contain no portal tracts. Many unpaired arteries are present. Clinically, DNs and most of early HCCs are found as hypo- or isovascular lesions and receive portal blood supply through the intratumoural portal tracts as well. Small HCCs of the distinctly nodular type and all of moderately differentiated HCCs are hypervascular and show 'washout' on contrast images. DNs could be interpreted as pre-malignant lesions, well-differentiated HCC of the vaguely nodular type are early HCC, and small HCCs of the distinctly nodular type are advanced HCC.

International Working Party Classification rationalised the nomenclature of early hepatocellular neoplasia by referring to pre-malignant neoplastic nodules as LGDN and HGDN [7]. This terminology has been widely accepted. In order to obtain an international consensus on the pathological diagnosis of equivocal lesions, such as DNs and early HCC, an International Consensus Group for Hepatocellular Neoplasia was convened in April 2002 in Kurume, Japan. The group met several times subsequently after April 2002 up to July 2007 in Leuven, Belgium, Bordeaux, France and Tessaloniki, Greece, respectively, culminating a consensus document that was reported in Hepatology in 2009 [8]. A very important feature that differentiates HGDN from early HCC is stromal invasion in portal tracts, which are still present in early HCC, albeit at low number. A panel of molecular markers are now also used for the diagnosis of early HCC, namely glypican-3, heat shock protein 70 and glutamine synthetase. If two of these three markers are positive, a sensitivity of 72% and specificity of 100% is reached for the diagnosis of HCC.

Diagnosis of primary liver cancer: HCC, cholangiocarcinoma or mixed phenotypes

Once the diagnosis of malignancy is established, primary liver carcinoma is classically classified as HCC or cholangiocarcinoma (CC) as the main categories, and also according to degree of cellular differentiation. While this differentiation may be of prognostic relevance, problems remain because of the marked degree of heterogeneity in both HCC and CC. Although a mixed HCC/CC category is recognised in the WHO classification, confusing terminology has been generated to describe different overlapping entities (e.g. intermediate cell tumours, progenitor cell tumours, mixed tumours, small cell HCC, cholangiocellular carcinomas), showing features of both HCC and CC or of cells intermediate between hepatocytes and cholangiocytes. The variously proposed terminology reflects our increasing knowledge on the pathogenesis of liver cancer and possible cellular precursors. In fact, there is growing evidence for the concept of a stem/progenitor cell origin of liver cancer, as was proposed in animal models and human tumours showing a whole range of immunophenotypical traits of hepatocytes, cholangiocytes and progenitor cells [9–12] (Figure 7.2). In essence, in humans, the so-called transit amplifying cells of the liver (hepatic progenitor cells, HPC) have been localised in the canals of Hering [13–16]. These are cells that have a higher probability of undergoing terminal differentiation than self-renewal. Among other properties, these cells have been shown to be capable of differentiating into hepatocytes and cholangiocytes and of expressing multidrug resistance proteins, including Breast Cancer Related Protein. The latter causes resistance to various disadvantageous survival conditions, including toxic drugs [17,18]. These cells are activated in the majority of chronic human liver diseases [19–21]. Chronic liver disease and specifically cirrhosis is a major risk factor for HCC development. In the cirrhotic stage of chronic liver disease, mature hepatocytes are known to become senescent [22]. Inhibition of replication of hepatocytes is the perfect trigger for activation of progenitor cells [16,19,23,24]. As such, activated progenitor cells may form target cells for subsequent initiation of carcinogenesis [10,11,25,26].

The presence of progenitor cell features in a tumour can be explained in two ways: either the cell of origin is a progenitor cell (maturation arrest theory) or, alternatively, tumours dedifferentiate and acquire progenitor cell features during carcinogenesis (dedifferentiation theory) (Figure 7.2). When progenitor cells are the cell of origin of a subtype of primary liver tumours, one would expect that the earlier pre-malignant precursor lesions would also consist of progenitor cells and their progeny. This is indeed the case: 55% of small cell dysplastic foci (<1 mm), the earliest pre-malignant lesions known to-date in humans, consist of progenitor cells and intermediate hepatocytes [29]. This is a very strong argument in favour of the progenitor cell origin of at least some of the HCCs.

An often-emphasised concept is that of the cancer stem cell, which is the cell renewal source of a neoplasm and the seed for metastasis [30], which expresses similar toxic drug-exporting protein pumps as the non-neoplastic stem cell. According to this concept, a tumour consists of a hierarchy of cell populations, of which the very small cancer stem cell population is the one that has the growth and metastatic potential of the tumour. The other neoplastic cells are offspring of the cancer stem cells and each can differentiate a little differently, according to the local micro-environment in each part of the tumour. This explains the enormous heterogeneity of the phenotype of a neoplasm in different areas. How do liver stem cells drive cancer initiation? By using microdissection and analysis of the molecular pathways of activated progenitor cells, we could show that Wnt signalling plays an pivotal role in expansion of non-neoplastic human progenitor cells, while notch activation is important for biliary differentiation and notch inhibition is necessary to have hepatocyte differentiation [31]. An excessive and persistent self-renewal signal, involving Wnt/beta-catenin and BMI-1 is also one of the key events in early carcinogenesis [32–35]. Therefore, targeting the liver cancer stem cells should be the ideal treatment for liver cancer.

Immunophenotype of primary liver carcinoma

Mature hepatocytes express keratins (K) 8 and 18 in the cytoplasm, CD10 and CD66e (detectable by polyclonal anti-CEA antibody) in canaliculi (Figure 6a) and Hep-Par-1 Ag in cytoplasmic granules. This profile contrasts with that of mature cholangiocytes, which express K7 and K19, in addition to K8 and K18. HPC present K19, a very early hepatoblast marker (Figure 7.1), and K7, K8 and K18, while some subpopulations express epithelial cell adhesion molecule (EpCAM), CD133, c-kit, CD34 and CD90.

As in rodents, HCC and CC evolve from focal precursor lesions that reflect the stages of multistep carcinogenesis [5,6,36]. Most tumours show still phenotypical features of their cell of origin, and the histopathological classification of tumours is largely based on this. A considerable number of human HCCs (diagnosed according to WHO criteria on hematoxylin-eosin (HE) staining) express markers of progenitor/biliary cells such as K7, K19 and OV6 [9,37–44] (Figure 7.2). Morphologically, these tumours consist of cells with a very immature phenotype as well as a range of cells with intermediate phenotypes in between progenitor cells and hepatocytes. One common feature of all these tumours was decreased survival of patients; in fact, survival of patients with these tumours was close to the known poor survival of patients with CC [9,37–42,44].

Wu et al. observed a significantly shorter survival in patients with HCCs expressing AE1-AE3 and K19 without any treatment (than in AE-1-AE3 and K19 negative tumours) [40]. Uenishi et al. reported that HCCs expressing K19 and K7 have a lower tumour-free survival rate after curative resection (than for K19 and K17 negative lesions) and demonstrated that K19 expression was an independent predictor of post-operative recurrence [38]. In a study by

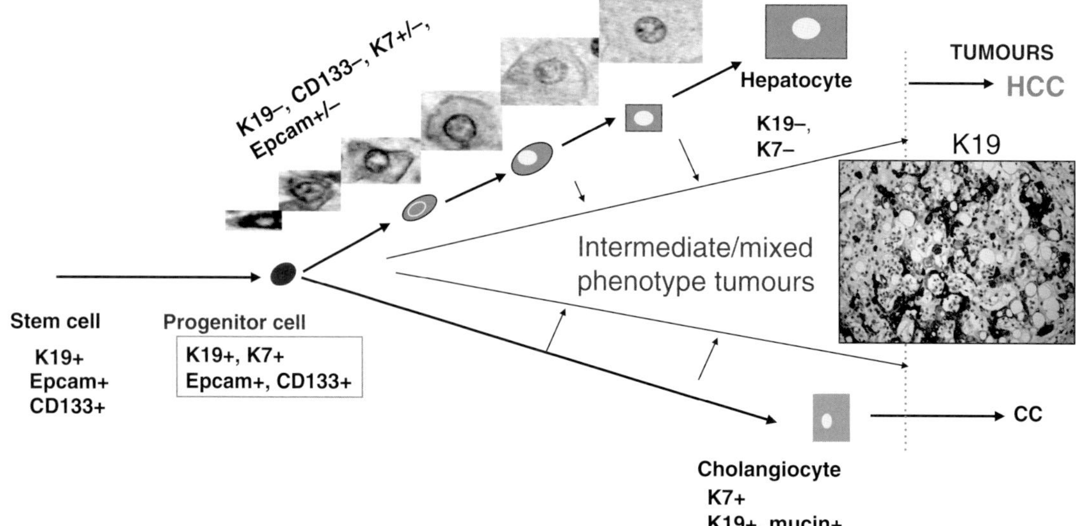

FIG 7.2 Possible cancer phenotypes originating from a progenitor cell. Progenitor cells can differentiate into hepatocytes and cholangiocytes, which in turn can give rise to HCC/cholangiocellular carcinoma. When a progenitor cell on its way to differentiation, develops into cancer (maturation arrest), this can give rise to tumours with a whole range of phenotypes with varying hepatocellular and cholangiocellular differentiation characteristics. Cytokeratin 19 stain is suggested as a progenitor cell/bililary marker. The inset shows a K19 staining of a hepatocellular carcinoma with small-undifferentiated progenitor cells and a range of intermediate phenotypes in between hepatocytes and progenitor/biliary cells. Several studies show that a cut-off of 5% CK19 reactive cells already influences the outcome of the patient. These hepatocellular carcinomas with progenitor cell features have more and faster recurrence of disease after surgical treatment.

Ding et al., over-expression of K19 corrected with HCC metastasis [45]. In a consecutive series of 109 HCCs in Caucasians, K19-positive tumours (K19+ in more than 5% of tumour cells) had a higher rate of tumour recurrence after liver transplantation compared with patients with K19-negative HCCs [41]. K19 expression was significantly associated with elevated serum alpha-fetoprotein (AFP > 400 ng/mL), and expression of AFP by the tumour. The authors concluded that the association with AFP, a marker of hepatic progenitor cells, is compatible with a progenitor cell origin of these tumours. Aishima et al. [46] studied 35 small (<3 cm) HCC with biliary differentiation based on morphology, K19 immunoexpression and mucin secretion and compared them with 61 ordinary HCC. They found that extrahepatic recurrence was more common in K19(+) than in K19(−) HCC and that patients with K19(+)/mucin(+) HCC had the worst survival. More recently, Zhuang et al. [42] recognised two pathologic types of HCC in terms of lymph node metastasis based on their K19-immunophenotype. They studied 172 HCC with or without positive lymph nodes and showed that K19 immunoreactivity was an independent prognostic factor for development of lymph node metastasis. Moreover, in the subgroup of lymph node metastatic HCC, patients with K19-expressing HCC had shorter overall survival.

The prognostic value of K19 expression in HCC was further supported by micro-array-based gene expression profiling. Study of the global gene expression pattern in 91 HCCs from China and Belgium revealed two distinctive subclasses (A and B) that were highly associated with patient survival [47]. A subsequent integrative functional genomics study compared the gene expression data of an independent set of 61 HCCs with rat foetal hepatoblasts and adult hepatocytes, and with mouse HCCs from different experimental models. Individuals with HCC who shared a gene expression pattern with foetal hepatoblasts (hepatoblast signature) belonged to subclass A with poor prognosis and the profile that included markers of hepatic progenitor cells (K19, K7, vimentin) suggested that HCC of this subtype may arise from progenitor cells [48]. Yamashita et al. [43] used cDNA micro-arrays to study 238 HCC and identified a subset of EpCAM-positive HCC with worse prognosis, which displayed a unique molecular signature with features of HPC including the presence of K19 expression. In the current WHO guidelines, K19 is, therefore, included as a prognostic marker for HCC.

Potential liver cancer stem cell markers

Several liver stem cell markers have been proposed. Given the similarities between normal stem cells and cancer stem cells, it is reasonable to assume that the phenotype of liver cancer stem cells resembles that of normal stem/progenitor cells.

As described above, K19 is a very early hepatoblast marker and marker of normal adult liver progenitor cells and is associated with worse prognosis of HCC. OV6, a rodent progenitor cell marker, recognises K19 and K14 in rat and as such is the rodent equivalent of K19. Yang et al. [35] have demonstrated that OV6(+) HCC cells posses greater tumourigenic ability and chemoresistance to standard chemotherapy when compared with OV6(−) cells. The wnt/beta-catenin pathway plays a key role in the expansion of progenitor cells in human HCC, similar to its role in expansion of non-neoplastic progenitor cells in acute and chronic liver diseases [31].

Ma et al. [49] discovered that prominin-1, the murine homologue of human CD133, was significantly upregulated in liver regeneration. In subsequent functional studies on sorted HCC cells, $CD133^+$ cells displayed cancer stem cell properties. $CD133^+$ cells had greater tumourigenicity than $CD133^-$ cells in immunodeficient mice, higher colony-forming capacity and proliferation ability in vitro and could be induced into non-hepatocyte-like lineages, showing multipotency. The expression of 'stemness' genes were higher in $CD133^+$ cells then in $CD133^-$ cells. Further studies showed $CD133^+$ cells are resistance to conventional chemotherapy [50].

CD90 has been suggested as a putative marker for liver cancer stem cells. This marker is expressed on hepatic progenitor cells during development [51] and CD90 expression correlates with tumourigenic potential in a panel of liver cell lines [52]. Further characterisation with cell sorting for CD45 resulted in a population of $CD90^+CD45^-$ cells of which the majority also expressed CD44 [53]. CD44 is a cell surface receptor for hyaluronic acid and its blockade with neutralising antibodies induced apoptosis of $CD90^+$ cells and prevented tumour formation in mice [53].

EpCAM has been suggested as cancer stem cell marker, since $EpCAM^+$ HCC cells were found to be more tumourigenic than $EpCAM^-$ cells [54]. Interestingly, EpCAM is a direct transcriptional target in the wnt/beta-catenin pathway and hence could serve as a biomarker for the activation of this pathway [55].

Normal human progenitor cells have certain subtypes of active transmembrane adenosine triphosphate-binding cassette (ABC) transporters, such as MDR1, ABCG2 and ABCC2 [17,18,56], rendering them resistant to oxidative stress, and toxic substances, including chemotherapy agents. These transporters also efflux the DNA-binding dye Hoechst 33342 and hence 'side sort' in fluorescence-activated cell sorting. It was shown that side population cells from HCC cell lines harbour cancer stem cell-like properties; they were highly proliferative and chemoresistant in vitro [57] whereas non-side population cells did not. The increased tumourigenic potential of side population cells was shown in vivo in SCID mice, where 103 side populations cells consistently led to tumour formation whereas 10^6 non-side population did not. In addition, it was found that side population cells isolated from HCC cell lines may be related to the metastatic potential of HCC [58]. MRP1 expression correlated with a more aggressive tumour phenotype and with K19 expression [59]. High expression of ABC transporters renders the cells resistant to chemotherapy, including cisplatin and doxorubicin. Inhibition of MDR1 [60], ABCG2 [61] and ABCC2 [62] by inhibitors or using an antisense approach can reverse this chemoresistance.

Conclusions

An East–West consensus on the definition of dysplastic versus (early) neoplastic liver lesions has been reached. Molecular markers (glypican-3, HSP-70, glutamine synthetase) and stromal invasion are used for the differential diagnosis. A better understanding of signalling pathways in HCC pathogenesis has led to targeted therapies against HCC, using drugs like sorafenib, erlotinib and bevacizumab [63]. These therapies target the major cell populations of rapidly growing differentiated tumour cells [63]. However, increasing evidence for the existence of cancer stem cells suggests the possibility of targeting the undifferentiated cancer stem cells that only constitute a small proportion of the tumour. The identification of liver cancer stem cell markers and their related pathways is one of the important goals of liver cancer research. Therefore, understanding the mechanisms of activation and differentiation of non-neoplastic stem/progenitor cells and especially the differences with their malignant counterparts should also be a top priority. New therapies should ideally target cancer stem cells and *not* normal stem/progenitor cells, since these are very important in regeneration and repair mechanisms. Individualised HCC therapy will require better definition of patient subgroups that benefit most or should be protected from therapy failure and unwanted side effects; for example, biliary/progenitor cell features in an HCC render these tumours more resistant to chemotherapy. For all these reasons, tumour tissue acquisition should be mandatory, reversing the practice that was established years ago when no targeted HCC therapy was available.

References

1. Bruix J, Llovet JM. Two decades of advances in hepatocellular carcinoma research. *Semin Liver Dis* 2010; 30:1–2.
2. Hayashi PH, Trotter JF, Forman L, et al. Impact of pretransplant diagnosis of hepatocellular carcinoma on cadveric liver allocation in the era of MELD. *Liver Transpl* 2004; 10:42–48.
3. Wiesner RH, Freeman RB, Mulligan DC. Liver transplantation for hepatocellular cancer: the impact of the MELD allocation policy. *Gastroenterology* 2004; 127: S261–S267.
4. Compagnon P, Grandadam S, Lorho R, et al. Liver transplantation for hepatocellular carcinoma without preoperative tumor biopsy. *Transplantation* 2008; 86:1068–1076.
5. Kojiro M, Roskams T. Early hepatocellular carcinoma and dysplastic nodules. *Semin Liver Dis* 2005; 25:133–142.
6. Roskams T, Kojiro M. Pathology of early hepatocellular carcinoma: conventional and molecular diagnosis. *Semin Liver Dis* 2010; 30:17–25.
7. Party IW. Terminology of nodular hepatocellular lesions. *Hepatology* 1995; 22:983–993.
8. International Consensus Group for Hepatocellular Neoplasia. Pathologic diagnosis of early hepatocellular carcinoma: a report of the international consensus group for hepatocellular neoplasm. *Hepatology* 2009; 49:658–664.
9. Yoon DS, Jeong J, Park YN, et al. Expression of biliary antigen and its clinical significance in hepatocellular carcinoma. *Yonsei Med J* 1999; 40:472–477.
10. Roskams T. Liver stem cells and their implication in hepatocellular and cholangiocarcinoma. *Oncogene* 2006; 25:3818–3822.
11. Alison MR, Lovell MJ. Liver cancer: the role of stem cells. *Cell Prolif* 2005; 38:407–421.
12. Theise ND, Yao JL, Harada K, et al. Hepatic 'stem cell' malignancies in adults: four cases. *Histopathology* 2003; 43:263–271.
13. Theise ND, Saxena R, Portmann BC, et al. The canals of Hering and hepatic stem cells in humans. *Hepatology* 1999; 30:1425–1433.
14. Kuwahara R, Kofman AV, Landis CS, Swenson ES, Barendswaard E, Theise ND. The hepatic stem cell niche:

identification by label-retaining cell assay. *Hepatology* 2008; 47(6):1994–2002.
15. Roskams TA, Theise ND, Balabaud C, et al. Nomenclature of the finer branches of the biliary tree: canals, ductules, and ductular reactions in human livers. *Hepatology* 2004; 39:1739–1745.
16. Roskams T. Different types of liver progenitor cells and their niches. *J Hepatol* 2006; 45:1–4.
17. Ros JE, Libbrecht L, Geuken M, Jansen PL, Roskams TA. High expression of MDR1, MRP1, and MRP3 in the hepatic progenitor cell compartment and hepatocytes in severe human liver disease. *J Pathol* 2003; 200:553–560.
18. Vander Borght S, Libbrecht L, Katoonizadeh A, et al. Breast cancer resistance protein (BCRP/ABCG2) is expressed by progenitor cells/reactive ductules and hepatocytes and its expression pattern is influenced by disease etiology and species type: possible functional consequences. *J Histochem Cytochem* 2006; 54:1051–1059.
19. Falkowski O, An HJ, Ianus IA, et al. Regeneration of hepatocyte 'buds' in cirrhosis from intrabiliary stem cells. *J Hepatol* 2003; 39:357–364.
20. Libbrecht L, Desmet V, Van Damme B, Roskams T. Deep intralobular extension of human hepatic 'progenitor cells' correlates with parenchymal inflammation in chronic viral hepatitis: can 'progenitor cells' migrate? *J Pathol* 2000; 192:373–378.
21. Roskams T. Progenitor cell involvement in cirrhotic human liver diseases: from controversy to consensus. *J Hepatol* 2003; 39:431–434.
22. Wiemann SU, Satyanarayana A, Tsahuridu M, et al. Hepatocyte telomere shortening and senescence are general markers of human liver cirrhosis. *Faseb J* 2002; 16:935–942.
23. Lowes KN, Brennan BA, Yeoh GC, Olynyk JK. Oval cell numbers in human chronic liver diseases are directly related to disease severity. *Am J Pathol* 1999; 154:537–541.
24. Lowes KN, Croager EJ, Olynyk JK, Abraham LJ, Yeoh GC. Oval cell-mediated liver regeneration: role of cytokines and growth factors. *J Gastroenterol Hepatol* 2003; 18:4–12.
25. Roskams TA, Libbrecht L, Desmet VJ. Progenitor cells in diseased human liver. *Semin Liver Dis* 2003; 23: 385–396.
26. Roskams T, Yang SQ, Koteish A, et al. Oxidative stress and oval cell accumulation in mice and humans with alcoholic and nonalcoholic fatty liver disease. *Am J Pathol* 2003; 163:1301–1311.
27. Hixson DC, Brown J, McBride AC, Affigne S. Differentiation status of rat ductal cells and ethionine-induced hepatic carcinomas defined with surface-reactive monoclonal antibodies. *Exp Mol Pathol* 2000; 68:152–169.
28. Dumble ML, Croager EJ, Yeoh GC, Quail EA. Generation and characterization of p53 null transformed hepatic progenitor cells: oval cells give rise to hepatocellular carcinoma. *Carcinogenesis* 2002; 23:435–445.
29. Libbrecht L, Desmet V, Van Damme B, Roskams T. The immunohistochemical phenotype of dysplastic foci in human liver: correlation with putative progenitor cells. *J Hepatol* 2000; 33:76–84.
30. Hamburger AW, Salmon SE. Primary bioassay of human tumor stem cells. *Scie:ıce* 1977; 197:461–463.
31. Spee B, Carpino G, Schotanus BA, et al. Characterisation of the liver progenitor cell niche in liver doseases: potential involvement of Wnt and Notch signalling. *Gut* 2010; 59(2):247–257.
32. Wicha MS, Liu S, Dontu G. Cancer stem cells: an old idea – a paradigm shift. *Cancer Res* 2006; 66:1883–1890; discussion 1895–1886.
33. Taniguchi H, Chiba T. Stem cells and cancer in the liver. *Dis Markers* 2008; 24:223–229.
34. Armengol C, Cairo S, Fabre M, Buendia MA. Wnt signaling and hepatocarcinogenesis: the hepatoblastoma model. *Int J Biochem Cell Biol* 2011; 43(2):265–270.
35. Yang W, Yan HX, Chen L, et al. Wnt/beta-catenin signaling contributes to activation of normal and tumorigenic liver progenitor cells. *Cancer Res* 2008; 68:4287–4295.
36. Libbrecht L, Desmet V, Roskams T. Preneoplastic lesions in human hepatocarcinogenesis. *Liver Int* 2005; 25:16–27.
37. Hsia CC, Evarts RP, Nakatsukasa H, Marsden ER, Thorgeirsson SS. Occurrence of oval-type cells in hepatitis B virus-associated human hepatocarcinogenesis. *Hepatology* 1992; 16:1327–1333.
38. Uenishi T, Kubo S, Yamamoto T, et al. Cytokeratin 19 expression in hepatocellular carcinoma predicts early postoperative recurrence. *Cancer Sci* 2003; 94:851–857.
39. Van Eyken P, Sciot R, Paterson A, Callea F, Kew MC, Desmet VJ. Cytokeratin expression in hepatocellular carcinoma: an immunohistochemical study. *Hum Pathol* 1988; 12:562–568.
40. Wu PC, Lai VC, Fang JW, Gerber MA, Lai CL, Lau JY. Hepatocellular carcinoma expressing both hepatocellular and biliary markers also expresses cytokeratin 14, a marker of bipotential progenitor cells. *J Hepatol* 1999; 31: 965–966.
41. Durnez A, Verslype C, Nevens F, et al. The clinicopathological and prognostic relevance of cytokeratin 7 and 19 expression in hepatocellular carcinoma. A possible progenitor cell origin. *Histopathology* 2006; 49:138–151.
42. Zhuang PY, Zhang JB, Zhu XD, et al. Two pathologic types of hepatocellular carcinoma with lymph node metastasis with distinct prognosis on the basis of CK19 expression in tumor. *Cancer* 2008; 112(12):2740–2748.
43. Yamashita T, Forgues M, Wang W, et al. EpCAM and alpha-fetoprotein expression defines novel prognostic subtypes of hepatocellular carcinoma. *Cancer Res* 2008; 68:1451–1461.

44. Aishima S, Kuroda Y, Nishihara Y, et al. Proposal of progression model for intrahepatic cholangiocarcinoma: clinicopathologic differences between hilar type and peripheral type. *Am J Surg Pathol* 2007; 31:1059–1067.
45. Ding SJ, Li Y, Tan YX, et al. From proteomic analysis to clinical significance: overexpression of cytokeratin 19 correlates with hepatocellular carcinoma metastasis. *Mol Cell Proteomics* 2004; 3:73–81.
46. Aishima S, Nishihara Y, Kuroda Y, et al. Histologic characteristics and prognostic significance in small hepatocellular carcinoma with biliary differentiation: subdivision and comparison with ordinary hepatocellular carcinoma. *Am J Surg Pathol* 2007; 31:783–791.
47. Lee JS, Chu IS, Heo J, et al. Classification and prediction of survival in hepatocellular carcinoma by gene expression profiling. *Hepatology* 2004; 40:667–676.
48. Lee JS, Heo J, Libbrecht L, et al. A novel prognostic subtype of human hepatocellular carcinoma derived from hepatic progenitor cells. *Nat Med* 2006; 12(4):410–416.
49. Ma S, Chan KW, Hu L, et al. Identification and characterization of tumorigenic liver cancer stem/progenitor cells. *Gastroenterology* 2007; 132:2542–2556.
50. Ma S, Lee TK, Zheng BJ, Chan KW, Guan XY. CD133+ HCC cancer stem cells confer chemoresistance by preferential expression of the Akt/PKB survival pathway. *Oncogene* 2008; 27:1749–1758.
51. Dan YY, Riehle KJ, Lazaro C, et al. Isolation of multipotent progenitor cells from human fetal liver capable of differentiating into liver and mesenchymal lineages. *Proc Natl Acad Sci USA* 2006; 103:9912–9917.
52. Yang ZF, Ho DW, Ng MN, et al. Significance of CD90+ cancer stem cells in human liver cancer. *Cancer Cell* 2008; 13:153–166.
53. Yang ZF, Ngai P, Ho DW, et al. Identification of local and circulating cancer stem cells in human liver cancer. *Hepatology* 2008; 47:919–928.
54. Yamashita T, Ji J, Budhu A, et al. EpCAM-positive hepatocellular carcinoma cells are tumor-initiating cells with stem/progenitor cell features. *Gastroenterology* 2009; 136:1012–1024.
55. Yamashita T, Budhu A, Forgues M, Wang XW. Activation of hepatic stem cell marker EpCAM by Wnt-beta-catenin signaling in hepatocellular carcinoma. *Cancer Res* 2007; 67:10831–10839.
56. Ros JE, Libbrecht L, Geuken M, Jansen PL, Roskams TA. High expression of MDR1, MRP1, and MRP3 in the hepatic progenitor cell compartment and hepatocytes in severe human liver disease. *J Pathol* 2003; 200(5):553–560.
57. Chiba T, Kita K, Zheng YW, et al. Side population purified from hepatocellular carcinoma cells harbors cancer stem cell-like properties. *Hepatology* 2006; 44:240–251.
58. Shi GM, Xu Y, Fan J, et al. Identification of side population cells in human hepatocellular carcinoma cell lines with stepwise metastatic potentials. *J Cancer Res Clin Oncol* 2008; 134:1155–1163.
59. Vander Borght S, Komuta M, Libbrecht L, et al. Expression of multidrug resistance-associated protein 1 in hepatocellular carcinoma is associated with a more aggressive tumour phenotype and may reflect a progenitor cell origin. *Liver Int* 2008; 28:1370–1380.
60. Wakamatsu T, Nakahashi Y, Hachimine D, Seki T, Okazaki K. The combination of glycyrrhizin and lamivudine can reverse the cisplatin resistance in hepatocellular carcinoma cells through inhibition of multidrug resistance-associated proteins. *Int J Oncol* 2007; 31:1465–1472.
61. Hu C, Li H, Li J, et al. Analysis of ABCG2 expression and side population identifies intrinsic drug efflux in the HCC cell line MHCC-97L and its modulation by Akt signaling. *Carcinogenesis* 2008; 29:2289–2297.
62. Folmer Y, Schneider M, Blum HE, Hafkemeyer P. Reversal of drug resistance of hepatocellular carcinoma cells by adenoviral delivery of anti-ABCC2 antisense constructs. *Cancer Gene Ther* 2007; 14:875–884.
63. Siegel A. Moving targets in hepatocellular carcinoma: hepatic progenitor cells as novel targets for tyrosine kinase inhibitors. *Gastroenterology* 2008; 135:733–735.

8 Not to forget the unusual tumour

Bernard C. Portmann
King's College Medical School, University of London, London, UK

LEARNING POINTS

- *Combined hepatocellular carcinoma and cholangiocarcinoma* (cHCC-CC) may be difficult to diagnose prior to surgical excision. Even a retrospective diagnosis will help understanding the natural history of this uncommon variant whose overall prognosis appears poorer than that of common hepatocellular carcinoma (HCC)
- K7 expression is not uncommon in HCC. K19 appears a more specific marker of progenitor cells/biliary differentiation, but the threshold associated with a more aggressive tumour behaviour remains to be determined
- A diagnosis of *fibrolamellar hepatocellular carcinoma* (FL-HCC) should include both histological appearances and the demographic context of young age, alpha-fetoprotein (AFP) negativity and absent cirrhosis. Fibrolamellar foci in otherwise common HCC or the rare sclerosing or scirrhous HCC lack the lenient prognosis of timely diagnosed FL-HCC
- Metastatic deposit of *hepatoid adenocarcinoma* (HAC) may be histologically identical to HCC. Multiple nodules on a non-cirrhotic liver and old patient age should arise suspicion of a possible occult primary site, most often in stomach
- Amongst metastatic deposits that may mimic HCC, *clear cell renal carcinoma, amelanotic melanoma* and *neuroendocrine neoplasms* are most important to exclude in view of their different therapeutic options and prognosis. This can easily be achieved in applying relevant immunohistochemical techniques
- Conventional histology of *epithelioid angiomyolipoma* (AML), an essentially benign neoplasm, may easily been misdiagnosed as HCC. The clinical context, pathologist awareness and HMB-45 immunostaining performed on a biopsy specimen are diagnostic and will avoid unnecessarily aggressive surgery or chemotherapy

Introduction

On histology, HCC generally recapitulates its tissue of origin in both cell morphology and architectural pattern. In essence, the tumour cells, like hepatocytes, are large with abundant eosinophilic, clear or fatty cytoplasm and centrally placed nuclei containing a prominent nucleolus. The cells form several cell-thick trabeculae separated by thin endothelium-lined channels reminiscent of hepatic sinusoids. A pseudoglandular growth pattern is also well recognised with prominent lumens that variably contain amorphous eosinophilic, bile-stained or colloid-like material. In most instances, the histological diagnosis is straightforward, especially when bile pigment can be identified, but in a significant number of cases that depart from this basic histology, the diagnostic has to be supported by immunohistochemical staining using polyclonal carcinoembryonic antigen (pCEA) or CD10 antibodies that highlight canalicular structures or hepatocyte specific antibodies (HepPar1), whose positivity, although not entirely specific will strongly favour HCC, whereas tissue staining for AFP is often

Clinical Dilemmas in Primary Liver Cancer, First Edition. Edited by Roger Williams and Simon D. Taylor-Robinson.

unreliable. Diagnostic problems arise with poorly differentiated HCC or at the other end of the spectrum with well-differentiated tumour that may be difficult to differentiate from hepatocellular adenoma (HCA).

In less than 5% of HCC, distinctive features allow tumour sub-grouping whose recognition has prognostic and management implications. These include mixed or combined HCC-cholangiocellular carcinoma and the fibrolamellar variant of HCC, which will be considered first.

Conversely, metastatic deposits may mimic HCC, in particular hepatoid carcinoma, clear cell renal carcinoma, malignant melanoma and some endocrine neoplasms. Benign lesions such as AML and adrenal gland inclusions may occasionally be misdiagnosed as HCC, and finally, rare cases of splenosis have been clinically confused with HCC.

Variants of HCC

Combined hepatocellular and cholangiocellular carcinoma

cHCC-CC with features of both hepatocellular and biliary epithelial differentiation remains an uncommon form of primary liver cancer, although the broader use of immunohistochemistry and genetic profiling has lead to a better recognition of biliary features in HCC and an increasing number of lesions are now reallocated to this subgroup.

Aberrant expression of keratin 7 (K7) is a common finding in both acute and chronic liver disorders and not surprisingly patchy staining may be found in about a third of HCC [1], whereas cells expressing K19, a more selective biliary/progenitor cell marker, seem associated with poor differentiation and a more aggressive tumour behaviour [2]. A threshold of K7/19 expression that may impart to the lesion such an adverse prognosis is not clearly defined. As gene expression profiling is not routinely performed in clinical practice, one can only speculate that some of these cases may represent the novel cholangiocarcinoma-like HCC subtype identified by Woo et al., which expresses cholangiocarcinoma-like traits (CC signature) linked with an aggressive tumour phenotype [3].

Based on histological appearances and immunostaining cases actually diagnosed as cHCC-CC accounts for some 1% of primary liver tumours. In cHCC-CC portions of the tumour consist of smaller and more basophilic cells forming distorted glandular structures set in a sclerosing stroma, a pattern reminiscent of CC (Plate 8.1). This component expresses K7/19, MOC31 [4], may show a diffuse pattern of staining with pCEA and a variable expression of Ca19-9 and CC apomucins. The HCC component is confirmed by HepPar 1 immunostaining, the demonstration of canalicular structures highlighted by pCEA or CD10, AFP, whose sensitivity in tissue is very low, glypican-3 [5] and thyroid transcription factor (TTF)-1, which may be misleading [6]. In situ hybridisation for albumin mRNA is also used [7]. The two components of cHCC-CC vary in their extent and may occur side by side or be intimately intermingled. Rarely HCC and CCA occur separately (coincidental or collision tumours).

Due to the mixed histological features, a pre-operative diagnosis is rarely achieved with tumour markers in the serum or cross-sectional abdominal imaging [8]. This makes the natural history of this infrequent neoplasm incompletely studied. Although the cHCC-CC patients show greater similarity with HCC patients with regard to male/female ratio, status of hepatitis viral infection, serum AFP level and background liver [9], all published series agree that tumour progression, recurrence after surgery and metastatisation are higher for cHCC-CC than for HCC, the prognosis being even poorer than that of CC occurring alone [8–12]. However, in one recent series of liver transplant (LT) recipients for cHCC-CC, 1-, 3- and 5-year cumulative survival probabilities were 79%, 66% and 16%, respectively, with a 5-year survival comparable to or better than LT for intrahepatic CC but lower than LT for HCC following the Milan criteria. The cholangiocarcinoma component seems to explain the poor outcome for this rare tumour as suggested by a high CA-19-9 serum levels associated with a poorer prognosis in one study [11]. Good long-term survival after transplantation is recorded in an isolated case [13]. By multivariate analysis of overall survival in another study, lymph node metastasis, histological subgroup, and vascular invasion were significant independent prognostic factors; a large CC component and presence of rare *sarcomatous* areas correlated with particularly aggressive tumours [14].

Carcinosarcoma

Foci of vimentin or S-100 positive spindle cells are occasionally detected in HCC and cHCC-CC [15], but extremely rare is a true carcinosarcoma in which a carcinoma element sharing features of HCC or cHCC-CC occur alongside differentiated sarcomatous elements, such as chondrosarcoma, osteosarcoma, leiomyosarcoma or malignant schwanoma.

The prognosis is very poor with a less than 6 months survival [16], a single case with an encapsulated lesion having had a tumour free survival of 30 months following partial hepatectomy [17].

Fibrolamellar hepatocellular carcinoma

This variant of HCC recognised as a distinct clinicopathological entity in 1980 affects young, AFP seronegative, non-cirrhotic patients in the absence of known risk factors for HCC.

The tumour often bears a characteristic central scar with discrete radiating septa reminiscent of focal nodular hyperplasia, which may lead to misleading interpretation on imaging (Plate 8.2A). Microscopically, FL-HCC is characterised by large hepatoid cells with deeply eosinophilic and granular cytoplasm due to the presence of a large number of mitochondria. Hyaline globular inclusions, usually PAS positive, react with alpha1-antitrypsin, and ground glass-like cytoplasmic inclusions may represent fibrinogen retention. Tumour cell nuclei are large, hyperchromatic and vesicular, and have prominent eosinophilic, nucleoli. The fibrous stroma that gives the lesion its name consists of thick bundles of hyaline collagen often forming parallel lamellae (Plate 8.2B). As expected, the tumour cells react with HepPar1, and also express the macrophages marker CD68, a transmembrane glycoprotein located within lysosomes/endosomes [18]. K7 staining is more prominent in FL-HCC than in classic HCC, whereas glypican-3 is prevalent in the latter [19]. Differentiation from sclerosing foci that may occur in otherwise classical HCC, from some CC with a trabecular pattern and from scirrhous HCC is important in term of prognosis and may require immunohistochemistry [20]; scirrhous HCC have a preferentially sub-capsular location and an increased content in hepatic stellate cells, but in all other aspects they are similar to classical HCC [21].

FL-HCC carries a high resectability rate and an excellent prognosis, if an early diagnosis can be achieved [21]. However, advanced disease has a high recurrence rate after either resection or transplantation. In fact, post-transplant immunosuppression seems to enhance tumour progression, particularly in patients with lymph nodes involvement at the time of surgery. Whether the better prognosis is due to a peculiar tumour biology or the absence of cirrhosis in the background liver remains uncertain [22]. Recent data suggest that limited differentiation and cell cycle arrest may underpin the indolent nature and relative chemoresistance of FL-HCC [23]. The vitamin B12 binding protein haptocorrin has been advocated as a suitable marker of disease recurrence and progression. Given the lack of effective treatment repeat resections for recurrent tumour has been advocated [21]. In one series, an early detection of relapse combined with multimodality therapy including re-resection, systemic chemotherapy and radiotherapy resulted in a prolonged median survival of 9.3 years [24].

Clear cell HCC

This rare histological variant of HCC, which cannot be diagnosed pre-operatively apparently, shares the same clinical characteristics as that of common HCC according to a recent survey from the Far East [25]. Clear cell change reflects either lipid or glycogen overload. The importance of the lesion lies in its differential diagnosis from metastatic clear cell neoplasm (see the following). Clear cell HCC is generally positive for HepPar1 and canaliculi can be demonstrated with pCEA, but in situ hybridisation for albumin mRNA is the most specific and sensitive technique [26]. An isolated case developed 25 years after successful treatment of a hepatoblastoma [27].

Well-differentiated HCC adenoma

Distinction of HCA from well-differentiated HCC can be difficult and sometimes impossible. Features of malignancy, including high nuclear/cytoplasmic ratios and nuclear irregularities are helpful, but these may be present to some extent in tumours associated with a prolonged intake of oestrogenic or C17-alkylated steroids (Plate 8.3), a history that is most important in evaluating these tumours. A positive immunostaining for glypican-3 support HCC, but results are often negative in well-differentiated HCC [28]. Similarly, markers of nuclear proliferation (Ki67) and endothelial differentiation (CD34) are more strongly expressed in HCC, but identical staining may be obtained in some HCA. It must be mentioned that immunohistochemistry showing translocation ofbeta-catenin to the nuclei and a strong cytoplasmic expression of glutamine synthetase in HCA are predictors of beta-catenin-activating mutations that bear an increased risk of HCC transformation irrespective of the presence of atypical features [29].

Metastatic deposits that may mimic HCC

Distinguishing poorly differentiated HCC from other malignancies, especially metastases, and also from poorly differentiated cholangiocarcinoma may at times be problematic. A large cell with eosinophilic cytoplasm, prominent nuclei and nucleoli and scanty vascular stroma suggests HCC. In most instances, definite evidence of hepatocellular differentiation such as bile in canaliculi recognisable on haematoxylin and eosin sections, canaliculi demonstrated by pCEA or CD10 immunostaining, a positive granular staining with HepPar-1 will confirm HCC, except for the rare cases of liver metastasis from a gastrointestinal adenocarcinoma with hepatoid features that can be similarly positive. When doubt subsists, additional immunohistochemistry may allow us either to rule out HCC and/or to characterise the nature of metastatic deposit whose appearances imitate HCC.

Hepatoid adenocarcinoma

HAC is a rare and aggressive extrahepatic tumour morphologically mimicking HCC. Liver metastases occur as multiple nodules, which may be a first manifestation in AFP sero-positive patients who are generally older than patients with HCC. In a literature review of 261 cases, the most common primary locations of HAC were stomach (63%), ovaries (10%), lung (5%), gallbladder (4%), pancreas (4%) and uterus (4%), which may be occult at the time liver metastases are detected [30]. Gastric HAC has a higher rate of vascular invasion, lymph node and liver metastases than non-HAC gastric adenocarcinoma, with a 5-year survival rate of 9% for HAC versus 44% for ordinary adenocarcinoma [31]. Rare cases of pancreatic primary associated with neuroendocrine carcinoma seem to have a slightly better prognosis [32].

Histologically, the tumour shares features and immunomarkers of HCC, but unlike HCC, HAC may express EpCAM antibodies HEA125 or MOC31 [30]. SALL4, an oncofetal protein that is expressed in foetal stomach up to gestational week 9 and may reappear in intestinal metaplastic mucosa, has recently been found not only to co-localise with glypican-3 and AFP in tumour cells but also to discriminate HAC from HCC, the latter being SALL4 negative [33]. ATP-binding cassette transporters, in particular P-glycoprotein, multidrug resistant-associated protein (MRP)1, MRP2 and MRP6 that play a role in the ATP-dependent outward efflux of drugs are expressed in gastric HAC, possibly explaining the mechanisms of tumour chemoresistance [34].

Renal clear cell carcinoma

As alluded to in the preceding text, clear cell HCC may closely resemble a metastatic deposit of renal clear cell carcinoma (RCC) because of cell size and appearances, which may include hyaline globules [35] and a scanty vascular stroma. Hepatocyte markers, in particular HepPar1 and pCEA, and more specifically in situ hybridisation for albumin mRNA [26] will generally allow the differential diagnosis, but when negative or doubtful, the use of RCC markers that are negative in HCC such as vimentin, epithelial membrane antigen, Leu M-1, pancytokeratin and RCC antigen [36] are recommended, as positive staining will allow further investigation and avoid unnecessary and potentially life-shortening liver replacement.

Adrenocortical carcinoma may rarely enter the differential diagnosis as immunomarkers may somewhat overlap with HCC; positive inhibin-1 and melan A (A103) have been found as reliable discriminants [37].

Metastatic *melanoma*, especially when amelanotic and not associated with a history of previously removed skin or ocular lesions, may be overlooked and misdiagnosed as poorly differentiated HCC, but HMB-45, S100 and/or melan A are positive in melanoma and negative in HCC. A diagnosis of melanoma may lead to newly applied therapy such as surgery followed by tumour infiltrating lymphocytes, although promising results remain to be confirmed [38].

Neuroendocrine neoplasms metastatic to liver may resemble HCC, in particular variants with small uniform eosinophilic or clear cells in, respectively, a macronodular or an acinar growth pattern (Plate 8.4A) [39]. The latter have to be ruled out using neuroendocrine markers such as CD56, chromogranin and synaptophysin (Plate 8.4B) as the prognosis and management of endocrine neoplasms differ dramatically from that of HCC. Positive results will warrant an octreotid scan to seek for an occult primary site. HCC expressing neuroendocrine markers or neuroendocrine neoplasms apparently primary in the liver have been occasionally recorded.

Rare benign lesions with overlapping features

Angiomyolipoma

AML is a benign tumour composed of variable admixtures of thick-walled blood vessels, smooth muscle (spindle or epithelioid) and adipose tissue leading to a broad lesion spectrum [40]. It matches that observed in renal AML which is more common than liver AML. The variant with a marked predominance of myomatous elements frequently exhibits trabecular, discohesive or pelioid growth patterns and variably pleomorphic epithelioid cells that may be clear or oncocytic (Plate 8.5A). It is the type most frequently mistaken for HCC [41]. Unlike its renal counterpart, hepatic AML often shows haemopoietic foci.

The neoplasm is thought to arise from putative perivascular epithelioid cells, which may be found forming perivascular aggregates in various organs of patients with tuberous sclerosis. Tuberous sclerosis is associated more rarely with hepatic than renal AML (6% vs. 40–50%), and when it occurs the patients have coexisting renal AML and often multiple liver tumours. The cells express both melanic (HMB-45) (Plate 8.5B) and variably smooth muscle makers (alpha-smooth muscle actin and desmin).

Radiological features of AML are inconsistent due to the immense diversity in the composition of these lesions, but the presence of early draining vein connecting with prominent tumour vessels and absence of capsule were useful CT findings to differentiate fat-deficient AML from HCC in non-cirrhotic liver [42].

Hepatic AML should be suspected in liver tumour patients with a normal AFP levels, an absence of underlying liver disease or risk factors for HCC and the CT characteristics mentioned above. Percutaneous fine-needle biopsy is the diagnostic method of choice, provided pathologists are aware of AML variants with a deceptive epithelial appearance. HepPar1 negativity and HMB-45 (Plate 8.5A) confirm the diagnosis which is essential to avoid an unduly aggressive surgical procedure. Malignant transformation of AML appears extremely rare [43].

Adrenal rest tumour

Adrenal-rest tumours may be non-functioning clinically and enter the differential diagnosis of hypervascular fatty liver masses. Histologically, the mass is composed of pale cells resembling adrenal cortex and immunohistochemistry for adrenal 4-binding protein and enzymes involved in the synthesis of adrenocortical steroids may confirm the origin [44].

Splenosis

Heterotopic splenic tissue generally occurs after traumatic rupture of the spleen or surgical manipulation during splenectomy. It is well recognised in both the abdominal and thoracic cavities as multiple nodules, which may also affect solid organs [45]. Splenosis is rare in the liver, where it may become manifest many years after splenectomy and raise the differential diagnosis of mass lesions [46]. Appearances on contrast-enhanced ultrasound [47], a sub-capsular location and history of splenectomy assist in differentiating splenosis from malignancy in particular HCC. However, some cases are not diagnosed prior to biopsy or excision of the lesion.

References

1. Durnez A, Verslype C, Nevens F, et al. The clinicopathological and prognostic relevance of cytokeratin 7 and 19 expression in hepatocellular carcinoma. A possible progenitor cell origin. *Histopathology* 2006; 49:138–151.
2. van Sprundel RG, van den Ingh TS, Desmet VJ, et al. Keratin 19 marks poor differentiation and a more aggressive behaviour in canine and human hepatocellular tumours. *Comp Hepatol* 2010; 9:4.
3. Woo HG, Lee JH, Yoon JH, et al. Identification of a cholangiocarcinoma-like gene expression trait in hepatocellular carcinoma. *Cancer Res* 2010; 70:3034–3041.
4. Porcell AI, De Young BR, Proca DM, Frankel WL. Immunohistochemical analysis of hepatocellular and adenocarcinoma in the liver: MOC31 compares favorably with other putative markers. *Mod Pathol* 2000; 13:773–778.
5. Shirakawa H, Kuronuma T, Nishimura Y, et al. Glypican-3 is a useful diagnostic marker for a component of hepatocellular carcinoma in human liver cancer. *Int J Oncol.* 2009; 34:649–656.
6. Lei JY, Bourne PA, diSant'Agnese PA, Huang J. Cytoplasmic staining of TTF-1 in the differential diagnosis of hepatocellular carcinoma vs cholangiocarcinoma and metastatic carcinoma of the liver. *Am J Clin Pathol* 2006; 125:519–525.
7. Tickoo SK, Zee SY, Obiekwe S, et al. Combined hepatocellular-cholangiocarcinoma: a histopathologic, immunohistochemical, and in situ hybridization study. *Am J Surg Pathol* 2002; 26:989–997.
8. Panjala C, Senecal DL, Bridges MD, et al. The diagnostic conundrum and liver transplantation outcome for combined hepatocellular-cholangiocarcinoma. *Am J Transplant* 2010; 10:1263–1267.
9. Yano Y, Yamamoto J, Kosuge T, et al. Combined hepatocellular and cholangiocarcinoma: a clinicopathologic study of 26 resected cases. *Jpn J Clin Oncol* 2003; 33:283–287.
10. Lee JH, Chung GE, Yu SJ, et al. Long-term prognosis of combined hepatocellular and cholangiocarcinoma after curative resection comparison with hepatocellular carcinoma and cholangiocarcinoma. *J Clin Gastroenterol* 2011; 45:69–75.

11. Kim KH, Lee SG, Park EH, et al. Surgical treatments and prognoses of patients with combined hepatocellular carcinoma and cholangiocarcinoma. *Ann Surg Oncol* 2009; 16:623–629.
12. Zuo HQ, Yan LN, Zeng Y, et al. Clinicopathological characteristics of 15 patients with combined hepatocellular carcinoma and cholangiocarcinoma. *Hepatobiliary Pancreat Dis Int* 2007; 6:161–165.
13. Maganty K, Levi D, Moon J, et al. Combined hepatocellular carcinoma and intrahepatic cholangiocarcinoma: outcome after liver transplantation. *Dig Dis Sci* 2010; 55:3597–3601.
14. Aishima S, Kuroda Y, Asayama Y, et al. Prognostic impact of cholangiocellular and sarcomatous components in combined hepatocellular and cholangiocarcinoma. *Hum Pathol* 2006; 37:283–291.
15. Papotti M, Sambataro D, Marchesa P, Negro F. A combined hepatocellular/cholangiocellular carcinoma with sarcomatoid features. *Liver* 1997; 17:47–52.
16. Goto H, Tanaka A, Kondo F, et al. Carcinosarcoma of the liver. *Intern Med* 2010; 49:2577–2582.
17. Yamamoto Y, Ojima H, Shimada K, et al. Long-term recurrence-free survival in a patient with primary hepatic carcinosarcoma: case report with a literature review. *Jpn J Clin Oncol* 2010; 40:166–173.
18. Ross HM, Daniel HD, Vivekanandan P, et al. Fibrolamellar carcinomas are positive for CD68. *Mod Pathol* 2011; 24(3):390–395.
19. Abdul-Al HM, Wang G, Makhlouf HR, Goodman ZD. Fibrolamellar hepatocellular carcinoma: an immunohistochemical comparison with conventional hepatocellular carcinoma. *Int J Surg Pathol* 2010; 18:313–318.
20. Kurogi M, Nakashima O, Miyaaki H, Fujimoto M, Kojiro M. Clinicopathological study of scirrhous hepatocellular carcinoma. *J Gastroenterol Hepatol* 2006; 21:1470–1477.
21. Stipa F, Yoon SS, Liau KH, et al. Outcome of patients with fibrolamellar hepatocellular carcinoma. *Cancer* 2006; 106:1331–1338.
22. Kakar S, Burgart LJ, Batts KP, Garcia J, Jain D, Ferrell LD. Clinicopathologic features and survival in fibrolamellar carcinoma: comparison with conventional hepatocellular carcinoma with and without cirrhosis. *Mod Pathol* 2005; 18:1417–1423.
23. Dhingra S, Li W, Tan D, Zenali M, Zhang H, Brown RE. Cell cycle biology of fibrolamellar hepatocellular carcinoma. *Int J Clin Exp Pathol* 2010; 3:792–797.
24. Maniaci V, Davidson BR, Rolles K, et al. Fibrolamellar hepatocellular carcinoma: prolonged survival with multimodality therapy. *Eur J Surg Oncol* 2009; 35:617–621.
25. Ye XP, Li LQ, Peng T, et al. Diagnosis and treatment of primary clear cell carcinoma of the liver. *Zhonghua Zhong Liu Za Zhi* 2010; 32:64–66.
26. Oliveira AM, Erickson LA, Burgart LJ, Lloyd RV. Differentiation of primary and metastatic clear cell tumors in the liver by in situ hybridization for albumin messenger RNA. *Am J Surg Pathol* 2000; 24:177–182.
27. Basile J, Caldwell S, Nolan N, Hammerle C. Clear cell hepatocellular carcinoma arising 25 years after the successful treatment of an infantile hepatoblastoma. *Ann Hepatol.* 2010; 9:465–467.
28. Shafizadeh N, Ferrell LD, Kakar S. Utility and limitations of glypican-3 expression for the diagnosis of hepatocellular carcinoma at both ends of the differentiation spectrum. *Mod Pathol* 2008; 21:1011–1018.
29. Bioulac-Sage P, Rebouissou S, Thomas C, et al. Hepatocellular adenoma subtype classification using molecular markers and immunohistochemistry. *Hepatology* 2007; 46:740–748.
30. Metzgeroth G, Ströbel P, Baumbusch T, Reiter A, Hastka J. Hepatoid adenocarcinoma – review of the literature illustrated by a rare case originating in the peritoneal cavity. *Onkologie* 2010; 33:263–269.
31. Liu X, Cheng Y, Sheng W, et al. Analysis of clinicopathologic features and prognostic factors in hepatoid adenocarcinoma of the stomach. *Am J Surg Pathol* 2010; 34:1465–1471.
32. Jung JY, Kim YJ, Kim HM, et al. Hepatoid carcinoma of the pancreas combined with neuroendocrine carcinoma. *Gut Liver* 2010; 4:98–102.
33. Ushiku T, Shinozaki A, Shibahara J, et al. SALL4 represents fetal gut differentiation of gastric cancer, and is diagnostically useful in distinguishing hepatoid gastric carcinoma from hepatocellular carcinoma. *Am J Surg Pathol* 2010; 34:533–540.
34. Kamata S, Kishimoto T, Kobayashi S, Miyazaki M. Expression and localization of ATP binding cassette (ABC) family of drug transporters in gastric hepatoid adenocarcinomas. *Histopathology* 2008; 52:747–754.
35. Nayar R, Bourtsos E, DeFrias DV. Hyaline globules in renal cell carcinoma and hepatocellular carcinoma. A clue or a diagnostic pitfall on fine-needle aspiration? *Am J Clin Pathol.* 2000; 114:576–582.
36. Murakata LA, Ishak KG, Nzeako UC. Clear cell carcinoma of the liver: a comparative immunohistochemical study with renal clear cell carcinoma. *Mod Pathol* 2000; 13:874–881.
37. Pan CC, Chen PC, Tsay SH, Ho DM. Differential immunoprofiles of hepatocellular carcinoma, renal cell carcinoma, and adrenocortical carcinoma: a systemic immunohistochemical survey using tissue array technique. *Appl Immunohistochem Mol Morphol* 2005; 13:347–352.
38. Ripley RT, Davis JL, Klapper JA, et al. Liver resection for metastatic melanoma with postoperative tumor-infiltrating lymphocyte therapy. *Ann Surg Oncol* 2010; 17:163–170.
39. Arista-Nasr J, Fernández-Amador JA, Martínez-Benítez B, de Anda-González J, Bornstein-Quevedo L. Neuroendocrine

metastatic tumors of the liver resembling hepatocellular carcinoma. *Ann Hepatol.* 2010; 9:186–191.

40. Zeng JP, Dong JH, Zhang WZ, Wang J, Pang XP. Hepatic angiomyolipoma: a clinical experience in diagnosis and treatment. *Dig Dis Sci* 2010; 55:3235–3240.
41. Tsui WM, Colombari R, Portmann BC, et al. Hepatic angiomyolipoma: a clinicopathologic study of 30 cases and delineation of unusual morphologic variants. *Am J Surg Pathol* 1999; 23:34–48.
42. Jeon TY, Kim SH, Lim HK, Lee WJ. Assessment of triple-phase CT findings for the differentiation of fat-deficient hepatic angiomyolipoma from hepatocellular carcinoma in non-cirrhotic liver. *Eur J Radiol* 2010; 73:601–606.
43. Nguyen TT, Gorman B, Shields D, Goodman Z. Malignant hepatic angiomyolipoma: report of a case and review of literature. *Am J Surg Pathol* 2008; 32:793–798.
44. Baba Y, Beppu T, Imai K, et al. A case of adrenal rest tumor of the liver: radiological imaging and immunohistochemical study of steroidogenic enzymes. *Hepatol Res* 2008; 38:1154–1158.
45. Wedemeyer J, Gratz KF, Soudah B, et al. Splenosis – important differential diagnosis in splenectomized patients presenting with abdominal masses of unknown origin. *Z Gastroenterol* 2005; 43:1225–1229.
46. Yoshimitsu K, Aibe H, Nobe T, et al. Intrahepatic splenosis mimicking a liver tumor. *Abdom Imaging* 1993; 18:156–158.
47. Bertolotto M, Quaia E, Zappetti R, Cester G, Turoldo A. Differential diagnosis between splenic nodules and peritoneal metastases with contrast-enhanced ultrasound based on signal-intensity characteristics during the late phase. *Radiol Med* 2009; 114:42–51.

9 What can be learned from molecular diagnostic techniques and genetic signatures?

Tariq Moatter[1], Saeed Hamid[2]

[1]Department of Pathology and Microbiology, Aga Khan University, Karachi, Pakistan
[2]Department of Medicine, Aga Khan University, Karachi, Pakistan

LEARNING POINTS

- Several genes and signalling pathways involved in cell proliferation, and differentiation, have been implicated in the pathogenesis of hepatocellular carcinoma (HCC)
- Unique gene expressions have been reported that can be used not only for diagnosis but also for prognosis
- mRNA signatures can also be useful for predicting HCC recurrence and metastasis

Introduction

Conventionally, poor prognostic factors in HCC are vascular invasion, tumour multiplicity and tumour size above 5 cm. On the basis of these parameters, staging systems for HCC like Okuda, Cancer of the Liver Italian Program (CLIP) and Barcelona Clinic Liver Cancer (BCLC) were developed, as considered elsewhere in this book, to predict prognosis and to determine the outcome of various treatment modalities while providing a treatment algorithm based on the clinical characteristics of HCC at the time of diagnosis. However, none of the systems take into account tumour biology, which could significantly impact on the patient's prognosis. Even standard biopsy examination of the tumour tissue, whether obtained by a percutaneous biopsy or by examination of resected material, has its prognostic limitations. Hence, these factors are not always commensurate with the disease state, and this is particularly so with respect to recurrence of the tumour. For example, with surgical resections of the tumour, in almost 80% of the patients intrahepatic reappearance of tumour occurs and half of those die within 5 years [1]. Vascular invasion is an established marker of metastatic recurrence of HCC and is considered to be a poor prognostic factor if present at the time of tumour resection. Although macrovascular invasion can be determined by gross examination of the liver by radiologic and other imaging systems, microscopic invasion into smaller vessels is difficult to identify at assessment time [2]. Another challenge in treating HCC is the presence of patho-genetically different tumour subtypes, which cannot be deciphered on the basis of current diagnostic techniques. Gene expression profiling, an innovative and promising tool, can simultaneously analyse thousands of genes in tumour samples with a lower detection limit of around 10 copies of mRNA per cell [3].

Gene expression and genetic signatures

A gene expression pattern represents a tumour phenotype and its cross-talk with the surrounding microenvironment. According to published studies, differential patterns of gene expression can be associated with differing tumour behaviour and disease states. In tumours, gene expression patterns can be linked to regulatory mechanisms or biochemical pathways involved in carcinogenesis. Furthermore, gene expression patterns can uncover occult tumour subtypes that arise because of tumour evolution

Clinical Dilemmas in Primary Liver Cancer, First Edition. Edited by Roger Williams and Simon D. Taylor-Robinson.

and its interaction with the micro-environment. On a similar note, gene expression technology is also useful for the identification of new targets for therapeutic interventions; for example, genes associated with poor outcomes or failure to treatment response may become potential therapeutic targets.

Methods used for the interpretation of gene expression data

The two most successful micro-array platforms in use for this technology are the spotted cDNA micro-array and high-density oligonucleotide micro-array [4]. Although both techniques in principle are different, they provide effective data for tumour classification. However, a major challenge to micro-array-based techniques is the statistical analysis of image data. There are two main types of statistical methods, that is, supervised and unsupervised [5]. Raw data are first normalised to counter variations caused by differences in experimental design. Following normalisation of the data, supervised methods are generally applied. If the class label is known for each sample, for example if the histopathological grade or clinical outcome is known, supervised analysis techniques are used for the identification of differentially expressed genes between groups of samples. A training set comprising a large number of unknown samples is first analysed to develop a classifier. Expression signatures deduced from the classifier are then tested for their significance in tumour classification or for the prediction of disease outcome against independent samples. A variety of mathematical methods are used for classifying tumours on the basis of gene expression profiles, including maximum likelihood statements, k-nearest neighbour, support vector machines and weighted voted machines [6]. On the other hand, unsupervised methods (clustering) explore previously unknown relationships between samples. Methods for cluster analysis include hierarchical clustering or κ-means clustering. Hierarchical cluster analysis is used to create tree maps that assemble genes in groups according to similarities in their expression profiles; furthermore, for better visual acuity, expression levels are represented with coloured boxes. For the analysis of time-course micro-array experiments, a clustering method termed 'self-organising map' is commonly used. Some other unsupervised methods include principle component analysis and relevance networks [7,8].

Gene signatures for disease progression

The transition from mild to moderate hepatic fibrosis consequent on disease progression is a major step in development of HCC. Expression profiles that can predict transition of hepatic fibrosis from the mild to the moderate grade were developed using an 11-gene signature, which could discriminate mild from moderate fibrosis with 78% accuracy. The investigators found a different panel of gene dysregulation in the transition from normal to mild compared with mild to moderate. The genes that were dysregulated in the expression signature were mainly responsible for immune system functioning and matrix turnover. The expression of keratin 19 (*KRT19*), *STMN2/SCG10* and *COL1A1* were up-regulated. In alcoholic liver disease KRT19 has been linked with the appearance of Mallory bodies and liver damage, whereas COL1A1 has been associated with matrix turnover. In addition, increased levels of STMN2/SCG10 are implicated in liver fibrogenesis through activation of sympathetic neurotransmitter. In addition, genes up-regulated in mild fibrosis were mainly interferon-inducible genes and differed with mild to moderate fibrosis transition. Whereas genes up-regulated with more advanced fibrosis coded for molecules implicated in both Th1 and Th2 immune responses [9].

Several gene signatures have been published that have claimed to distinguish between dysplasia and early HCC. A molecular signature consisting of 120 genes was proposed to separate dysplastic tumours from early HCC tumours in both HBV- and HCV-positive patients. In one study, authors have reported a three-gene panel to distinguish between small nodules of HCC, median size of 18–22 mm, and dysplastic nodules of ~10 mm in size. The three-gene expression signature gave an accurate distinction (94% accuracy). The panel consisted of glypican-3 (*GPC3*), survivin (*BIRC5*) and *LYVE1* (*XLKD1*) as the leading genes. *GPC3* and survivin were highly up-regulated in early HCC compared with the dysplastic nodules. *GPC3* is a heparin sulfate proteoglycan that augments growth of HCC through Wnt signalling pathway. Wnt proteins belong to the class of signalling-molecules that regulate cell-to-cell interactions during embryogenesis. Mutations in Wnt genes are also responsible for development of various human diseases, including hepatocellular cancer [10]. Both mechanisms, proliferation and inhibition of apoptosis, potentiate HCC growth. This expression analysis in combination with clinical and pathological findings can serve as a useful tool for evaluating the nature of hepatic lesions.

Gene signature data for tumour recurrence

Some of the recently published gene expression studies have successfully predicted the likelihood of recurrence of HCC following surgery. On the basis of the findings of Lee et al., HCC patients can be separated in good and poor prognosis groups according to their gene expression profiles [11]. In one study, Wang et al. have used a 57-gene expression signature to successfully predict recurrence in 84% of the HCC patients who have undergone surgical resection. This 57-gene profile evolved from a cohort of HCC patients diagnosed with either vascular tumour invasion or underlying cirrhosis. A 22-gene panel recurrence signature was identified from the larger signature that was consistently elevated in liver biopsy specimens and that was involved in a wide array of cellular functions. USH1C and Rac GTPAse-activating gene products were noted to be the most up-regulated genes. Rac GTPase-activating protein is known for its central role in cell–cell contact and can cause malignant transformation. Although, vascular invasion or the presence of cirrhosis cannot independently predict HCC recurrence, gene signatures incorporated with the clinicopathological findings can predict HCC recurrence with a greater accuracy [12].

Similarly, by using a random permutation test, Kurokawa et al. have developed a 20-gene expression signature to classify HCC patients on the basis of the expression patterns in the early recurrence and non-recurrence groups. However, its accuracy in predicting the recurrence outcome was limited to 72.5%. In this signature, *CDH1* was down-regulated, which encodes to cell adhesion molecule E-cadherin, and loss of *CDH1* expression can lead to progression of the disease and to tumour recurrence by growth invasion and metastasis [13]. Several other studies have attempted to predict HCC recurrence on the basis of gene expression patterns. Intrahepatic recurrence was more accurately predicted by a 12-gene signature, which correctly classified 92% of almost all early intrahepatic HCC. Biologically, some genes identified in the 12-gene signature were involved in the modulation of the immune system. For instance, *TNF* induces apoptosis in immune cells, which is inhibited by *TNFAIP3*. Removal of *TNFAIP3* signal leads to withdrawal of the immune system and increase venous invasion by tumour cells. Similarly, down-regulation of other immune system modulators human leukocyte antigen DRα and TRIM22 expression, which were also noted in the recurrent group, triggers a diminished immune response against tumour cell escape [14]. Recent research has also led to the view that the recurrence signature is embedded in the surrounding tissue and not in the tumour itself. Two signatures associated with the recurrence phenotype were identified: a good prognosis signature (no recurrence) was associated with the gene expression observed with normal liver function. In contrast, poor signature (recurrence) gene products were responsible for inflammation such as NFkβ signalling and TNFα [15]. However, a correlation between the expression profiles of tumours and the patient's outcome was not evident.

Gene signatures for metastasis

Metastasis in HCC is dependent on a multitude of factors, including proliferation of cancer colonies, survival advantage, acquiring invasive potential and formation of new vasculature. HCC tumours are highly vascular, which increases their ability to spread and invade into the surrounding tissue and distant sites [16]. There is a general debate whether metastatic attributes are inherited at an early stage of tumour formation or formulated by host genetic background where the micro-environment modulates tumour metastatic potential. Chronic hepatitis leads to inflamed liver infiltrated with lymphocytes, where the interaction between the immune cells and the micro-environment surrounding the tumour may influence tumour cell predisposition to metastasis. A recent study has attempted to predict the role of hepatic micro-environment with distinction of a metastasis inclined micro-environment and a metastasis adverse micro-environment in tumorigenesis by using a 17-gene unique signature. This signature was utilised to successfully predict with 92% accuracy both venous metastasis and extrahepatic metastases. The genes that primarily constituted the signature were involved in the cellular immune and inflammatory responses. Pro-inflammatory cytokines were down-regulated while anti-inflammatory mediators were elevated in patients with metastatic HCC [16]. It was proposed that the patient's genetic makeup can influence immune system elements and thus engendering tumour promoting effects. Other studies have concluded that gene expression signatures of the metastatic tumour and primary tumour were close to each other. However, gene expression signatures of metastasis-free HCC and that of HCC associated with intrahepatic metastasis were shown to be disparate. The signature predictive of distant metastasis developed many years after resection. Secondly, it is a general impression that metastasis occurs late, and tumours acquire this potential by accumulating genetic aberrations over a period of time. Therefore, analysis of primary tumour is not pertinent for predicting metastatic potential of the tumour. Recently, this established view was challenged by a new theory, which suggests that metastatic potential is not acquired during late phase but is embedded in the primary tumour [1]. It is suggested that a gene expression profile distinctive for metastasis can be detected in the primary tumour. In contrast, Hoshida et al. showed that early recurrence of HCC was associated with gene expression profile of the surrounding tissue and not the tumour itself [15].

Limitations of the gene expression technology

However, despite these remarkable attributes, the successful adaptation of expression technology into clinical practice requires the standardisation of data analysis procedures along with quality control guidelines.

That HCC can have diverse aetiologies, which is evident from difference in gene expression patterns [17]. Gene expression signatures can vary depending upon the aetiology of the underlying disease and other host factors. Application of gene expression profiling in association with the aetiological factors and disease state for accurate classification of HCC patients has been documented in recent literature. However, the utility of gene expression technology for grouping HCC into clinically useful subtypes or predicting HCC recurrence is limited because of the involvement of a wide variety of factors, such as viral, environmental and host genetics, which can modulate the development of HCC. Several studies utilising gene expression techniques have claimed to predict HCC recurrence; however, the confirmation of these results in sufficiently large patient populations remains pending. In addition, other studies have reported an association between expression patterns and clinical outcomes. A well-known obstacle to micro-array-based expression profiling studies is the dependence upon fresh or frozen tissue samples. This limits access to a large number of suitable patients' specimens, since in hospitals and tissue banks, specimens with clinical and other laboratory data are archived as formalin-fixed paraffin-embedded blocks.

References

1. Yoshioka S, Takemasa I, Nagano H, et al. Molecular prediction of early recurrence after resection of hepatocellular carcinoma. *Eur J Cancer* 2009; 45:881–889.
2. Tanaka S, Mogushi K, Yasen M, et al. Gene-expression phenotypes for vascular invasiveness of hepatocellular carcinomas. *Surgery* 2009; 147:405–414.
3. Tarca AL, Romero R, Draghici S. Analysis of microarray experiments of gene expression profiling. *Am J Obstet Gynecol* 2006; 195:373–388.
4. Schulze A, Downward J. Navigating gene expression using microarrays – a technology review. *Nat Cell Biol* 2001; 3: E190–E195.
5. Belacel N, Wang Q, Cuperlovic-Culf M. Clustering methods for microarray gene expression data. *Omics* 2006; 10: 507–531.
6. Brown MP, Grundy WN, Lin D, et al. Knowledge-based analysis of microarray gene expression data by using support vector machines. *Proc Natl Acad Sci USA* 2000; 97:262–267.
7. Dysvik B, Jonassen I. J-Express: exploring gene expression data using Java. *Bioinformatics* 2001; 17:369–370.
8. Sturn A, Quackenbush J, Trajanoski Z. Genesis: cluster analysis of microarray data. *Bioinformatics* 2002; 18:207–208.
9. Asselah T, Bieche I, Laurendeau I, et al. Liver gene expression signature of mild fibrosis in patients with chronic hepatitis C. *Gastroenterology* 2005; 129:2064–2075.
10. Llovet JM, Chen Y, Wurmbach E, et al. A molecular signature to discriminate dysplastic nodules from early hepatocellular carcinoma in HCV cirrhosis. *Gastroenterology* 2006; 131:1758–1767.
11. Lee JS, Chu IS, Heo J, et al. Classification and prediction of survival in hepatocellular carcinoma by gene expression profiling. *Hepatology* 2004; 40:667–676.
12. Wang SM, Ooi LL, Hui KM. Identification and validation of a novel gene signature associated with the recurrence of human hepatocellular carcinoma. *Clin Cancer Res* 2007; 13: 6275–6283.
13. Kurokawa Y, Matoba R, Takemasa I, et al. Molecular-based prediction of early recurrence in hepatocellular carcinoma. *J Hepatol* 2004; 41:284–291.
14. Iizuka N, Oka M, Yamada-Okabe H, et al. Oligonucleotide microarray for prediction of early intrahepatic recurrence of hepatocellular carcinoma after curative resection. *Lancet* 2003; 361:923–929.

15. Hoshida Y, Villanueva A, Kobayashi M, et al. Gene expression in fixed tissues and outcome in hepatocellular carcinoma. *N Engl J Med* 2008; 359:1995–2004.
16. Budhu A, Forgues M, Ye QH, et al. Prediction of venous metastases, recurrence, and prognosis in hepatocellular carcinoma based on a unique immune response signature of the liver microenvironment. *Cancer Cell* 2006; 10:99–111.
17. Chang SH, Suh KS, Yi NJ, Lee KH, Kim BY, Jang JJ. Predicting the prognosis of hepatocellular carcinoma using gene expression. *J Surg Res* 2010; in press.

PART 3

Complexities of Patient Assessment and Scoring Systems

10 Looking after the liver as well as the tumour

Roger Williams
The Institute of Hepatology London and Foundation for Liver Research

LEARNING POINTS

- Importance of early diagnosis through surveillance programmes of patient groups at risk
- Essential matching of treatment modalities with stage of liver disease (Child-Pugh category)
- Prolonged survival and even cure obtained with treatment of liver nodules smaller than 3 cm in diameter
- Recurrence of tumour and new tumour development represent outstanding issues
- Key role of hepatologist/physician in multidisciplinary team of oncologists, surgeons, radiologists and histopathologists

Much success has attended efforts in recent years to put in place surveillance programmes for the detection of hepatocellular cancer (HCC) at an early stage, which allow certain treatment options, including liver resection, liver transplantation and radiofrequency ablation (RFA), to give long-term survival or even cure. Surveillance programmes and the monitoring of individual cases are essential in the care of the patient with cirrhosis or fibrosis in the liver as a consequence of hepatitis C virus (HCV), hepatitis B virus (HBV) or alcohol excess, the three commonest causes of primary HCC worldwide. HCC is unique amongst solid organ cancers in that the prognosis is dependent on both the degree of liver dysfunction consequent on the underlying liver condition and the oncological characteristics of the HCC. Of the latter, the best documented is size at the time of initial diagnosis. As size increases, so does the likelihood of vascular invasiveness with spread throughout the liver.

Looking after the liver disease is an important part of the equation that determines outcome of the various options available for treatment of the HCC. Thus, antiviral therapy for hepatitis B or C, when successful in controlling viral replication, can lead to an improvement in liver dysfunction, allowing greater opportunities for treatment of the HCC and a better tolerance to such treatments. Although such antiviral treatment constitutes an additional burden for the patient with HCC, it may also decrease the chances of tumour recurrence after treatment of the initial tumour nodule and further new tumour development within the cirrhotic or severely damaged liver. Of the various systems for the staging of HCC, the one in clinical practice, which is most widely used for equating the stage of the liver disease and that of the HCC with the most likely beneficial treatment option, is the Barcelona Clinic Liver Cancer (BCLC) strategy (Figure 10.1) [1].

Assessment of liver dysfunction

The Child-Pugh score with its A–D categories – reflecting increasing hepatic decompensation – is based on the scoring of clinical manifestations such as ascites and encephalopathy and is more relevant to HCC treatment than the Model for End-stage Liver Disease (MELD) score derived from laboratory measurements of liver dysfunction and coagulation disturbances. Furthermore, the MELD score does not give information on the presence and severity of portal hypertension, which is of considerable importance if surgical resection is one of the possible treatment options. Morbidity and mortality figures for surgical resection in

Clinical Dilemmas in Primary Liver Cancer, First Edition. Edited by Roger Williams and Simon D. Taylor-Robinson.

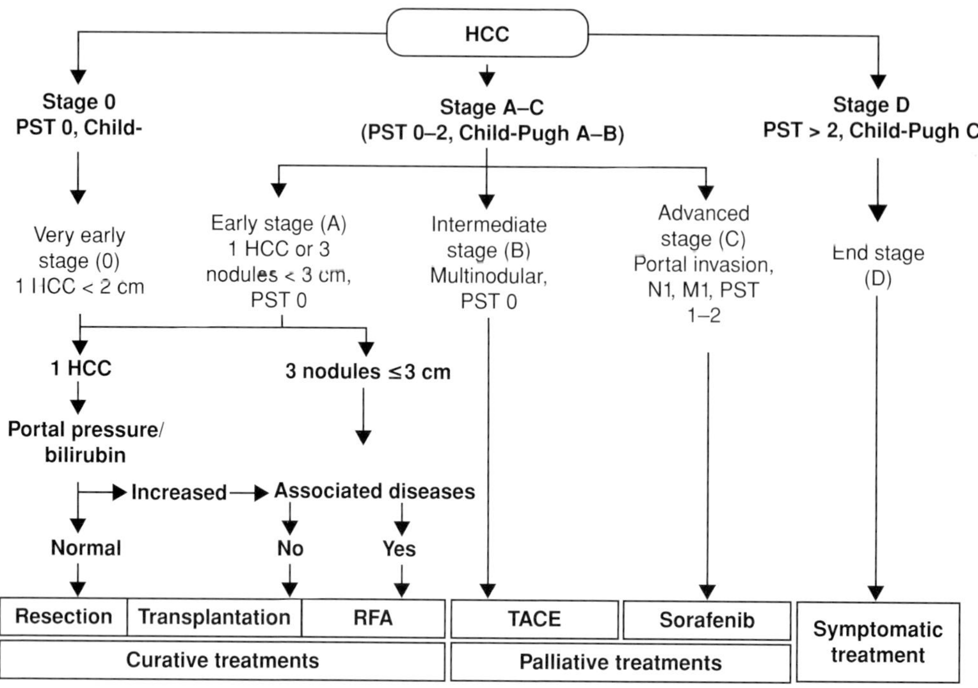

FIG 10.1 BCLC staging and treatment strategy showing the clinical decision-making process applied to stratify patients with HCC into very early or early, intermediate, advanced and end stage. (Tremosini S, Reig M, de Lope CR, et al. Treatment of early hepatocellular carcinoma: towards personalized therapy. *Dig Liver Dis* 2010; 42(suppl 3):S242–S248.)

patients with cirrhosis are substantially lower in the absence of portal hypertension, and the measurement of the wedged hepatic venous pressure (WHVP) gradient is an essential part of the pre-operative assessment of a patient for liver resection. Elevation of the WHVP gradient above 10 mmHg (normal range 1–5 mmHg) is associated with a higher risk of post-operative liver decompensation and of a poor long-term outcome. Measurement of indocyanine green clearance which gives an overall assessment of liver functional capacity is also used, along with calculation of liver volumes by computed tomography (CT), for determining the sufficiency of hepatic function of the remaining liver segments after the resection procedure (see Chapter 22).

Sophisticated imaging techniques are providing new information on the early stages of HCC development, and new knowledge is also accruing on the nature of the liver conditions underlying tumour formation. Thus, it is increasingly apparent that cirrhosis is not an essential prerequisite. A proportion of patients will have fibrosis of varying severity without nodular regeneration. This is so not only for HBV liver disease, where it is known that the virus can have a direct oncogenic action, but also for HCV-induced liver disease. With treatment options for the HCC dependent on the stage of underlying liver disease, the presence of fibrosis rather than cirrhosis is an important consideration. This is also relevant to a newly recognised occurrence of HCC in non-alcoholic fatty liver disease (NAFLD). In a series of patients with cirrhosis having liver resections for HCC, a comparison of those attributed to NAFLD and those having an overt cause for the cirrhosis showed that the number with F0–2 fibrosis was significantly higher in the NAFLD group (66% vs. 26%) [2]. There are also reports of HCC in patients with hepatic steatosis alone, and there appears to be a general increase in the risk of malignancy in obese subjects. In another series of NAFLD patients, it was shown that those who reported any regular alcoholic intake were at greater risk of developing HCC [3], and on this basis, abstinence and control of diabetes – another added risk factor for HCC development – as well as weight reduction might all be considered as part of expanded liver care for the patient with HCC. Visceral fat accumulation in a series of 62 patients with HCC from suspected NAFLD curatively treated by RFA was shown to be an independent risk factor for tumour recurrence – 69% at 3 years compared with 43% in the control group [4].

Place of liver biopsy and risk of seeding

Although obtaining the histological confirmation by biopsy is usually considered a mandatory investigation in a patient with possible malignancy, the place of liver biopsy currently in the assessment of a patient with HCC is limited. This is mainly because of the high diagnostic accuracy obtainable with dynamic radiological imaging and the purported high risk of tumour seeding during a biopsy procedure. Liver biopsy is indicated according to American Association for the Study of Liver Diseases (AASLD) and European Association for the Study of the Liver (EASL) guidelines for potential tumour nodules smaller than 2 cm in diameter unless positive diagnostic imaging by two techniques is obtainable. However, histological distinction of a small HCC from other nodular lesions including adenoma, focal nodular hyperplasia and particularly high-grade dysplastic nodules may be difficult. An expert histopathologist is required for interpretation, and accurate placement of a biopsy needle within a small lesion is not always possible. In a recent study, a positive diagnosis was obtained in only 70% of cases and the false negative rate for a second biopsy was 38.9% [5].

As to the risk of seeding of tumour cells, a recent PubMed review of both English and non-English literature gave a 2.92% risk following liver biopsy with figures of 0.72% and 0.61% for RFA with and without liver biopsy [6]. The time over which seeding occurred was wide, ranging from 1 to 58 months. Such seeding is of most concern in the context of patients who are being considered for transplantation, where there is the greatest chance of obtaining a complete cure. There may be a greater call for tissue assessment in the future with the more certain identification of genomic markers of importance in diagnosis and long-term prognosis. An alternative approach for the small <2 cm diameter nodule without positive diagnostic imaging is to allow a wait period of 2 months, by which time, if it is an HCC, repeat imaging with further growth of the nodule is likely to show the characteristic hypervascularisation picture. On the downside, any increase in size of the nodule, as already referred to, is accompanied by a greater risk of microvascular tissue invasion and, with this, risk of tumour recurrence following potentially curative treatment procedures.

Antiviral therapy for hepatitis B or C

Antiviral therapy has an important place in the management of a patient with HCC when the underlying cause of the liver disease is HBV or HCV infection. Obtaining a sustained virological response (SVR) in chronic HCV hepatitis will reduce the risk of progression of the liver disease, and the same applies to HBV-positive liver disease treated with antiviral agents. However, a long-term follow-up study of patients in whom there was complete control of HBV replication over a number of years showed a small risk of HCC remaining, particularly in those with decompensated cirrhosis (Figure 10.2) [7]. Interestingly, recent figures have shown that the number of transplants carried out in the United States for HBV-associated HCC increased by 72% over the past 7 years, whereas the number of decompensated end-stage hepatitis B cases transplanted decreased by 47% [8]. Improvement in the degree of hepatic decompensation with antiviral therapy, when there is evidence of active ongoing viral replication as shown by a significantly raised HBV DNA level (above 2000 IU/mL), may enable a patient to move to a better category within BCLC, thereby giving more options for treatment and possibly a lower risk of recurrent tumour. The latest antiviral agents for HBV infection, namely entecavir and tenofovir, are highly effective over a period of 4–8 weeks in reducing viral load with minimal toxicity for the patient.

Obtaining an SVR – virological cure – in the HCV-positive patients with continuing viral replication, and where in the context of complicating HCC the patient is more likely than the hepatitis B positive case to have severe fibrosis or cirrhosis, is more difficult. With any evidence of clinical decompensation, severe complications of treatment may occur. However, using a low-accelerating dose regime of pegylated interferon (PegIFN) and ribavirin, Everson and colleagues achieved an overall SVR of 24% in a series of cases with decompensated cirrhosis, resulting in a greatly improved tolerance [9]. Treatment of the tumour has to take priority when nodules are of 2–3 cm diameter and suitable for RFA, but for the HCV patient with a HCC fulfilling criteria for a liver transplant, there is every reason for initiating antiviral therapy during the waiting period. Complete clearance of the virus, or a substantial reduction in viraemia level before surgery, greatly lessens the chances of post-transplant recurrence of HCV infection and severe graft damage. Analysis of 150 such treated cases from six series gave an average of 34% HCV RNA negativity on the

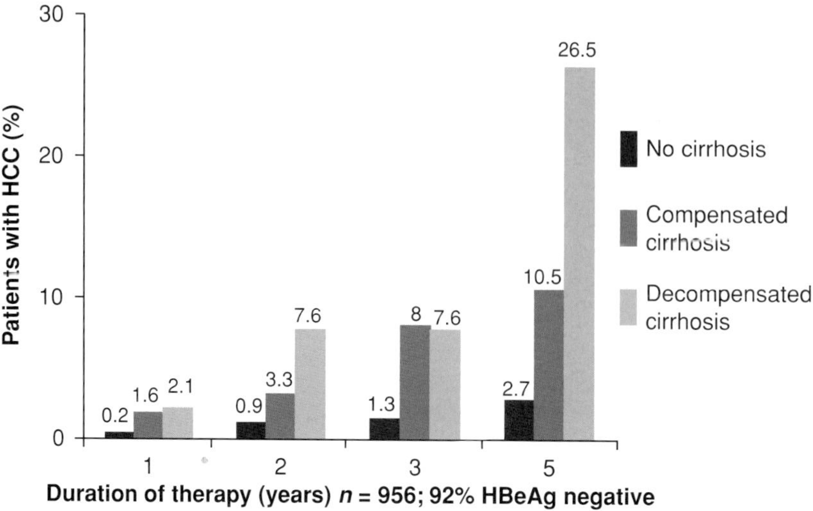

FIG 10.2 Risk of HCC during treatment with anti-HBV nuclosides over a 5-year period according to clinical stage of liver disease at start of treatment. (From Wiegand J, van Bömmel F, Berg T. Management of chronic hepatitis B: status and challenges beyond treatment guidelines. *Semin Liver Dis* 2010; 30(4):361–377, based on data of Papatheodoridis GV, Manolakopoulos S, Touloumi G, et al. Risk of hepatocellular carcinoma (HCC) in chronic hepatitis B (CHB) patients with or without cirrhosis treated with oral antivirals: results of the nationwide Hepnet. Greece Cohort Study. *Hepatology* 2009; 50(4): Suppl. 368–69A.)

day of transplant, with 21% remaining negative at 6 months after transplant [10]. This is to be compared with a 100% recurrence rate when transplantation is carried out at the time of HCV RNA positivity.

Similarly, transplantation in HBV-positive cases is less hazardous if viral replication has been successfully controlled with antiviral drugs by the time of the transplant. Transplantation carried out at the time of HBeAg positivity and a high viral load is known to be associated with early graft loss and poorer long-term outcome.

In cases of HCC being treated by surgical liver resection or RFA where there is a substantial risk by 5 years of HCC recurrence (30–50%), such use of antiviral therapy is unlikely to have an effect on already disseminated tumour clones that lead to early recurrence. To what extent it will reduce metachronous HCC, i.e. new tumour development in areas distant from initial tumour at a later date, requires further study.

The post-liver transplant period

Antiviral therapy also has an important place after liver transplantation. For the HCV transplanted patient with viral re-infection in the graft, there is a 25% chance of developing cirrhosis by 5 years after the transplant, with a dip downwards in the survival curve thereafter. Rather than treat all cases early in post-transplant period (a pre-emptive approach), which would include the 75% who are not at such risk, the approach usually adopted is to delay treatment until there is the histological evidence of a graft hepatitis, as determined by a protocol biopsy at 12 months, which cannot be attributed to acute rejection or other causes. Alternatively, antiviral treatment can be delayed until there is evidence of significant fibrosis, and in accurately predicting progression of hepatic fibrosis in the graft, serial measurements of the WHVP gradient have been shown to be superior to liver biopsy [11]. The results of treating recurrent HCV graft disease are more encouraging than is generally thought. In one randomised controlled trial, histological response was seen in 74% of treated cases compared with 30% in the non-treated arm with an overall SVR in the treated group of 48% [12]. Progression of fibrosis may be prevented with a decreased risk of graft failure, but whether tumour recurrence in the transplanted cases with HCC is also reduced is not proven. Of note, tumour recurrence occurs much less frequently after liver transplantation than after liver resection, even

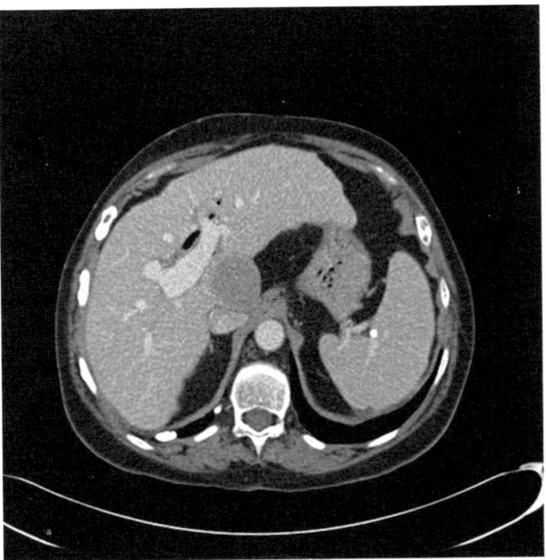

FIG 10.3 The 3-cm HCC in segment 1 shown in portal phase washout of CT scan examination was first detected in 2008 – 19 years after liver transplantation and 16 years after clearance of HCV with interferon therapy. Liver histology at that time showed severe bridging fibrosis.

though the Milan Criteria allow transplantation for nodules up to 5 cm diameter. New tumour formation may still occur, as in the transplant case illustrated in (Figure 10.3) where a 3 cm diameter HCC nodule was first detected 16 years after successful clearance of HCV with antiviral therapy.

For the HBV-positive transplant case – if there has been a breakthrough of prophylactic therapy with the well-established maintenance immunoglobulin regimes – treatment of recurrent disease is relatively straightforward with the efficacy and minimal toxicity of the new antiviral agents. Graft function is improved and progression of the disease prevented. In transplanted HBV-positive subjects, there is one study showing that HBV re-infection is significantly associated with the presence of HCC pre-transplant and the recurrence of HCC post-transplant [13].

Regular monitoring of immunosuppressive drug levels is essential during antiviral therapy in the transplanted patient as a response to it may lead to a fall in blood levels as a result of improved liver function and biotransformation. Precipitation of rejection by interferon in the HCV-positive liver transplant subject is another potential risk, although this is much less likely than with a kidney transplant. Distinction of rejection from recurrent HCV hepatitis may be difficult on histological examination, which may need to be repeated serially with different approaches to therapy. Regular ultrasound surveillance is also essential in cases transplanted for HCC if tumour recurrence is to be picked up at an early stage and treated successfully by RFA, or occasionally by a second transplant if the biological characteristics of the tumour, i.e. a long interval between transplantation and tumour recurrence, are favourable.

The patient on sorafenib

The new treatment option of sorafenib is shown in the BCLC staging system as appropriate for those with advanced stage C tumour with portal invasion and some impairment in performance staging tests but still remaining within Child-Pugh A and B categories. The initial controlled trials of sorafenib showing a significant improvement in survival times restricted entry to those with well-preserved liver function and excellent performance status. Whether sorafenib will give similar benefit in those with an advanced BCLC stage C tumour and whether it has additional value in patients treated by ablation or chemoembolisation or as adjuvant therapy after liver resection is uncertain at present and will have to await the results of ongoing controlled clinical trials.

In the writer's experience, patients given sorafenib can feel generally unwell even if they do not have the more serious side effects reported with the agent and are often unwilling to take the full dose of 800 mg daily. In this context, a recently published paper describing tolerance and outcome of 50 patients with unresectable HCC treated with sorafenib is of interest [14]. Sixty-six per cent of the patients were Child-Pugh A and 34% in Child-Pugh B category. Although the occurrence of adverse events were similar in both categories, the duration of treatment until discontinuation on account of poor tolerance was lower in the Child-Pugh B group – 5 versus 7.8 months with a correspondingly low survival (1.8 months only) – and the authors questioned the use of sorafenib in this category of patient.

An ongoing phase III trial of sorafenib plus doxorubicin versus sorafenib alone is based on the concept of synergism between sorafenib and doxorubicin [15], but such combinations of treatment will require considerable care of the patient as drug toxicity is likely to be high. This also applies to the randomised phase II trial now underway comparing sorafenib alone with sorafenib plus GEMOX. A recent case report described a complete remission with GEMOX in a 35-year-old with poorly differentiated HCC in a non-fibrotic liver and metastatic tumour deposits [16]. What will be important in these further clinical trials is a better documentation of tumour response in addition to the current single outcome measure of survival time. The Response Evaluation Criteria in Solid Tumours (RECIST) guideline gives an overall index of tumour response based on an assessment of the response of a chosen target lesion as shown by changes in imaging characteristics and measurements of viable tumour size [17].

Conclusion – role of hepatologist/physician

In 'looking after the liver as well as the tumour', the hepatologist/physician has a key role in the multidisciplinary team of radiologists, oncologists, surgeons and histopathologists involved in the care of patients with HCC developing as a consequence of chronic liver disease. He/she will have the primary responsibility for the initial assessment of the patient's liver disease and of the staging of the HCC relevant to the options for treatment. Throughout the course of the illness, the hepatologist/physician is responsible for the continuing care of the patients' liver disease including the optimal use of antiviral therapy and the management of often complex side effects resulting from the different methods of treatment.

References

1. Tremosini S, Reig M, de Lope CR, et al. Treatment of early hepatocellular carcinoma: towards personalized therapy. *Dig Liver Dis* 2010; 42(suppl 3):S242–S248.
2. Paradis V, Zalinski S, Chelbi E, et al. Hepatocellular carcinomas in patients with metabolic syndrome often develop without significant liver fibrosis: a pathological analysis. *Hepatology* 2009; 49(3):851–859.
3. Ascha MS, Hanouneh IA, Lopez R, et al. The incidence and risk factors of hepatocellular carcinoma in patients with nonalcoholic steatohepatitis. *Hepatology* 2010; 51(6):1972–1978.
4. Ohki T, Tateishi R, Shiina S, et al. Visceral fat accumulation is an independent risk factor for hepatocellular carcinoma recurrence after curative treatment in patients with suspected NASH. *Gut* 2009; 58(6):839–844.
5. Forner A, Vilana R, Ayuso C, et al. Diagnosis of hepatic nodules 20 mm or smaller in cirrhosis: prospective validation of the noninvasive diagnostic criteria for hepatocellular carcinoma. *Hepatology* 2008; 47(1):97–104. Erratum in: *Hepatology* 2008; 47(2):769.
6. Stigliano R, Marelli L, Yu D, et al. Seeding following percutaneous diagnostic and therapeutic approaches for hepatocellular carcinoma. What is the risk and the outcome? Seeding risk for percutaneous approach of HCC. *Cancer Treat Rev* 2007; 33(5):437–447.
7. Wiegand J, van Bömmel F, Berg T. Management of chronic hepatitis B: status and challenges beyond treatment guidelines. *Semin Liver Dis* 2010; 30(4):361–377.
8. Kim WR, Terrault NA, Pedersen RA, et al. Trends in waiting list registration for liver transplantation for viral hepatitis in the United States. *Gastroenterology* 2009; 137(5):1680–1686.
9. Everson GT, Trotter J, Forman L, et al. Treatment of advanced hepatitis C with a low accelerating dosage regimen of antiviral therapy. *Hepatology* 2005; 42(2):255–262.
10. Fortune BE, Forman LM. HCV in liver transplant recipients: how do you approach them? In: GR Foster, KR Reddy (eds) *Clinical Dilemmas in Viral Liver Disease*. Blackwell Publishing Ltd, Oxford; 2010, pp. 110–114.
11. Samonakis DN, Cholongitas E, Thalheimer U, et al. Hepatic venous pressure gradient to assess fibrosis and its progression after liver transplantation for HCV cirrhosis. *Liver Transpl* 2007; 13(9):1305–1311.
12. Carrión JA, Navasa M, García-Retortillo M, et al. Efficacy of antiviral therapy on hepatitis C recurrence after liver transplantation: a randomized controlled study. *Gastroenterology* 2007; 132(5):1746–1756.
13. Saab S, Yeganeh M, Nguyen K, et al. Recurrence of hepatocellular carcinoma and hepatitis B reinfection in hepatitis B surface antigen-positive patients after liver transplantation. *Liver Transpl* 2009; 15(11):1525–1534.
14. Ozenne V, Paradis V, Pernot S, et al. Tolerance and outcome of patients with unresectable hepatocellular carcinoma treated with sorafenib. *Eur J Gastroenterol Hepatol* 2010; 22(9):1106–1110.
15. Abou-Alfa GK, Johnson P, Knox JJ, et al. Doxorubicin plus sorafenib vs doxorubicin alone in patients with advanced hepatocellular carcinoma: a randomized trial. *JAMA* 2010; 304(19):2154–2160.
16. Boschetti G, Walter T, Hervieu V, et al. Complete response of hepatocellular carcinoma with systemic combination chemotherapy: not to get out the chemotherapy? *Eur J Gastroenterol Hepatol* 2010; 22(8):1015–1018.
17. Lencioni R, Llovet JM. Modified RECIST (mRECIST) assessment for hepatocellular carcinoma. *Semin Liver Dis* 2010; 30(1):52–60.

11 Comparative performances of staging systems for hepatocellular cancer: early HCC considerations

Peter D. Peng, Timothy M. Pawlik
Johns Hopkins Hospital, Baltimore, MD, USA

LEARNING POINTS

- Both tumour- and liver-specific factors impact prognosis of patients with hepatocellular carcinoma (HCC)
- The major tumour-specific factors associated with HCC prognosis include tumour size, tumour number, and the presence of vascular invasion
- For patients with advanced HCC and those patients undergoing locoregional therapy, the CLIP staging system appears to perform well
- For patients with intermediate or advanced HCC who undergo resection/transplantation, the American Joint Committee on Cancer/Union Internationale Contre le Cancer (AJCC/UICC) is probably the most utilised and favoured staging system
- Most major HCC staging systems perform poorly in staging patients with early HCC. For early HCC tumours, tumour size larger than 2 cm for both solitary and multifocal tumours and microscopic vascular invasion for multifocal tumours have prognostic impact

Introduction

The objective of cancer staging is to stratify patients into groups for guiding treatment recommendations, predicting prognosis and assessing enrolment in investigational therapies. Staging can be broadly divided into clinical staging, which determines the pre-procedural tumour stage usually by exam, laboratory tests and imaging, versus pathologic staging, which assesses tumour stage after operative resection or exploration. Traditionally, pathologic staging systems have provided more accurate prognostic information and have been used to help guide patient selection for surveillance, prognosis and adjuvant therapies. Although a number of clinical and pathologic staging systems have been proposed for HCC, there is continued debate regarding which staging system is the most useful/accurate.

Establishing an accurate staging system for HCC is complicated by a number of factors. Unlike many other tumours, HCC commonly arises in a pre-neoplastic cirrhotic liver that can itself be associated with significant mortality. Both liver- and tumour-specific factors should ideally be integrated into disease staging for accurate recommendations and prognosis. Additionally, up to 60–80% of patients who present with HCC have unresectable disease. As such, any staging system for HCC needs to incorporate factors applicable to patients with both early and late stage presentations.

A number of staging systems for HCC have been proposed over the last two decades. The clinical staging systems include the Okada staging system, Cancer of the Liver Italian Program (CLIP) and Barcelona Clinic Liver Cancer (BCLC) system. The pathologic staging systems are dependent on data after resection or transplantation and include the Liver Cancer Study Group of Japan (LCSGJ) system, Japanese Integrated Staging (JIS) score, Chinese University Prognostic Index (CUPI) and AJCC/UICC system. We herein review the various staging systems, provide comparative data, and highlight the performance of the staging systems for early HCC.

Clinical Dilemmas in Primary Liver Cancer, First Edition. Edited by Roger Williams and Simon D. Taylor-Robinson.

Okuda staging system

Introduced in 1985 from a retrospective analysis of 850 patients with HCC, the Okuda staging system is based on tumour size, ascites, jaundice and serum albumin. Scoring is based on the following factors: tumour burden >50% of liver, ascites, serum albumin <3 g/dL and serum bilirubin ≥3 mg/dL [1]. Patients are assigned one point for each factor. Stage I disease is defined as 0 points, stage II defined as 1–2 points and stage III defined as 3–4 points. Although it was an early attempt to account for both tumour and liver factors, it has subsequently been criticised for including only a single tumour factor. As the Okuda staging system utilises a 50% tumour burden cut-off, the prognostic discrimination for early stage HCC is insufficient and the Okuda staging system is not particularly useful in patients with early HCC disease.

Cancer of the Liver Italian Program score

The CLIP score was developed from a study of 435 Italian patients as an attempt to address some of the criticisms of the Okuda staging system and thereby allow for better prognostic stratification of early tumours [2]. The CLIP score incorporates Child-Pugh score, tumour morphology (<50% tumour burden involvement is subdivided into uninodular vs. multinodular), alpha-fetoprotein (AFP) >400 and portal vein thrombosis. Several validation studies have demonstrated that the CLIP outperforms the Okuda staging among HCC patients undergoing a wide range of therapies [3–5]. An early prospective validation study enrolled 196 HCC patients with cirrhosis and found the CLIP score to provide more accurate prognostic information with greater predictive power when compared with the Okuda system [3]. In a separate retrospective analysis of 662 Japanese patients that examined the CLIP, Okuda and the fifth edition AJCC staging systems, the authors found CLIP to have the best ability to stratify patients undergoing surgery, transcatheter arterial chemoembolisation (TACE) and percutaneous ethanol injections [4].

Several additional studies have noted CLIP to have particular prognostic accuracy among HCC patients undergoing catheter-based therapies. A case-control study of 56 patients undergoing TACE reported that CLIP, but not Okuda, staging provided accurate survival stratification [6]. In a different retrospective study of 200 patients undergoing 425 transcatheter treatments, the authors noted that on multivariate analysis CLIP score <2 was predictive of response and longer survival, while neither Okuda and BCLC were informative [7]. While these studies indicate that CLIP staging provides accurate prognostic stratification in patients with advanced disease undergoing catheter-based therapies, the accuracy of the CLIP score for early stage lesions remains poorly defined. In fact, similar to the Okuda staging system, the CLIP score can be criticised for inadequate differentiation of smaller tumours as it still largely defines extent of disease using a 50% cut-off value. As such, while the CLIP score includes tumour number (e.g. uninodular disease vs. multinodular disease), it remains relatively crude in its ability to stratify patients with early stage HCC.

Barcelona Clinic Liver Cancer staging system

The BCLC staging system was introduced in 1999 to improve on the prognostic stratification of the previous staging systems by incorporating additional tumour, liver and patient factors. Specifically, the BCLC includes factors related to tumour size, number, liver function, level of portal hypertension and vascular involvement [8]. Unlike the Okuda or CLIP staging systems, the BCLC not only attempts to stratify patients according to prognosis but also provides treatment recommendations. Patients are stratified into five stages: very early, early, intermediate, advanced and end-stage according to liver function, tumour burden and functional status, which in turn are associated with curative, non-curative or symptomatic treatment recommendations. Several validation studies have demonstrated the prognostic utility of the BCLC. Specifically, one retrospective study of 187 patients found that the BCLC outperformed Okuda, CLIP and CUPI staging systems for the entire patient population, including both surgical and non-surgical subgroups [9]. A subsequent prospective study by the same group undertaken in 195 consecutive HCC patients found that the BCLC staging system had better prognostic ability than Okuda, CLIP, AJCC sixth edition (2002) and JIS [10]. However, the study deviated from treatment recommendations and nodule size and number were not used to exclude curative therapies and resection. Another retrospective study of 400 surgical patients again found that BCLC demonstrated improved prognostic ability when compared with Okuda, CLIP, AJCC sixth edition (2002) and JIS score. However, the BCLC algorithm has been criticised for being too restrictive and exclusionary in its recommendation for curative intent therapies such as surgical resection. Both resection and ablative therapies have been shown to be safe and effective in prolonging survival among a wider group of patients than perhaps suggested in the BCLC algorithm. As such, the BCLC may be overly conservative in its recommendations for patients with both early as well as intermediate stage HCC.

Liver Cancer Study Group of Japan staging system

The International Hepato-Pancreato-Biliary Association and the LCSGJ used data from 21,711 Japanese patients who underwent liver resection for HCC to develop the LCSGJ staging system [11]. The LCSGJ uses as a standard tumour-node metastasis (TNM) classification schema. The T category is stratified according to several factors: (1) solitary lesions, (2) lesion <2 cm and (3) absence of vascular invasion of portal vein, hepatic vein and bile duct. Staging is classified as T1, all three factors; T2, two factors; T3, one factor and T4, no factors. Nodal status is scored as N0 for no lymph-node metastasis versus N1 for lymph-node metastasis. Metastatic disease is likewise scored as M0 for no distant metastatic disease versus M1 for distant metastatic disease present.

Several important criticisms have called the utility and accuracy of the LCSGJ staging system into question. While the LCSGJ staging system aims to account for additional tumour factors, the equal weighting of these tumour-specific factors may be problematic. For example, giving the same prognostic weight to tumour size and major vascular invasion may be inaccurate and inappropriate. In addition, the LCSGJ staging system does not take into account underlying liver function and does not differentiate microscopic from major vascular invasion.

Japanese Integrated Staging score

The JIS score integrates the Child-Pugh score with the LCSGJ staging system to address the specific deficiency of the LCSGJ for not having included liver function evaluation [12]. Two validation studies appeared to indicate JIS superiority to the CLIP staging system [12,13]. The other limitations inherent in the LCSGJ staging system, such as inaccurate weighting of size and vascular involvement, as well as the lack of incorporation of microscopic pathology information, remain.

Chinese University Prognostic Index

The CUPI staging system is a TNM-based system with the addition of several liver- and tumour-specific factors in an attempt to better stratify patients with regard to their disease. On the basis of data derived from a review of 926 Chinese patients primarily with hepatitis B associated HCC, the authors derived a staging system that included such factors as total bilirubin, ascites, alkaline phosphatase, AFP and asymptomatic disease on presentation [14]. One weakness of the CUPI may be the homogeneity of the hepatitis B-related HCC patient population on which it is based [15–17]. In comparison to other staging systems, the CUPI has not shown a prognostic advantage over other staging systems and the CUPI has failed to gain widespread acceptance or usage.

American Joint Committee on Cancer/International Union Against Cancer staging system (sixth and seventh editions)

The sixth edition AJCC/UICC TNM staging system was based on an international multicentre study of 591 patients who had undergone resection of HCC [18]. Centralised pathologic review provided data on tumour size, microscopic or macroscopic vascular invasion, and degree of fibrosis. In the sixth edition AJCC/UICC staging, T stage is classified as T0, no evidence of primary tumour; T1, solitary tumour without vascular invasion; T2, solitary tumour with vascular invasion or multiple tumours less than 5 cm; T3, multiple tumours larger than 5 cm or involvement of major branch or portal or hepatic veins and T4, tumour with direct invasion of adjacent organs. Nodal disease and metastatic disease are scored 0 for absence and 1 for presence. In addition to tumour-specific factors, the presence of fibrosis is included based on the Ishak histological grading system. Specifically, a score of F0 is given for Ishak grades 0–4 fibrosis versus F1 for Ishak grades 5–6 [19]. The sixth edition AJCC/UICC staging system has been independently validated in several studies including a hepatitis-B dominant HCC Chinese population [20] and among patients undergoing liver transplantation [21].

The recently updated seventh edition has been revised to further distinguish large tumours from those with major vascular involvement by subdividing the T3 subgroup. Specifically, in the T3 category, patients with invasion of major vessels are distinguished from patients with multiple tumours, of which any are >5 cm but lack major vessel invasion. As such, T3a patients are those with multiple tumours, any >5 cm while T3b are those with tumours of any size involving a major portal vein or hepatic vein. These subgroups form the new stage IIIA and IIIB. T4 disease with direct tumour invasion of surrounding organs is designated stage IIIC. Inferior phrenic nodes are now classified as N1 and any N1 nodal involvement now is designated stage IV disease. Distant metastatic disease distinguishes stage IVB from IVA. The new changes to the seventh edition of the AJCC/UICC staging system focus, however, on further refinement in prognostic stratification of patients with intermediate and advanced HCC. For patients with early stage HCC, the applicability of the AJCC/UICC staging system remains poorly defined.

Comparative performance of staging systems: early HCC considerations

In examining the comparative performance of the HCC staging systems for early disease, attention must be paid to the patient cohort, underlying liver function and treatment modalities being employed in the study population. In one single institution study of 239 patients with cirrhosis and HCC, BCLC outperformed the Okuda, CLIP, and JIS systems [22]. However, the patients were treated according to the proposed treatment algorithm with a surprisingly low percentage undergoing surgical resection (4%) [23,24]. In another study of 195 HCC patients with earlier stage disease found that the BCLC outperformed Okuda, CLIP, JIS and AJCC/UICC sixth edition staging systems [10]. Interestingly in this study, a significant number of patients were treated outside the recommended algorithm with 27% undergoing operative resection, again suggesting the BCLC treatment guidelines may be too conservative. Several other studies have noted the CLIP staging system to be superior to other staging systems [25–27]. A retrospective study of 1713 HCC patients with HCC, which included both surgical and non-surgical cases, found the CLIP staging system to be the best prognostic staging system independent of treatment strategy [28]. The CLIP seems to perform particularly well among patients with advanced disease as one retrospective study of 953 patients noted that the CLIP outperformed JIS, BCLC, MELD and the sixth edition AJCC/UICC in predicting 3-month mortality among non-surgical patients [29]. While the CLIP may perform well among patients with advanced HCC, the structure of the staging system seems to suggest that other systems including the LCSJG and AJCC/UICC, with greater stratification of early tumours, may have greater utility for predicting outcome among patients with early HCC. In one study of 234 patients undergoing curative resection of HCC, the sixth edition AJCC/UICC was noted to be superior to the Okuda, CLIP and CUPI [16]. In another study, the AJCC/UICC was compared with the LCSJG staging system and was again noted to be superior [20]. However, a major critique of this latter study was that it included mostly patients with large tumour and some have suggested that the LCSJG may be a better staging system among patients with smaller tumours and earlier stage disease.

To better evaluate predictors of survival after resection, Nathan and colleagues examined a large cohort of patients exclusively with early HCC [30]. In this study, the authors sought to specifically identify those clinicopathologic factors that predict survival following hepatectomy in patients with early HCC – defined as HCC with tumour size ≤5 cm and no nodal involvement, metastases or major vascular invasion. The authors utilised the Surveillance, Epidemiology and End Results (SEER) database to identify patients with histologically confirmed early HCC. The study included 788 patients with a median tumour size of 3.2 cm, and 20% of patients had tumours ≤2 cm. Most lesions were solitary (74%) and had no evidence of vascular invasion (82%). Among patients with early HCC, median survival and 5-year survival were 45 months and 39%, respectively. On the basis of multivariate analyses, the authors identified several factors that were associated with survival including tumour size >2 cm, multifocality, and vascular invasion. On the basis of these findings, the authors proposed a prognostic scoring system for early HCC that allotted 1 point each for these factors (Table 11.1). Patients could be stratified into three distinct prognostic groups (median and 5-year survival): 0 points (70 months, 55%), 1 point (52 months, 42%) and ≥2 points (24 months, 29%) ($p < 0.001$). On the basis of these data, the authors concluded that while early HCC is generally associated with a good prognosis, pathologic factors can still be used to stratify patients with respect to survival. Furthermore, these data underscore the

TABLE 11.1 Survival statistics by early HCC prognostic score[a]

		Median survival		5-year survival		Cox analysis		
Variable	***N***	**Months**	**95% CI**	**Per cent**	**95% CI**	**HR**	**95% CI**	***p***
Overall score	788	45	38–52	39	35–44	–	–	–
								<0.001
0	105	70	58–00	55	40–68	Ref.	–	
1	410	52	41–60	42	36–49	1.67	1.15–2.44	
2–3	273	24	19–32	29	22–36	2.66	1.82–3.90	

Source: From Nathan H, Schulick RD, Choti MA, Pawlik TM. Predictors of survival after resection of early hepatocellular carcinoma. *Ann Surg* 2009; 249(5):799–805.
CI, confidence interval; Ref, referent.
[a]One point allotted for each of tumour size > 2 cm, multifocality and vascular invasion.

importance of accurate staging even among patients with early HCC.

In a subsequent study, the same group of investigators compared the prognostic accuracy of several staging systems for patients with early stage HCC [31]. While many previous studies had evaluated the relative comparative performance of HCC staging systems, few – if any – had evaluated the comparative performance of HCC staging systems exclusively in patients with early HCC. In this study, 379 patients with early HCC who underwent liver resection or liver transplantation for HCC at one of six major hepatobiliary centres in the United States or Europe were evaluated. The staging systems evaluated were the Okuda, CLIP, BCLC, JIS and the sixth edition AJCC/UICC, as well as the newly proposed early HCC prognostic scoring system [31]. The discriminative abilities of the staging systems were evaluated with Cox proportional hazard models and concordance index (*c*). Interestingly, most staging systems demonstrated poor discriminatory power ($c \approx 0.5$) and an inability to separate patients into distinct prognostic groups (Figure 11.1). While the sixth edition AJCC/UICC staging system did stratify patients, it was only into two distinct groups. In contrast, the new proposed early HCC scoring system clearly stratified patients the best and identified three distinct prognostic groups. The main difference between these two staging systems is that the early HCC prognostic score allows patients with solitary tumours to be stratified with respect to both tumour size (>2 cm vs. ≤2 cm) and the presence of microvascular invasion, whereas the AJCC/UICC system does not consider size to be a prognostic factor for solitary tumours. Other data have suggested that further stratification of solitary tumours without vascular invasion based on a 2 cm cut-off size can enhance the predictive ability of the standard AJCC/UICC staging system [32]. Specifically, for early HCC tumours, the addition of tumour size > 2 cm for both solitary and multifocal tumours and the inclusion of microscopic vascular invasion for multifocal tumours can add prognostic impact. In sum, these data have important implications as they demonstrated that most major HCC staging systems perform poorly in staging patients with early HCC.

Conclusions

For patients with HCC, survival is dependent on a number of different tumour factors as well as underlying liver function. In turn, there are many different staging systems for HCC.

For patients with advanced HCC and those patients undergoing locoregional therapy, the CLIP staging system appears to perform well. In contrast, for patients with intermediate or advanced HCC who undergo resection, the AJCC/UICC is probably the most utilised and favoured staging system. However, for those patients with early stage HCC, recent data have shown that virtually all traditional staging systems perform poorly with inadequate discriminatory ability. Instead, a recently proposed early HCC prognostic scoring system that incorporates tumour size (≥ 2 cm), multifocality and the presence of vascular invasion provides a simple and accurate method to predict survival of patients with early HCC. As more patients are

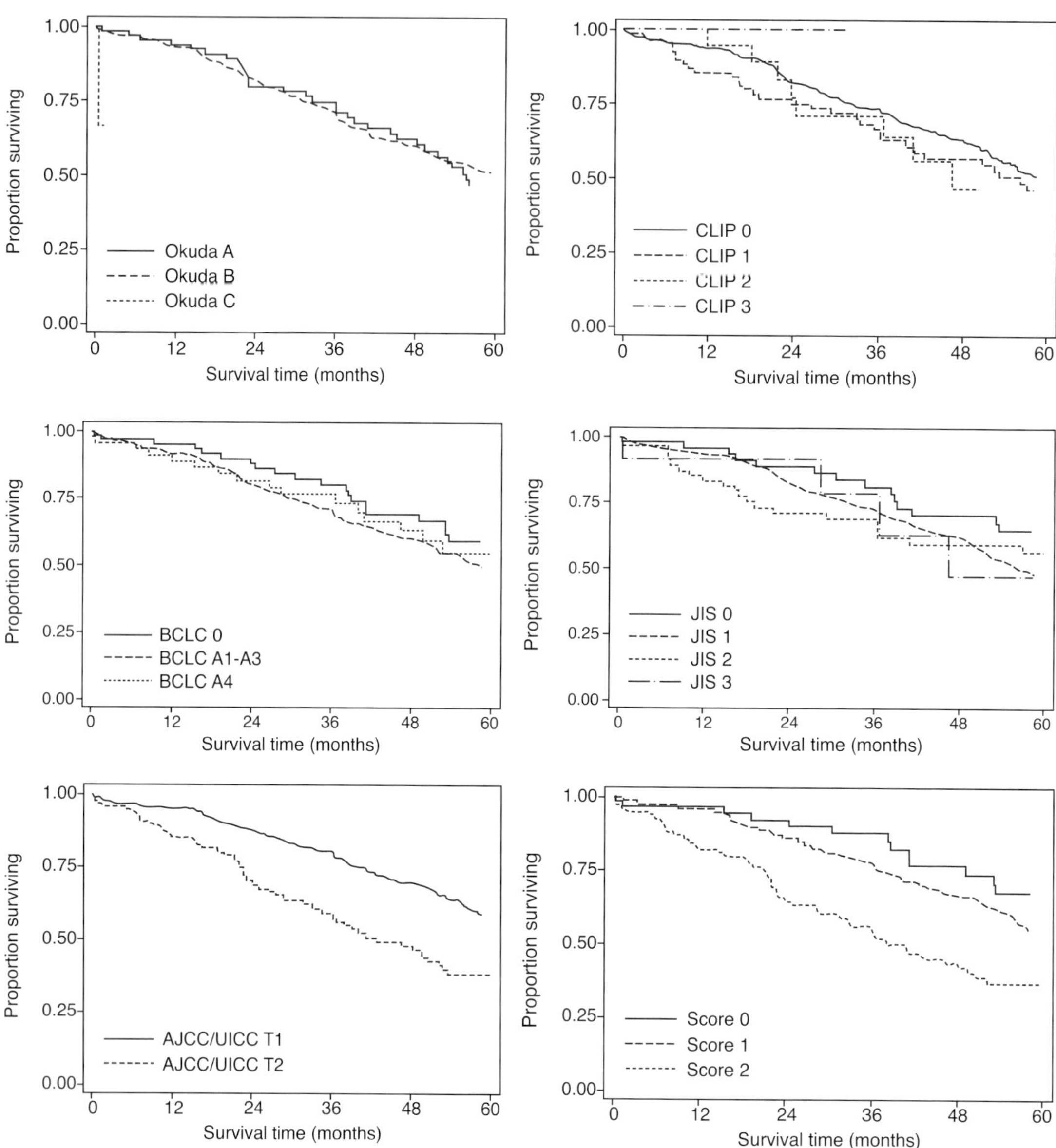

FIG 11.1 Comparative performances of staging systems for early hepatocellular carcinoma. (Used with permission, Nathan H, Mentha G, Marques HP, et al. Comparative performances of staging systems for early hepatocellular carcinoma. *HPB (Oxford)* 2009; 11(5):382–390.)

diagnosed with early HCC, it will be critically important to accurately stage this group of patients. As such, future studies will need to continue to define and refine the predictive factors associated with outcome in this specific cohort of patients.

References

1. Okuda K, Ohtsuki T, Obata H, et al. Natural history of hepatocellular carcinoma and prognosis in relation to treatment. Study of 850 patients. *Cancer* 1985; 56(4):918–928.

2. The Cancer of the Liver Italian Program (CLIP) investigators. A new prognostic system for hepatocellular carcinoma: a retrospective study of 435 patients. *Hepatology* 1998; 28(3):751–755.
3. Llovet JM, Bruix J. Prospective validation of the Cancer of the Liver Italian Program (CLIP) score: a new prognostic system for patients with cirrhosis and hepatocellular carcinoma. *Hepatology* 2000; 32(3):679–680.
4. Ueno S, Tanabe G, Sako K, et al. Discrimination value of the new western prognostic system (CLIP score) for hepatocellular carcinoma in 662 Japanese patients. Cancer of the Liver Italian Program. *Hepatology* 2001; 34(3):529–534.
5. Levy I, Sherman M. Staging of hepatocellular carcinoma: assessment of the CLIP, Okuda, and Child–Pugh staging systems in a cohort of 257 patients in Toronto. *Gut* 2002; 50(6):881–885.
6. Biselli M, Andreone P, Gramenzi A, et al. Transcatheter arterial chemoembolization therapy for patients with hepatocellular carcinoma: a case-controlled study. *Clin Gastroenterol Hepatol* 2005; 3(9):918–925.
7. Miraglia R, Pietrosi G, Maruzzelli L, et al. Predictive factors of tumor response to trans-catheter treatment in cirrhotic patients with hepatocellular carcinoma: a multivariate analysis of pre-treatment findings. *World J Gastroenterol* 2007; 13(45):6022–6026.
8. Llovet JM, Bru C, Bruix J. Prognosis of hepatocellular carcinoma: the BCLC staging classification. *Semin Liver Dis* 1999; 19(3):329–338.
9. Cillo U, Bassanello M, Vitale A, et al. The critical issue of hepatocellular carcinoma prognostic classification: which is the best tool available? *J Hepatol* 2004; 40(1):124–131.
10. Cillo U, Vitale A, Grigoletto F, et al. Prospective validation of the Barcelona Clinic Liver Cancer staging system. *J Hepatol* 2006; 44(4):723–731.
11. Makuuchi M, Belghiti J, Belli G, et al. IHPBA concordant classification of primary liver cancer: working group report. *J Hepatobiliary Pancreat Surg* 2003; 10(1):26–30.
12. Kudo M, Chung H, Osaki Y. Prognostic staging system for hepatocellular carcinoma (CLIP score): its value and limitations, and a proposal for a new staging system, the Japan Integrated Staging Score (JIS score). *J Gastroenterol* 2003; 38(3):207–215.
13. Kudo M, Chung H, Haji S, et al. Validation of a new prognostic staging system for hepatocellular carcinoma: the JIS score compared with the CLIP score. *Hepatology* 2004; 40(6):1396–1405.
14. Leung TW, Tang AM, Zee B, et al. Construction of the Chinese University Prognostic Index for hepatocellular carcinoma and comparison with the TNM staging system, the Okuda staging system, and the Cancer of the Liver Italian Program staging system: a study based on 926 patients. *Cancer* 2002; 94(6):1760–1769.
15. Kondo K, Chijiiwa K, Nagano M, et al. Comparison of seven prognostic staging systems in patients who undergo hepatectomy for hepatocellular carcinoma. *Hepatogastroenterology* 2007; 54(77):1534–1538.
16. Lu W, Dong J, Huang Z, et al. Comparison of four current staging systems for Chinese patients with hepatocellular carcinoma undergoing curative resection: Okuda, CLIP, TNM and CUPI. *J Gastroenterol Hepatol* 2008; 23(12):1874–1878.
17. Huitzil-Melendez FD, Capanu M, O'Reilly EM, et al. Advanced hepatocellular carcinoma: which staging systems best predict prognosis? *J Clin Oncol 2010*; 28(17):2889–2895.
18. Vauthey JN, Lauwers GY, Esnaola NF, et al. Simplified staging for hepatocellular carcinoma. *J Clin Oncol* 2002; 20(6):1527–1536.
19. Ishak K, Baptista A, Bianchi L, et al. Histological grading and staging of chronic hepatitis. *J Hepatol* 1995; 22(6):696–699.
20. Poon RT, Fan ST. Evaluation of the new AJCC/UICC staging system for hepatocellular carcinoma after hepatic resection in Chinese patients. *Surg Oncol Clin N Am* 2003; 12(1):35–50, viii.
21. Vauthey JN, Ribero D, Abdalla EK, et al. Outcomes of liver transplantation in 490 patients with hepatocellular carcinoma: validation of a uniform staging after surgical treatment. *J Am Coll Surg* 2007; 204(5):1016–1027; discussion 1027–1028.
22. Marrero JA, Fontana RJ, Barrat A, et al. Prognosis of hepatocellular carcinoma: comparison of 7 staging systems in an American cohort. *Hepatology* 2005; 41(4):707–716.
23. Pawlik TM, Abdalla EK, Thomas M, et al. Staging of hepatocellular carcinoma. *Hepatology* 2005; 42(3):738–739; author reply 739–740.
24. Huo TI, Wu JC, Lee SD. Comparison of staging systems for HCC: one more positive answer or mission impossible? *Hepatology* 2005; 42(1):238–239.
25. Tateishi R, Yoshida H, Shiina S, et al. Proposal of a new prognostic model for hepatocellular carcinoma: an analysis of 403 patients. *Gut* 2005; 54(3):419–425.
26. Toyoda H, Kumada T, Kiriyama S, et al. Comparison of the usefulness of three staging systems for hepatocellular carcinoma (CLIP, BCLC, and JIS) in Japan. *Am J Gastroenterol* 2005; 100(8):1764–1771.
27. Nanashima A, Omagari K, Tobinaga S, et al. Comparative study of survival of patients with hepatocellular carcinoma predicted by different staging systems using multivariate analysis. *Eur J Surg Oncol* 2005; 31(8):882–890.
28. Hsu CY, Hsia CY, Huang YH, et al. Selecting an optimal staging system for hepatocellular carcinoma: comparison of 5 currently used prognostic models. *Cancer* 2010; 116(12):3006–3014.

29. Huo TI, Hsia CY, Huang YH, et al. Selecting a short-term prognostic model for hepatocellular carcinoma: comparison between the model for end-stage liver disease (MELD), MELD-sodium, and five cancer staging systems. *J Clin Gastroenterol* 2009; 43(8):773–781.
30. Nathan H, Schulick RD, Choti MA, Pawlik TM. Predictors of survival after resection of early hepatocellular carcinoma. *Ann Surg* 2009; 249(5):799–805.
31. Nathan H, Mentha G, Marques HP, et al. Comparative performances of staging systems for early hepatocellular carcinoma. *HPB (Oxford)* 2009; 11(5):382–390.
32. Kee KM, Wang JH, Lee CM, et al. Validation of clinical AJCC/UICC TNM staging system for hepatocellular carcinoma: analysis of 5,613 cases from a medical center in southern Taiwan. *Int J Cancer* 2007; 120(12):2650–2655.

12 Rival scoring systems: do they offer more?

Angelo Sangiovanni[1], Massimo Colombo[2]

[1]A.M. & A. Migliavacca Center for Liver Disease, 1st Division of Gastroenterology, Fondazione IRCCS Ca' Granda Ospedale Maggiore Policlinico and University of Milan, Milan, Italy

[2]Department of Medicine, 1st Division of Gastroenterology, Fondazione IRCCS Ca' Granda Ospedale Maggiore Policlinico and University of Milan, Milan, Italy

LEARNING POINTS

- The ideal staging system should incorporate information on tumour burden, liver disease severity, comorbidities and variables predicting the biological aggressiveness of the tumour to assist clinicians with treatment choice
- None of the available scoring systems rival to Barcelona Clinic Liver Cancer (BCLC), including Okuda, GRoupe d'Etude et de Traitement du Carcinoma Hépatocellulaire (GRETCH), Cancer of the Liver Italian Program (CLIP), Chinese University Prognostic Index (CUPI), Japan Integrated Staging (JIS), tumour-node-metastasis (TNM) and Tokyo, are standardised and able to predict survival at individual level
- The comparison of the staging systems other than BCLC does not provide a winner, confirming that all staging systems unable to guide treatment choice do not positively impact the practice field practice in liver oncology

Introduction

Tumour staging is of strategic importance in the management of patients with a hepatocellular carcinoma (HCC), since it establishes prognosis by stratifying patients on the basis of disease severity and guides the selection of treatment, which is ultimately the determinant of patient survival. Furthermore, tumour staging provides a means of selecting for adjuvant therapy and for the design of studies aimed at evaluating new treatments for HCC. Since HCC is an epidemiologically and clinically heterogeneous disease, a single staging system is unlikely to be applicable efficiently worldwide, thus leaving open the issue on which system performs best at staging HCC. Currently available staging systems need to be improved, since a standardised test is not available to determine the burden and spread of HCC, while no serum biomarkers of prognosis have been validated to replace the current approach based on anatomical and functional criteria. The BCLC scoring system has been endorsed by European Association for the Study of the Liver (EASL) and American Association for the Study of Liver Diseases (AASLD), since it proved to be discriminant in stratifying HCC patients with respect to the available treatment options. One, of course, may wonder whether the performance of BCLC can be improved by the addition of biomarkers thought to predict the biological aggressiveness of the tumour, i.e. the propensity of cancer cells to infiltrate blood vessels to spread within and outside the liver. Among the many scoring systems that have been proposed, the more discriminant are those that are multidimensional, including variables like severity of liver disease, number and size of tumour nodules and cancer spread, whereas unidimensional staging systems like TNM found to perform well in tumours other than HCC are not sensitive enough to stage HCC, which cumulates the prognostic factors of the tumour and of the underlying liver disease (Table 12.1).

The Okuda staging system

Historically, the Okuda classification (Table 12.2) [1] was the first multidimensional system to stage HCC, being generated from a set of patients with advanced HCC from Japan. This system includes the rate of liver involvement by the tumour (±50% invasion assessed by CT scan) and

Clinical Dilemmas in Primary Liver Cancer, First Edition. Edited by Roger Williams and Simon D. Taylor-Robinson.

TABLE 12.1 Staging systems in hepatocellular carcinoma other than Barcelona Clinic Liver Cancer (BCLC)

Classification	Type		Stages
Okuda	System	3	Stages I, II, III
French	Score	3	A: 0 points B: 1-5 points C: ≥ 6 points
CLIP	Score	5	0, 1, 2, 3, 4–6
CUPI	Score	3	Low risk: score ≤ 1 Intermediate: score 2–7 High: score ≥ 8
TNM	System	4	Stages I, II, III, IV
JIS	Score	4	Stages I, II, III, IV
Tokyo	Score	6	0, 1, 2, 3, 4–6

functional parameters like serum levels of albumin and bilirubin, and ascites. Despite the relevant sample size of the cohort that generated the Okuda system, important predictors of patient survival like portal vein thrombosis, size and number of tumour nodes are missed. The 115 (13%) stage I patients who underwent surgery had a mean survival of 26 months, compared with the median survival of 9 months of the 124 (15%) stage I who received no surgery. The Okuda staging system is unfit for patients with early HCC with respect to the options for radical treatment, whereas it is better applicable to patients with an advanced or symptomatic tumours. All in all, this system is useful for identifying end-stage patients (Okuda stage III) unfit for trials designed to assess new therapeutic agents, owing to the poor survival likelihood of the patients. Following the implementation of surveillance programmes resulting in an increasing number of patients with an early cancer, the Okuda classification has been progressively abandoned by hepatologists as a tool for stratifying patients with respect to treatment options [2].

TABLE 12.2 The Okuda staging system

	Scores	
Variables	**0**	**1**
Liver involvement by tumour	<50%	>50%
Ascites	No	Yes
Albumin (g/dL)	≥3.0	<3.0
Bilirubin (mg/dL)	<3.0	>3.0

Source: Okuda K, Ohtsuki T, Obata H, et al. Natural history of hepatocellular carcinoma and prognosis in relation to treatment. *Cancer* 1985; 56:918–928.
Stage I, score 0; stage II, score 1 or 2; stage III, score 3 or 4.

The French classification (GRETCH)

The French classification (Table 12.3) [3] proposed by the GRoupe d'Etude et de Traitement du Carcinoma Hépatocellulaire (GRETCH) was formulated in 1998, utilising 761 patients with HCC who were enrolled from 24 Western medical centres, with the exclusion of 18 patients who underwent liver transplantation. Reflecting the epidemiology of HCC in Europe, 80% of patients had cirrhosis. While 360 (47%) patients received treatments for HCC, both as a single modality or in combination, ultimately 401 (53%) patients had been left untreated. After being assigned to either a training cohort ($n = 506$, with 418 deaths), or a test cohort ($n = 255$, with 200 deaths), a score was developed based on five variables Karnofsky Index, bilirubin, alkaline phosphatase, serum alpha-fetoprotein (AFP) and presence/absence of portal vein thrombosis at imaging techniques, which stratified patients into three strata with a 2-year survival rate of 51%, 16% and 3%. Since the relatively short survival in two out of three strata reflects the prevalence of advanced HCC in the cohort, this stage classification has a limited prognostic sensitivity for early HCC, as compared with other staging systems, thus explaining why GRETCH was rapidly abandoned in clinical practice [4].

TABLE 12.3 The Groupe d'Etude et de Traitement du Carcinome Hépatocellulaire (GRETCH) staging classification

	Scores			
Stage	**0**	**1**	**2**	**3**
KI (%)	≥80			<80
Bilirubin (μmol/L)	<50			≥50
ALP (ULN)	<2		≥2	
AFP (ng/dL)	<35		≥35	
Portal vein thrombosis	No	Yes		

Source: Chevret S, Trinchet JC, Mathieu D, et al. A new prognostic classification for predicting survival in patients with hepatocellular carcinoma. *J Hepatol* 1999; 31:133–141.
KI, Karnofsky index.
French scores: A, 0 point; B, 1–5 points; C, ≥6 points.

Cancer of the Liver Italian Program

CLIP score [5] (Table 12.4) was first constructed and subsequently both internally and externally validated [6] using a cohort of 435 patients in Italy (38% Child-Pugh A, 37% Okuda stage I, 41% with AFP values > 400 ng/mL). By combining four variables related to tumour morphology, liver function (Child-Pugh), serum AFP and radiological diagnosis of portal vein thrombosis, CLIP generates a seven-strata classification. To internally validate the system, the whole cohort was split into a training (67%) and in a testing cohort (33%) that demonstrated a better discriminatory power of CLIP in patients with advanced HCC, compared with Okuda and TNM. While the score system showed predictive power for survival in Western patients, this was not the case for studies in Asia, thus attenuating the clinical significance of the external validation [7]. One major weakness of CLIP was the combination of different prognostic factors, causing intrascore heterogeneity, whereby the lower the CLIP score, the higher the intrascore variability, which suggested heterogeneity of mortality risk within a given score. However, from a clinical point of view, the major weakness of CLIP was the poor predictive power of stage I, which allowed for tumours greater than 5 cm to be in the same stage bracket as early cancers potentially suitable to radical therapies. This clearly limits the applicability of CLIP to patients in geographical areas where 30% of all patients present with a small HCC identified with screening.

TABLE 12.4 The Cancer of the Liver Italian Program (CLIP) scoring system

	Points		
Variables	**0**	**1**	**2**
Tumour burden	Single <50%[a]	Multiple <50%	Massive or >50%
Child-Pugh score	A	B	C
AFP (ng/mL)	<400	≥400	
Portal vs. thrombosis	No	Yes	

Source: CLIP group (Cancer of the Liver Italian Programme). Tamoxifen in the treatment of hepatocellular carcinoma: a randomised controlled trial. *Lancet* 1998; 352:17–20.

[a]Per cent of liver involvement by the tumour.

CLIP scores: 0, 1, 2, 3, 4–6.

The Chinese University Prognostic Index

This staging system was developed in Hong Kong, China, by studying 926 patients, mostly (79%) with HBV-related chronic liver disease and cirrhosis [8], whereas only a minority (18%) had symptomatic disease on presentation. A peculiar feature of CUPI was that half of the patients had >500 ng/mL serum AFP levels. Considering six predictive variables such as TNM, asymptomatic ascites, AFP value, bilirubin and alkaline phosphatases, CUPI stratifies and divides patients into three stages (Table 12.5). The low-risk group includes patients with a 3-month probability of dying <30%, the intermediate group includes patients with a probability between 30% and 70%, and the high-risk group includes patients with a probability >70%. Through this staging system was internally validated providing a better estimate of survival than CLIP and Okuda stages, however, the fact that the best group of CUPI has a 1-year survival of only 50%, clearly indicates CUPI performs better among patients with advanced HCC than in patients with earlier cancer.

TABLE 12.5 The Chinese University Prognostic Index (CUPI)

Variable	CUPI score
TNM stages I & II	−3
III	−1
IV	0
Asymptomatic disease	−4
Ascites	3
AFP (500 ng/mL)	2
Bilirubin (<2 mg/dL)	0
2–3	3
>3	4
ALP (>200 IU/L)	3

CUPI score	Mortality risk at month 3
Low risk ≤1	<30%
Intermediate risk 2–7	30–70%
High risk ≥8	>70%

Source: Leung TW, Tang AM, Zee B, et al. Construction of the Chinese University Prognostic Index for hepatocellular carcinoma and comparison with the TNM staging system, the Okuda staging system, and the Cancer of the Liver Italian Program staging system: a study based on 926 patients. *Cancer* 2002; 94:1760–1769.

TABLE 12.6 The Union for International Cancer Control (UICC) TNM classification (7th edition, 2010)

Primary tumour (T)			
TX	Primary tumour cannot be assessed		
T0	No evidence of primary tumour		
T1	Solitary tumour without vascular invasion		
T2	Solitary tumour with vascular invasion or multiple tumours none more than 5 cm		
T3a	Multiple tumours more than 5 cm		
T3b	Single tumour or multiple tumours of any size involving a major branch of the portal vein or hepatic vein		
T4	Tumour(s) with direct invasion of adjacent organs other than the gallbladder or with perforation of visceral peritoneum		
Regional lymph nodes (N)			
NX	Regional lymph nodes cannot be assessed		
N0	No regional lymph node metastasis		
N1	Regional lymph node metastasis		
Distant metastasis (M)			
M0	No distant metastasis		
M1	Distant metastasis		
Fibrosis score (F)[a]			
F0	Fibrosis score 0–4 (none to moderate fibrosis)		
F1	Fibrosis score 5–6 (severe fibrosis or cirrhosis)		
Anatomic stage/prognostic groups			
Stage I	T1	N0	M0
Stage II	T2	N0	M0
Stage IIIA	T3a	N0	M0
Stage IIIB	T3b	N0	M0
Stage IIIC	T4	N0	M0
Stage IVA	Any T	N1	M0
Stage IVB	Any T	Any N	M1

Source: Sobin LH, Gospodarowicz MK, Wittekind C (eds). *TNM Classification of Malignant Tumors*, 7th ed. Blackwell Publishing Ltd, Oxford; 2009, pp. 110–113.
Note: cTNM is the clinical classification and pTNM is the pathologic classification.
[a]The fibrosis score as defined by Ishak is recommended because of its prognostic value in overall survival. This scoring system uses a 0–6 scale.

The AJCC/UICC tumour-node-metastasis staging system

The TNM seventh edition (Table 12.6) [9] provided by the Union Internationale Contre le Cancer (UICC) is a unidimensional system founded on variables related to the anatomical stage of the tumour, i.e. number and size of nodes, vascular invasion and distant metastases. It was endorsed by the American Joint Committee on Cancer (AJCC) [10]. Therefore, the ability of TNM to predict prognosis in HCC patients is limited by the lack of variables related to the status of the accompanying liver disease. The TNM classification implies both a clinical (cTNM) and a pathologic classification (pTNM), the latter obtained in patients treated surgically where TNM showed discriminatory ability [11], but not for those where medical treatment was indicated. TNM system is thus utilised for staging HCC in the explanted livers, only (Zurich Consensus 2010).

Japan Integrated Staging

The fourth TNM staging and liver damage grade adopted by the Liver Cancer Study Group of Japan (LCSGJ) was

TABLE 12.7 The Japan Integrated Staging (JIS) scoring system

	Points			
Variables	**0**	**1**	**2**	**3**
Child-Pugh	A	B	C	
TNM stage by LCSGJ[a]	I	II	III	IV

	Factors		
T classification	**I. Single**	**II. Size < 2 cm**	**III. No vessel invasion**
T1		Fulfilling three factors	
T2		Fulfilling two factors	
T3		Fulfilling one factor	
T4		Fulfilling 0 factor	
Stage			
I	T1 N0 M0		
II	T2 N0 M0		
III	T3 N0 M0		
IV-A	T4 N0 M0 or T1–T4N M0		
IV-B	T1–T4, N0 or N1, M		

Source: Kudo M, Chung H, Osaki Y. Prognostic staging system for hepatocellular carcinoma (CLIP score): its value and limitations, and a proposal for a new staging system, the Japan Integrated Staging Score (JIS score). *J Gastroenterol* 2003; 38:207–215.
[a]TNM classification and stage by the Liver Cancer Study Group of Japan (LCSGJ), fourth edition.

combined with the Child-Pugh classification to build the JIS score (Table 12.7) [12]. The system was built using 722 patients (70% Child-Pugh A, 32% CLIP 0) treated in two institutions in a 10-year period to provide four strata of patients: early (score 0), intermediate (scores 1 and 2), advanced (scores 3 and 4) and end-stage group (score 5). This staging system was validated in Japan, only, where it was shown to perform better than CLIP, whereas it lacks external validation in Western countries. Surprisingly, the JIS system was able to identify 14% of the patients with a score 0, a finding that contrasts with the high proportion (30–40%) of HCC patients presenting to the referral centres with an early tumour.

Tokyo score

Four hundred and three HCC patients, consecutively treated by percutaneous ablation in Japan between 1990 and 1997, were used as a training set to identify prognostic factors for HCC. The Tokyo score is based on four variables, i.e. serum albumin, bilirubin, size and number of tumours, generating six strata [13] (Table 12.8). The system was internally validated in 203 independent patients who underwent hepatectomy. In the original study, the 5-year survival was 79%, 62%, 40%, 28%, and 14% for Tokyo scores 0, 1, 2, 3, and cumulated 4–6 with evidence that it was as good as CLIP and stronger than BCLC in discriminating patients with a HCC, indicating that Tokyo score is fit for the prognostication of Japanese patients with HCC requiring radical therapy.

TABLE 12.8 The Tokyo score

	Points		
Variables	**0**	**1**	**2**
Albumin (g/dL)	3.5	2.8–3.5	2.8
Bilirubin (mg/dL)	<1	1–2	>2
Tumour size (cm)	<2	2–5	>5
Tumour no.	≤3		

Source: Tateishi R, Yoshida H, Shiina S, et al. Proposal of a new prognostic model for hepatocellular carcinoma: an analysis of 403 patients. *Gut* 2005; 54:419–425.
Tokyo score: 0, 1, 2, 3, 4–6.

The Model for End-Stage Liver Disease

The model for end-stage liver disease (MELD) [14] was originally developed to calculate short-term survival (3 months) of patients with cirrhosis, and it is not strictly considered a staging system. Though the MELD score was applied to calculate the probability of survival of patients with HCC, too, using the formula 3.8 × log (e) (bilirubin mg/dL) + 11.2 × log (e) (INR) + 9.6 log (e) (creatinine mg/dL), it is not adequate for prognostication of HCC patients, since it takes into account variables related to liver function without any prognostic factor for liver cancer.

Other staging systems

The oestrogen receptor classification is a molecular classification based on variant forms of the wild-type oestrogen receptor that may occur in patients with HCC, while they maintain constitutive transcriptional activity. Tumours containing this variant of oestrogen receptors tend to be more aggressive, with shorter doubling times than tumours lacking it. Through the presence of variant oestrogen receptors was a better predictor of an unfavourable prognosis compared with the CLIP and BCLC. ER classification is not used routinely, since it requires a liver tissue for the variant receptor [15].

The SLiDe scoring system [16] is based on three variables stage, liver damage and des-γ-carboxy prothrombin (DCP), using 'stage' and 'liver damage' of the fourth edition of the Japanese staging system edited by the LCSGJ [12]. The system assigns a linear four-grade score (0–1, 2, 3, 4–6), and it is useful for the assessment of the prognosis of patients with HCC, providing a better model than CLIP and JIS, as judged by the Akaike Information Criteria, which is measure of the goodness of fit of a statistical model (describing the trade-off between bias and variance in model construction, or loosely speaking between accuracy and complexity of the model). Limitations of the scoring system are the use of variables not routinely examined, such as DCP and stage by LCSGJ, as well as the lack of linkage to any treatment decision choice.

The BALAD score [17] is based on five serum markers: bilirubin, albumin, *Lens culinaris* agglutinin-reactive alpha-fetoprotein (AFP-L3), AFP and DCP. The bilirubin (<1, 1–2, >2 mg/dL) and albumin values (>3.5, 2.8–3.5, <2.8 mg/dL), combined with tumour marker (cut-off values 400 ng/dL for AFP, 15% for AFP-L3, 100 milli-arbitrary unit/mL for DCP) provide for classifying patients into six categories. The categories reflect patient survival with excellent discriminatory ability, but no indication for the choice of HCC treatment.

The Taipei integrated scoring system [18] is based on a retrospective analysis of 2030 Taiwanese HCC patients undergoing different treatment strategies. The total tumour volume, defined as the sum of the volume of each tumour, combined with the Child-Turcotte-Pugh and the AFP value, consistently showed a better prognostic ability in comparison to the current four staging systems: CLIP, Tokyo and JIS systems. The model, recently proposed, lacks of external validation outside Taiwan at the current time.

A new prognostic score for patients in the palliative setting [19] was developed in 2011 by *Tournoux-Facon* and colleagues on a set of 416 French HCC patients and it was validated on a second set of 271 patients. It is based on tumour morphology, portal vein obstruction, metastasis, ascites, jaundice, AFP and serum alkaline phosphatase. Three groups of increasing risk were defined. This score provides a better discriminatory ability than BCLC and CLIP in the original setting, but unfortunately, its absolute performance remains poor.

The TNM-Izumi classification [20] was proposed for patients undergoing hepatic resection and it is based on a modification of the current TNM classification in the 1994, incorporating clinical and pathological findings, such as vascular invasion and lobar distribution of the tumour. The classification was validated and supports the prognostic significance of pathologic evaluation, but is it may be not directly translated to the majority of the patients.

The Milan criteria [21] were proposed for predicting outcome after orthotopic liver transplantation (solitary tumour ≤5 cm, three or fewer nodules with the largest lesion ≤3 cm, and no macroscopic vascular invasion), as well as the *University of California, San Francisco (UCSF) criteria* [22] (solitary tumour < 6.5 cm, three or fewer nodules with the largest lesion <4.5 cm and a total number diameter < 8 cm, without gross vascular invasion), and the more recent 'metroticket' system [23] (up-to-seven criteria: HCCs with seven as the sum of the size of the largest tumour in cm, and the number of tumours).

Comparative studies

Studies assessing the prognosis of HCC patients are flawed by the lack of variables that adequately sense the

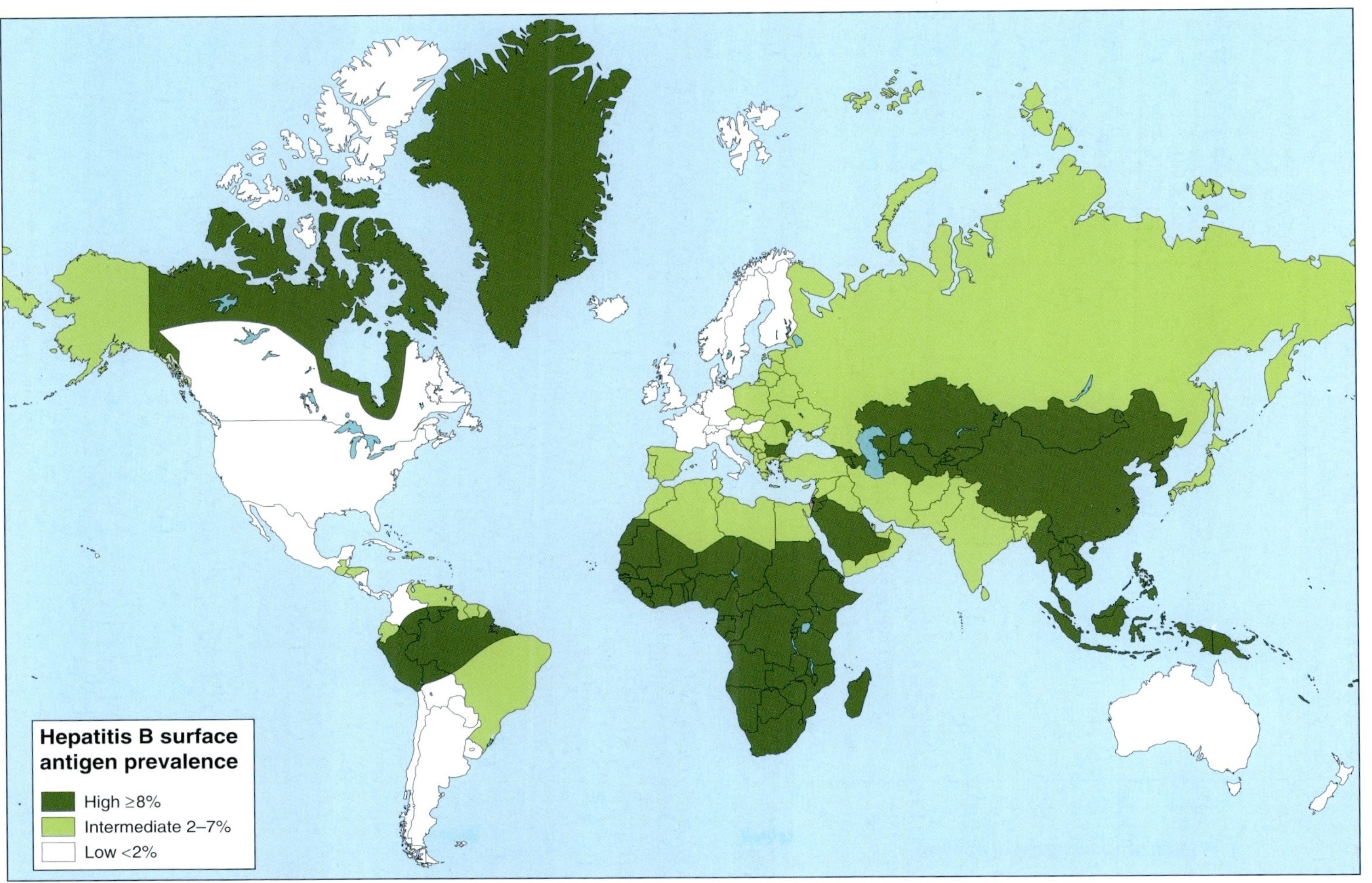

Plate 2.1 Global distribution of hepatitis B prevalence. (Reproduced by permission of WHO. Available from: http://www.who.int/csr/disease/hepatitis/HepatitisB_whocdscsrlyo2002_2.pdf. Accessed 20 October, 2010.)

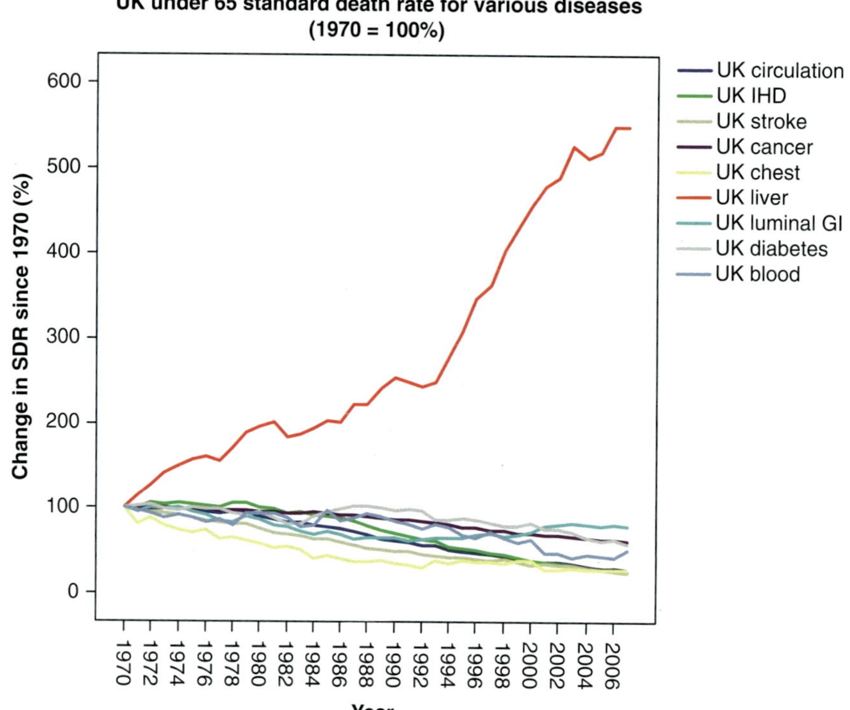

Plate 4.1 UK death rates for those under 65 from major diseases compared with 1970.

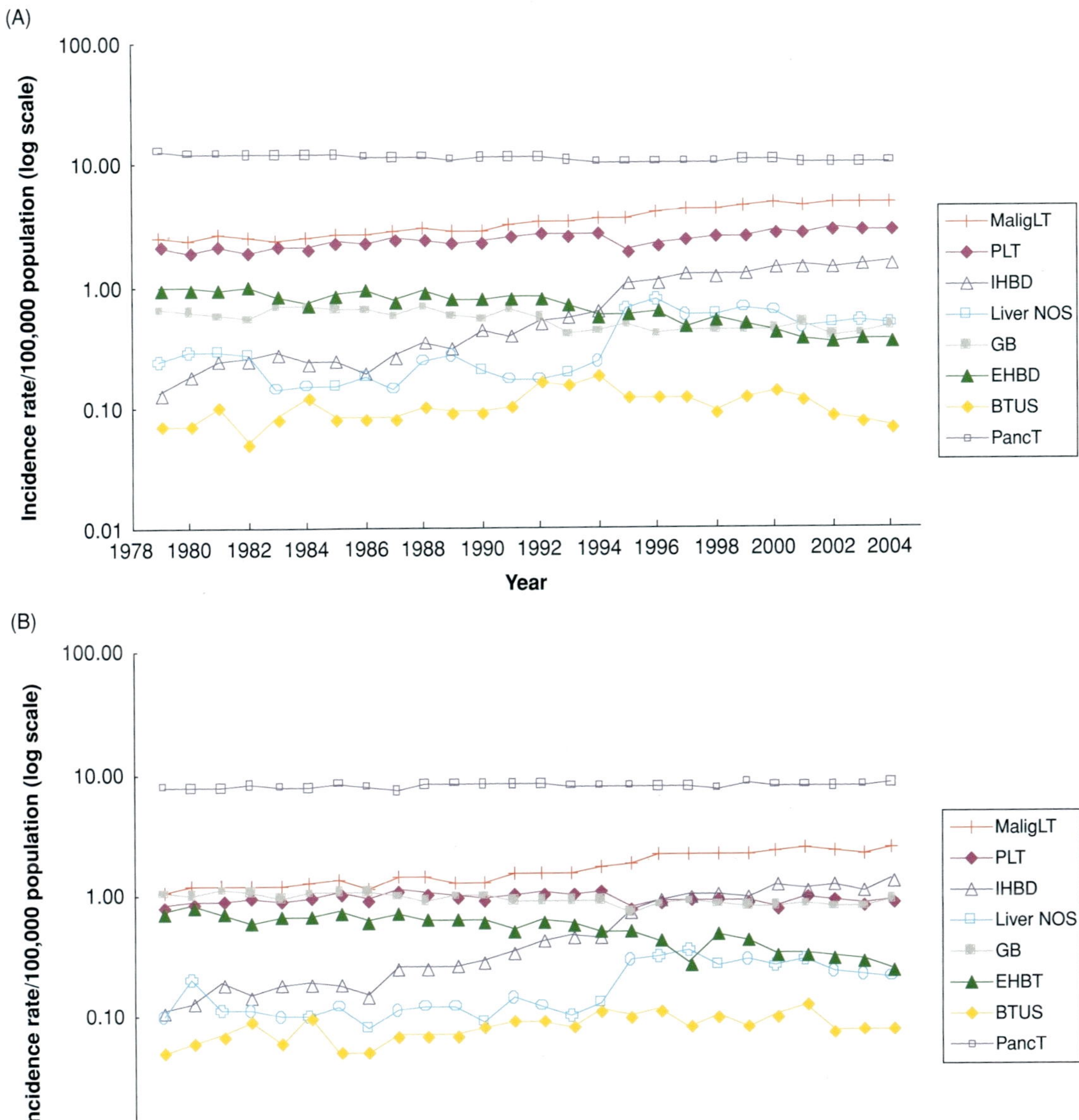

Plate 4.2 Age-standardised incidence rates per 100,000 population of England and Wales for selected hepatobiliary tumours in (A) males and (B) females, 1979–2004. MaligLT, all malignant liver tumours; PLT, primary liver tumours; IHBD, intrahepatic bile duct tumours; Liver NOS, unspecified liver tumours; GB, gall bladder tumours; EHBD, extrahepatic bile duct tumours; BTUS; PancT, pancreatic tumours.

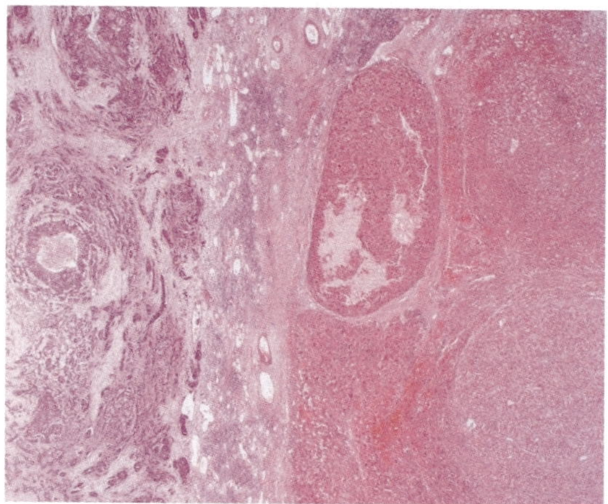

Plate 8.1 Combined HCC-CC. Cholangiocellular component with desmoplastic stroma (left) are separated from HCC nodules by a thin pseudocapsule (right).

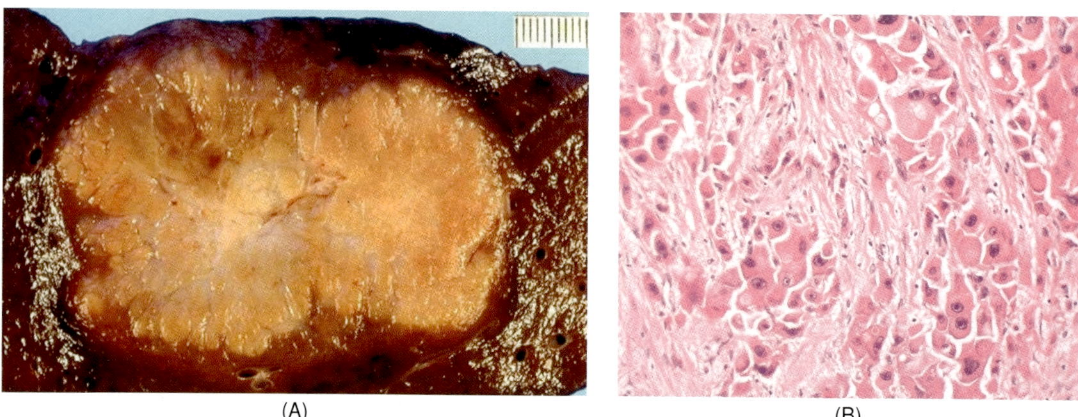

(A) (B)

Plate 8.2 Fibrolamellar HCC. (A) Gross appearance with central scarring resembling focal nodular hyperplasia. (B) Histology shows large eosinophilic cells separated by bands of lamellar collagen.

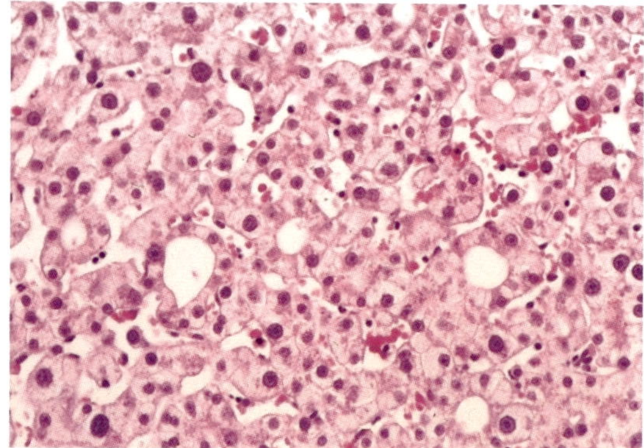

Plate 8.3 Large HCA associated with long exposure to danazol. Note a marked cellular atypia raising the differential diagnosis of well-differentiated HCC. A second nodule with similar histology on biopsy disappeared 6 months after drug withdrawal.

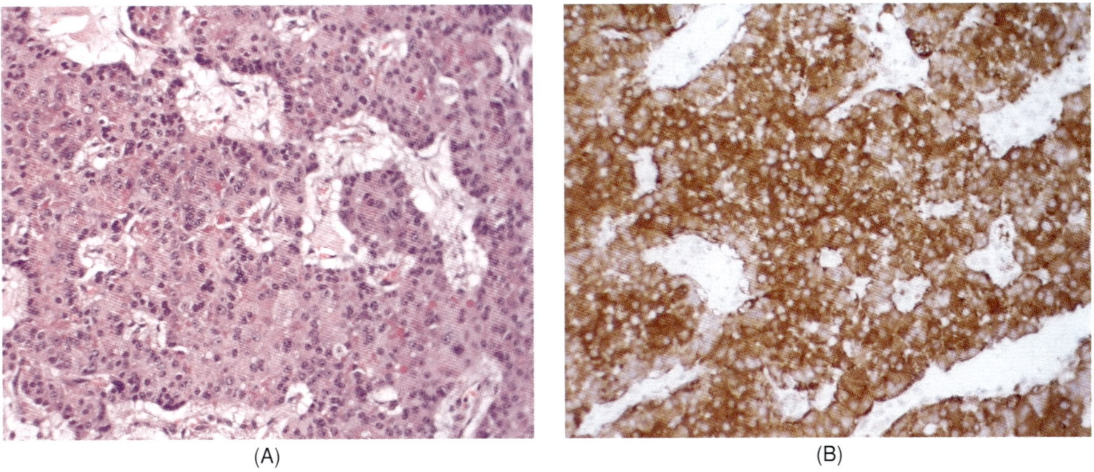

(A) (B)

Plate 8.4 (A) Endocrine neoplasm misdiagnosed as macrotrabecular, small-cell HCC. (B) Strong immunostaining for synaptophysin confirm the endocrine nature of the tumour.

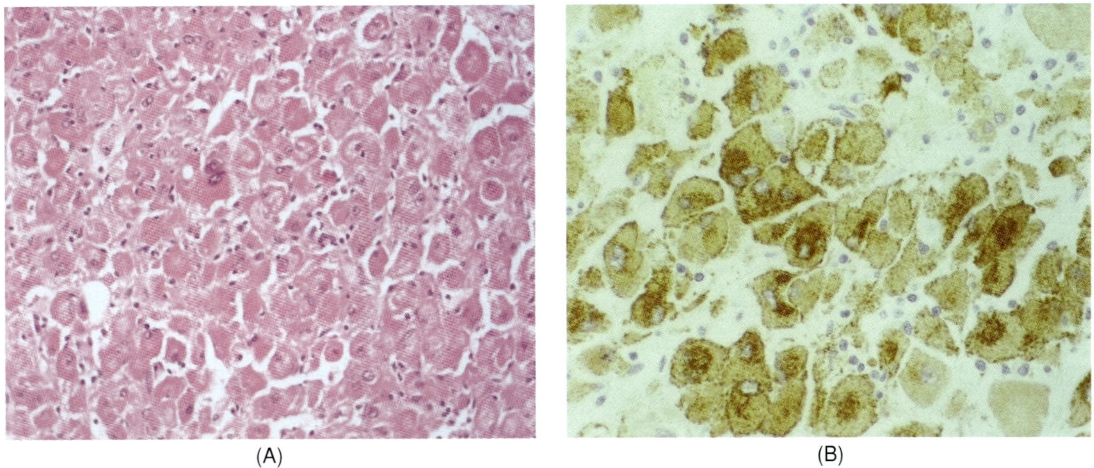

(A) (B)

Plate 8.5 Liver angiomyolipoma. (A) Predominantly myomatous tumour consists of large discohesive cells exhibiting with oncocytic cytoplasmic transformation. (B) Positive HMB-45 immunostaining confirms the diagnosis of AML.

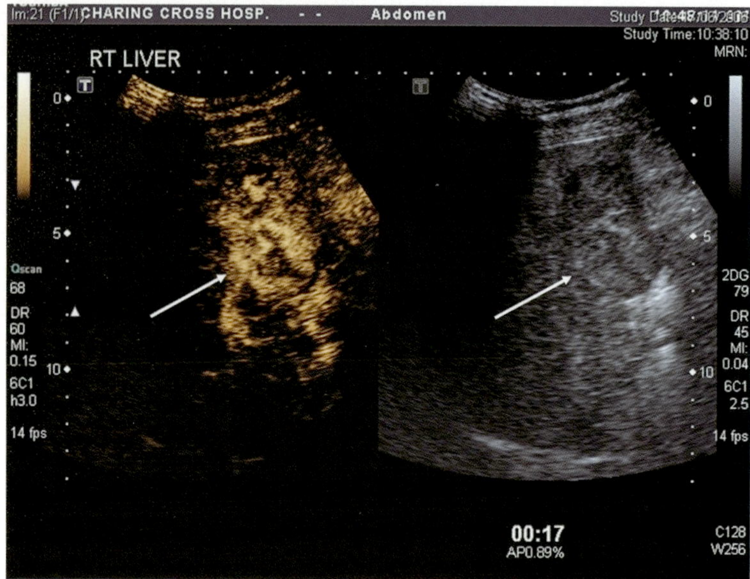

Plate 16.1 A CEUS image of a non-specific rounded hypoechoic lesion in a cirrhotic liver (left-hand image, arrow). The microbubble specific image in chrome is on the right and the arrow demonstrates that the lesion is hypervascular in the arterial phase (note timer at the bottom left-hand corner) with haphazard angiogenic vessels in a 'basket-weave' like pattern.

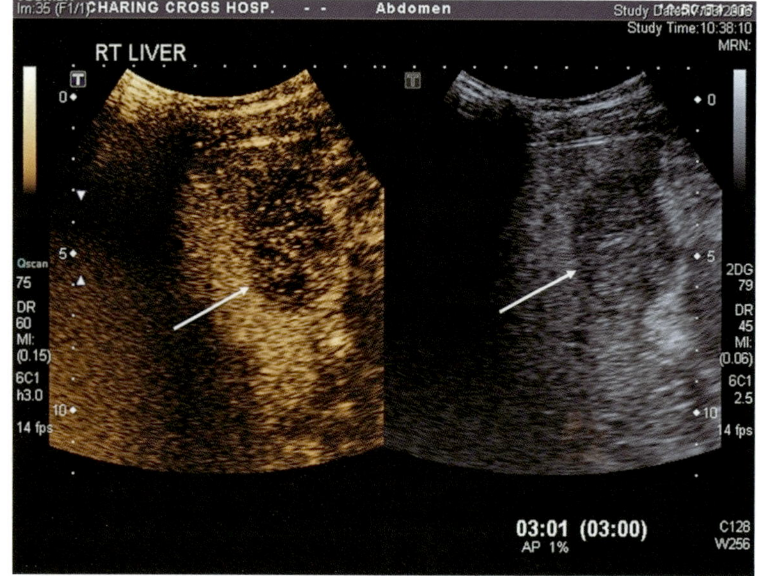

Plate 16.2 The same lesion demonstrating washout in the late phase at 3 minutes post-injection. This feature has a high sensitivity for detecting malignancy with CEUS. The overall enhancement characteristics would be compatible with a HCC.

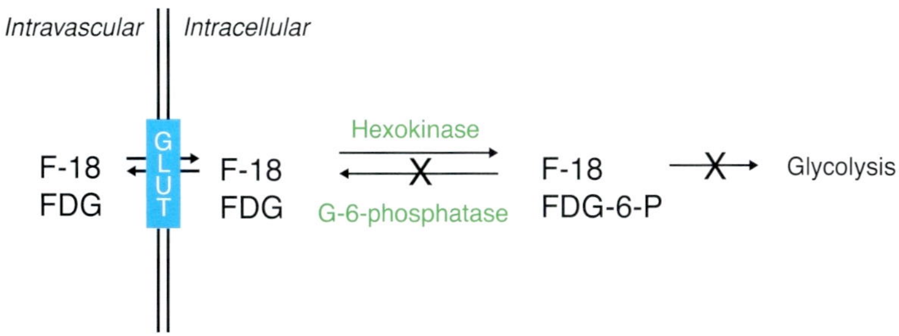

Plate 17.1 The metabolic pathway of F-18 FDG. F-18 FDG is actively transported into cells via GLUT membrane transporters and is phosphorylated by hexokinase to FDG glucose-6- phosphate (FDG-6-P). FDG-6-P is not a substrate for the next enzyme in the glycolysis pathway and also has a much slower rate of dephosphorylation, compared with glucose-6-phosphate and thus is progressively trapped within metabolically active cells.

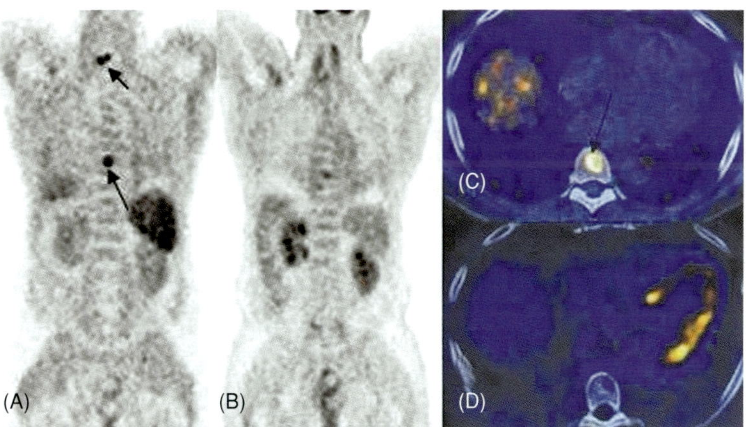

Plate 17.2 C-11 acetate and F-18 FDG PET/CT studies in a patient with metastatic HCC. (A) Coronal C11-acetate PET only image demonstrates bony metastases in the upper and lower thoracic spine (arrows) not clearly seen on the FDG-PET coronal image (B). (C) Fused C11-acetate image demonstrating the avid lytic metastasis (arrow) in the vertebral body, which is FDG negative on image (D). (Image courtesy of Professor S. Fanti.)

complexity of the HCC in its protean manifestations and diverse aetiology. If available, such variables could allow for an objective stratification of patients enrolled in interventional studies, quality of care evaluation and allocation of health care resources. The CLIP, GRETCH and CUPI scores were constituted, taking into account the variables selected by the multivariate analysis of survival factors in a cohorts of patients with HCC, causing these score systems to be applicable to the studied populations only, in the absence of any translational evidence and validation in independent cohorts. Further, investigating against the clinical predictivity of these staging systems is the fact that they do not incorporate all the component of tumour burden, hepatic function and performance status, while they miss any link to treatment options.

While the BCLC and CLIP systems are the most widely used among all the available prognostic scores having been extensively validated in different set of patients in various geographical areas, none of them, however, provided a confident prediction of survival in individual patients [24]. It should be outlined that are studies comparing various staging systems in different geographic area, invariably resulted in discordant results.

Studies in the West

When CLIP was evaluated in Italy against BCLC and GRETCH in a cohort of 406 cirrhotic patients with HCC (78% HCV, 44% treated) [24], CLIP showed the best discriminatory capacity in the entire cohort as well as in the advanced untreatable patients. Interestingly, BCLC predicted best the survival of treated patients. Overall, the predictive power of the three systems was not satisfactory, whereas none of the scoring systems provided confident prediction of survival in individual patients.

In a recent study comparing TNM sixth edition, Okuda, BCLC, CLIP, GRETCH, CUPI, JIS in 187 American patients (55% cirrhosis, 67% Child-Pugh A, 85% BCLC C) [25], CLIP, CUPI and GRETCH showed the greatest staging power, probably as a consequence of many patients having an advanced HCC.

The CLIP system was shown to be of limited value in determining prognosis of patients with HCC in other studies in the West [26,27], probably as a consequence of the lack of discriminatory power for patients with stages 1–3, the inclusion of AFP known to be an imperfect marker for HCC diagnosis, and the frequent interstrata overlap for treatment options.

When BCLC, Okuda classification, CLIP, GRETECH and CUPI were compared in patients treated with hepatic resection or percutaneous ablation [28], BCLC proved to be a superior prognosticator for the whole study group and for the two subgroups of surgical and non-surgical patients. However, it should be outlined that studies in surgical patients make the results not transferable to the general population of HCC patients.

When BCLC, Okuda, TNM, CLIP, CUPI, GRETECH and JIS were compared in a cohort of 239 consecutive patients with HCC recruited in a referral centre in the United States (62% HCV, 56% with more than 1 tumour nodule, 24% with portal vein thrombosis and 29% untreated), the 1- and 3-year survival rates were 58% and 29%, respectively [26]. The performance status ($p < 0.0001$), MELD greater than 10 ($p = 0.001$), portal vein thrombosis ($p = 0.0001$) and tumour diameter greater than 4 cm ($p = 0.001$) emerged as independent predictors of survival together with treatment of HCC. The BCLC staging system showed the best independent predictive power for survival when compared with the other six prognostic systems, showing that performance status, tumour extent, liver function and treatment were independent predictors of survival mostly in patients with cirrhosis and HCC, whereas it provided the best prognostic stratification for patients with HCC in Western countries.

When Okuda stage, TNM, BCLC, CLIP, GRETCH, CUPI and JIS were also compared in 112 Italian cirrhotic patients with HCC who underwent radiofrequency ablation with complete response in the 86% of them, it was shown that BCLC had a superior discriminatory ability, monotonicity of gradient ($p = 0.01$) and homogeneity ability than the other staging systems ($p = 0.008$) [29].

Studies in East Asia

Child-Pugh classification, Okuda stage, BCLC, CLIP, the MELD-based modified CLIP score, the JIS and the MELD-bases modified JIS were compared by Cho et al. in a cohort of 131 Korean patients who underwent chemoembolisation [30]. In this specific setting of patients, they found CLIP score to be superior to the other six prognostic systems in terms of discriminatory ability and monotonicity of the gradients.

More recently, a comparison study of TNM, BCLC, CLIP, GRETCH, CUPI, JIS and Tokyo score in 1713 patients in Taiwan [31] showed that CLIP staging system is the best long-term prognostic model for HCC in patients with early to advanced HCC (27% CLIP 0, 7% BCLC 0, 29% BCLC

A, 55% HBV infected), while it has a predictive accuracy independently on the treatment strategy.

When Chung et al. [32] compared BCLC, JIS and Tokyo in 290 patients with HCC, most on treated with radical therapies, JIS emerges as the staging system with the best prognostic power. Likewise, Toyoda [33] in study of 1508 Japanese patients recruited between 1976 and 2003 demonstrated CLIP to be more performant before 1991 compared with JIS, which was more efficient prognosticator after 1990. These data are contradicted by a retrospective study of 499 consecutive patients with HCC in Korea, which showed BCLC system to be the best predictor of survival in an HCC population treated with radical therapies compared with TNM, CLIP and UNOS system [34].

When 599 patients undergoing surgery in Taiwan were treated for CLIP, Okuda, TNM and JIS staging systems, Okuda and CLIP systems appeared not to be superior to TNM [35]. In a recent study [36], CLIP and JIS performed better than Okuda, TNM, BCLC, CUPI and MELD to predict survival. CLIP was a stronger predictor in patients treated with hepatectomy, whereas JIS was more performant in minor hepatectomy patients.

In a comparison study with BCLC and CLIP in 1679 patients in Japan (1976–2003) JIS was shown to be superior to the other two to predict of patient survival [37], but the lack of performance status, which is an essential prognostic factor of HCC, and of accurate estimates of tumour burden along with dramatic changes in treatment modalities occurred between 1976 and 2003, could have attenuated the sensitivity of this study. When the JIS was compared with CLIP in Japanese patients, the JIS system appeared to be superior in the prediction of outcome, though a significant overlap in the treatment offered to each JIS stratum was present [38]. Recently, the Tokyo prognostic score was developed for HCC patients, but without being validated in an external cohort of patients [32].

Do rival scores offer more than BCLC?

Advances in the treatment of HCC call for an accurate staging of patients with a HCC, which should incorporate guidance to treatment. Staging systems generated by studies of limited sample size that may reflect risk of patient misclassification because of referral bias, need to be validate by accurate investigation. This is particularly true for studies performed in the 1990s when the diagnostic window between radiological and pathological staging was greater than 15% [21].

Owing to the heterogeneous presentation of HCC reflecting differences in epidemiology and risk factors of the tumour in various geographical areas, studies of limited sample size together with the lack of serum biomarkers of predictive value fail to accurately predict survival at individual levels. Although the CUPI, CLIP and French systems been elaborated in patients with advanced HCC, they do not provide accuracy in the classification of patients with an early cancer. Such patients currently represent 30–50% of HCC patients seen in referral centres in the West. The fact that these systems consider an HCC burden in terms of 50% of liver involvement make it impossible to identify patients with an early tumour who are eligible for radical, potentially curative therapies. The new TNM classification by the AJCC, which has been internally validated only, is of limited application to patients indicated to hepatic resection, as is the case for JIS. In summary, staging systems that do not guide treatment choice are unlikely to positively impact on the practice in the field of liver oncology.

References

1. Okuda K, Ohtsuki T, Obata H, et al. Natural history of hepatocellular carcinoma and prognosis in relation to treatment. *Cancer* 1985; 56:918–928.
2. Giannini E, Risso D, Botta F, et al. Prognosis of hepatocellular carcinoma in anti-HCV positive cirrhotic patients: a single-centre comparison amongst four different staging systems. *J Intern Med* 2004; 255:399–408.
3. Chevret S, Trinchet JC, Mathieu D, et al. A new prognostic classification for predicting survival in patients with hepatocellular carcinoma. *J Hepatol* 1999; 31:133–141.
4. Cillo U, Bassanello M, Vitale A, et al. The critical issue of hepatocellular carcinoma prognostic classification: which is the best available? *J Hepatol* 2004; 40:124–131.
5. CLIP group (Cancer of the Liver Italian Programme). Tamoxifen in the treatment of hepatocellular carcinoma: a randomized controlled trial. *Lancet* 1998; 352:17–20.
6. The Cancer of the Liver Italian Program (CLIP) investigators. Prospective validation of the CLIP score: a new prognostic system for patients with cirrhosis and hepatocellular carcinoma. *Hepatology* 2000; 31:840–845.
7. Lin CY, Kee KM, Wang JH, et al. Is the Cancer of the Liver Italian Program system an adequate weighting for survival of hepatocellular carcinoma? Evaluation of intrascore prognostic value among 36 subgroups. *Liver Int* 2009; 29(1): 74–81.

8. Leung TW, Tang AM, Zee B, et al. Construction of the Chinese University Prognostic Index for hepatocellular carcinoma and comparison with the TNM staging system, the Okuda staging system, and the Cancer of the Liver Italian Program staging system: a study based on 926 patients. *Cancer* 2002; 94:1760–1769.
9. Sobin LH, Gospodarowicz MK, Wittekind C (eds). *TNM Classification of Malignant Tumors*, 7th ed. Blackwell Publishing Ltd, Oxford; 2009, pp. 110–113.
10. Edge SB, Byrd DR, Compton CC, Fritz AG, Greene FL, Trotti A (eds). *AJCC Cancer Staging Manual*, 7th ed. Springer, New York; 2010, pp. 191–195.
11. Vauthey J, Lauwers G, Esnaola N, et al. Simplified staging for hepatocellular carcinoma. *J Clin Oncol* 2002; 20:1527–1536.
12. Kudo M, Chung H, Osaki Y. Prognostic staging system for hepatocellular carcinoma (CLIP score): its value and limitations, and a proposal for a new staging system, the Japan Integrated Staging Score (JIS score). *J Gastroenterol* 2003; 38:207–215.
13. Tateishi R, Yoshida H, Shiina S, et al. Proposal of a new prognostic model for hepatocellular carcinoma: an analysis of 403 patients. *Gut* 2005; 54:419–425.
14. Kamath PS, Wiesner RH, Malinchoc M, et al. A model to predict survival in patients with end-stage liver disease. *Hepatology* 2001; 33:464–470.
15. Villa E, Colantoni A, Camma C, et al. Estrogen receptor classification for hepatocellular carcinoma: comparison with clinical staging systems. *J Clin Oncol* 2003; 21:441–446.
16. Omagari K, Honda S, Kadokawa Y, et al. Preliminary analysis of a newly proposed prognostic scoring system (SLiDe score) for hepatocellular carcinoma. *J Gastroenterol Hepatol* 2004; 19:805–811.
17. Toyoda H, Kumada T, Osaki Y, et al. Staging hepatocellular carcinoma by a novel scoring system (BALAD score) based on serum markers. *Clin Gastroenterol Hepatol* 2006; 4:1528–1536.
18. Hsu CY, Huang YH, Hsia CY, et al. A new prognostic model for hepatocellular carcinoma based on total tumor volume: the Taipei Integrated Scoring System. *J Hepatol* 2010; 53:108–117.
19. Tournoux-Facon C, Paoletti X, Barbare JC, et al. Development and validation of a new prognostic score of death for patients with hepatocellular carcinoma in palliative setting. *J Hepatol* 2011; 54:108–114.
20. Izumi R, Shimizu K, Ii T, et al. Prognostic factors of hepatocellular carcinoma in patients undergoing hepatic resection. *Gastroenterology* 1994; 106:720–727.
21. Mazzaferro V, Regalia E, Doci R, et al. Liver transplantation for the treatment of small hepatocellular carcinomas in patients with cirrhosis. *N Engl J Med* 1996; 334:693–699.
22. Yao FY, Ferrell L, Bass NM, et al. Liver transplantation for hepatocellular carcinoma: expansion of the tumor size limits does not adversely impact survival. *Hepatology* 2001; 33:1394–1403.
23. Mazzaferro V, Llovet JM, Miceli R, et al. Predicting survival after liver transplantation in patients with hepatocellular carcinoma beyond the Milan criteria: a retrospective, exploratory analysis. *Lancet Oncol* 2009; 10:35–43.
24. Cammà C, Di Marco V, Cabibbo G, et al. Survival of patients with hepatocellular carcinoma in cirrhosis: a comparison of BCLC, CLIP and GRETCH staging systems. *Aliment Pharmacol Ther* 2008; 28:62–75.
25. Huitzil-Melendez FD, Capanu M, O'Reilly EM, et al. Advanced hepatocellular carcinoma: which staging systems best predict prognosis? *J Clin Oncol* 2010; 28(17):2889–2895.
26. Marrero JA, Fontana RJ, Barrat A, et al. Prognosis of hepatocellular carcinoma: comparison of 7 staging systems in an American cohort. *Hepatology* 2005; 41:707–716.
27. Cillo U, Vitale A, Grigoletto F, et al. Prospective validation of the Barcelona Clinic Liver Cancer staging system. *J Hepatol* 2006; 44(4):723–731.
28. Cillo U, Bassanello M, Vitale A, et al. The critical issue of hepatocellular carcinoma prognostic classification: which is the best tool available? *J Hepatol* 2004; 40:124–131.
29. Guglielmi A, Ruzzenente A, Pachera S, et al. Comparison of seven staging systems in cirrhotic patients with hepatocellular carcinoma in a cohort of patients who underwent radiofrequency ablation with complete response. *Am J Gastroenterol* 2008; 103:597–604).
30. Cho YK, Chung JW, Kim JK, et al. Comparison of 7 staging systems for patients with hepatocellular carcinoma undergoing transarterial chemoembolization. *Cancer* 2008; 112:352–361.
31. Hsu CY, Hsia CY, Huang YH, et al. Selecting an optimal staging system for hepatocellular carcinoma: comparison of 5 currently used prognostic models. *Cancer* 2010; 116(12):3006–3014.
32. Chung H, Kudo M, Takahashi S, et al. Comparison of three current staging systems for hepatocellular carcinoma: Japan integrated staging score, new Barcelona Clinic Liver Cancer staging classification, and Tokyo score. *J Gastroenterol Hepatol* 2008; 23:445–452.
33. Toyoda H, Kumada T, Kiriyama S, et al. Comparison of the usefulness of three staging systems for hepatocellular carcinoma (CLIP, BCLC, and JIS) in Japan. *Am J Gastroenterol* 2005; 100:1764–1771.
34. Seo YS, Kim YJ, Um SH, et al. Evaluation of the prognostic powers of various tumor status grading scales in patients with hepatocellular carcinoma. *J Gastroenterol Hepatol* 2008; 23:1267–1275.

35. Huang YH, Chen CH, Chang TT, et al. Evaluation of predictive value of CLIP, Okuda, TNM and JIS staging systems for hepatocellular carcinoma patients undergoing surgery. *J Gastroenterol Hepatol* 2005; 20:765–771.
36. Chen TW, Chu CM, Yu JC, et al. Comparison of clinical staging systems in predicting survival of hepatocellular carcinoma patients receiving major or minor hepatectomy. *Eur J Surg Oncol* 2007; 33:480–487.
37. Toyoda H, Kumada T, Kiriyama S, et al. Comparison of the usefulness of three staging systems for hepatocellular carcinoma (CLIP, BCLC and JIS) in Japan. *Am J Gastroenterol* 2005; 100:1764–1771.
38. Kudo M, Chung H, Haji S, et al. Validation of a new prognostic staging system for hepatocellular carcinoma: the JIS score compared with the CLIP score. *Hepatology* 2004; 40(6):1396–1405.

13 Is it possible to detect early lesions effectively?

Ryota Masuzaki[1], Masao Omata[2]

[1]Department of Gastroenterology, Graduate School of Medicine, University of Tokyo, Tokyo, Japan
[2]Department of Gastroenterology, Yamanashi-Ken Hospital Organization, Yamanashi Japan /University of Tokyo, Japan

LEARNING POINTS

- The decision to enter a patient into a surveillance programme is determined by the risk of hepatocellular carcinoma (HCC) development
- Evaluation of the degree of liver fibrosis is of paramount importance in assessing the risk of HCC development in patients with chronic liver diseases of any aetiology
- To conduct surveillance of HCC in patients with chronic liver diseases, ultrasonography and tumour marker tests play important roles and are being widely used
- The early detection and diagnosis of HCC allow patients to be treated curatively. Nonetheless, whether routine screening and surveillance for HCC actually improve outcome would be best determined by prospective randomised controlled trials

Introduction

HCC is one of the most common cancers worldwide [1–5]. The majority of patients with HCC have a background of chronic liver disease, especially chronic hepatitis due to hepatitis C virus (HCV) or hepatitis B virus (HBV) infection [6,7]. Thus, at least some high-risk patients for HCC can be readily demarcated. Indeed, HCC surveillance is commonly performed as part of the standard clinical examination of patients with chronic viral hepatitis [8].

The primary objective of detecting small liver cancers at an early stage should be to reduce mortality as much as possible in the susceptible patient population, but in an acceptably cost-effective fashion. To this end, two distinct issues deserve detailed consideration: the target population and the mode of surveillance.

Target population

Surveillance is not recommended for the general population, given the low incidence of HCC among individuals with no risk factors. Thus, the first step in HCC screening should be the identification of patients at risk of HCC development. Since chronic viral hepatitis due either to HBV or HCV may be asymptomatic, mass screening for hepatitis virus infection of either the HBV or HCV type is justified if the prevalence of infection in the region is reasonably high.

Cirrhosis because of aetiologies other than chronic viral hepatitis also presents a risk for HCC development. Major aetiologies include alcoholic liver disease and non-alcoholic steatohepatitis (NASH) [9–11], the relative importance of which may differ geographically. Hassan et al. reported that alcoholic liver disease accounted for 32% of all cases of HCC in an Austrian cohort [12]. In the United States, the approximate hospitalisation rate for HCC related to alcoholic cirrhosis is 8–9 per 100,000 per year compared with about 7 per 100,000 per year for hepatitis C [13]. NASH is a chronic liver disease that is gaining increasing importance because of its high prevalence worldwide and its potential progression to cirrhosis, HCC and liver failure. Although NASH has been described in cohorts of patients with HCC [14,15], the incidence of HCC with respect to cirrhosis due to NASH is not well known.

In brief, evaluation of the degree of liver fibrosis is of paramount importance in assessing the risk of HCC development in patients with chronic liver diseases of any aetiology. Histological evaluation of liver biopsy samples has been considered the gold standard for the assessment of liver fibrosis, but the invasiveness accompanying liver

Clinical Dilemmas in Primary Liver Cancer, First Edition. Edited by Roger Williams and Simon D. Taylor-Robinson.

biopsy poses considerable limits to its clinical feasibility. In clinical practice, repeated assessment of liver fibrosis often will be required because non-fibrotic liver may become cirrhotic over time, sometimes rather rapidly. Consequently, the non-invasive evaluation of liver fibrosis is currently one of the main interests in hepatology.

Results obtained from the recently developed technique of ultrasound-based transient elastography correlate well with liver fibrosis stage, as determined histologically [16–18]. Transient elastography has a wide dynamic range within the cirrhotic stage, from the cut-off level from non-cirrhosis (12.5–14.9 kPa) to the upper measurement limit of the present device (75 kPa) [16,18]. We have shown the association between stiffness and the risk of HCC development in chronic hepatitis C patients [19]. The utility of transient elastography is not limited to a surrogate for liver biopsy, but can be applied as an indicator of the wide range of the risk of HCC development.

Patients who are considered to be at a non-negligible risk of developing HCC should participate in a surveillance programme, as discussed below. Possible exceptions may be patients with severe liver dysfunction who could not receive any treatment even if diagnosed with HCC, or those with other life-threatening diseases.

Surveillance methodology

Traditionally, two methodologies have been employed in HCC surveillance for high-risk patients: tumour marker determination, specifically serum alpha-fetoprotein (AFP) concentration and diagnostic imaging via liver ultrasonography. The utility of a surveillance programme should be evaluated, based on its beneficial effects in terms of outcome of patients diagnosed with HCC, relative to the cost. However, few prospective randomised trials have compared the outcome of patients with HCC, enrolled or not in a surveillance programme. Consequently, evidence regarding the benefits of surveillance on decreasing overall or disease-specific mortality has come mostly from retrospective or case-control studies.

Alpha-fetoprotein

Studies assessing the usefulness of AFP in HCC screening have varied widely in their design and in the characteristics of the targeted patients in terms of, for example, disease aetiology and severity of background liver diseases. Moreover, the reported specificity and sensitivity values inevitably vary depending on the cut-off level chosen for the diagnosis of HCC.

An intrinsic disadvantage of AFP as a tumour marker is the fact that serum AFP levels can increase in patients who have active hepatitis, but not HCC. This is partly due to the accelerated cellular proliferation during liver regeneration. An AFP concentration of 20 ng/mL is often adopted as the upper limit of normal, because this level is rarely exceeded in healthy people. However, slightly higher concentrations are hardly diagnostic of HCC among patients with chronic hepatitis, and the adoption of a cut-off value that is too low would result in an inappropriately low specificity. Moreover, an additional disadvantage exists in using AFP for HCC surveillance. Small HCC tumours, the detection of which is the primary objective of surveillance, are less likely to be AFP producing, but even if the marker is expressed by these tumours, the levels may not be high enough to result in a diagnosis of HCC.

For this and other reasons, AFP determination has been frequently dismissed as a screening test for HCC, except when ultrasonography is either not available or is such poor quality that lesions smaller than 2 cm in diameter cannot be detected. Moreover, as shown in HCC screening of Alaskan carriers of hepatitis B, AFP testing allowed the detection of tumours at an earlier, treatable stage [20], but although screened patients survived longer than their historic controls, the difference could be equally well explained by lead-time and length-time biases, which are inherent in retrospective studies on screening.

Ultrasonography

The resolution of ultrasonography in detecting small intrahepatic nodules has been greatly improved with technological developments. Ultrasound examination detects HCC nodules based on different echogenicity from the surrounding liver. Small tumour nodules are typically hypoechoic and become hyperechoic as they enlarge. The presence of a capsule may also be noted. Although confirmatory diagnosis of HCC usually depends on contrast-enhanced computed tomography (CT) or magnetic resonance imaging (MRI), colour Doppler ultrasonography and ultrasonography using contrast agents may provide additional qualitative information. Several new contrast agents are being evaluated as an aid to diagnose HCC or evaluate the effectiveness of ablation or assistance for ultrasonography-guided ablation therapy [21,22]. In particular, Sonazoid™ (Daiichi Sankyo, Tokyo, Japan), a new contrast agent commercially available in Japan since 2007, is very useful in detecting malignant liver tumours, including metastatic tumours, owing to the long duration of Kupffer imaging.

In a study on nodules that were 2 cm or smaller in diameter in patients with chronic hepatitis, the ability of ultrasonography to detect nodular lesions, adenomatous hyperplasia, and well-differentiated HCC was better than that of CT or MRI [23]. Thus, the non-invasiveness and relatively low cost of ultrasonography make it indispensable in HCC screening. Nonetheless, a definite diagnosis of HCC depends on the evaluation of tumour vascularity, which is not possible with conventional ultrasonography. Therefore, CT or MRI studies with contrast enhancement usually follow ultrasonography when the latter raises suspicion of HCC.

Ultrasonography, when conducted by less-experienced operators, has blind spots. Moreover, the resolution may not be satisfactory in patients with cirrhosis who show rough echo patterns in the background liver. While it may be expected that the detection capability of HCC would improve with the use of CT or MRI in combination with ultrasonography, few studies have reported on HCC surveillance in which either one of these modalities was employed.

Combined alpha-fetoprotein measurement and ultrasonography

In HCC screening, serum AFP measurement is less sensitive than ultrasonography, but its specificity may be comparable if the appropriate cut-off values are used. Screening by a combination of ultrasonography and AFP may improve HCC detection, but the results described in previous reports were generally negative [24–27]. However, in a non-randomised study of patients with cirrhosis, the sensitivity of detection increased when both ultrasonography and AFP measurements were conducted as compared with either screening approach alone [25].

Recently, a randomised trial was carried out in which 18,000 Chinese patients with HBV infection were either screened every 6 months for HCC or not by AFP measurements and ultrasonography. The results indicated that more cases of HCC were diagnosed in the screened group than in the non-screened group (86 vs. 67) and overall survival was better: 65.9%, 52.6% and 46.4% at 1, 3 and 5 years, respectively, compared with 31.2%, 7.2% and 0%.

A retrospective study assessed HCC screening in 367 patients aged 70 years or older, with AFP measurements and ultrasonography carried out every 6 or 12 months. Screening allowed more frequent diagnosis of HCC at an early stage, increased the proportion of patients able to be treated curatively and improved the prognosis of these patients compared with those who had not been screened. The apparent survival benefit was restricted to the first 3 years after HCC detection, probably because of the shorter life expectancy of this elderly population [28].

New serum markers and new methods

Recent developments in gene-expression micro-arrays, proteomics and tumour immunology now permit thousands of genes and proteins to be screened simultaneously. Furthermore, new biomarkers are expected to be established in the next decade for the screening of many cancers, including HCC.

The detection sensitivities of dynamic CT and dynamic MRI are high for hypervascular HCC. Considering that patients with HCC undergo repeated imaging examinations and that the diagnostic capabilities of the two imaging modalities are almost the same, dynamic MRI, which does not involve X-ray exposure, may be more advantageous. The development of multidetector computed tomography (MDCT) has dramatically accelerated scan acquisition in liver CT [29]. With MDCT, high-speed volume coverage of the entire liver is possible in 4–10 seconds, which allows the acquisition of two separate series of scans in the arterial phase, termed early arterial and late arterial phase scans [30,31]. MRI may be the diagnostic procedure of choice for HCC depending on its availability. Recent advances in MRI technology include scanner hardware, software and new contrast agents. A hepatocyte-specific contrast agent, gadolinium ethoxybenzyl diethylenetriamine pentaacetic acid (Gd-EOB-DTPA), was approved in Japan in 2008. This contrast agent enhances the blood pool and also is hepatocyte specific: it is taken up by hepatocytes and excreted into the biliary tract. The liver parenchyma is strongly stained white in the hepatocyte phase on T_1-weighted images, 20 minutes after the intravenous injection. Nodules that are lacking normal hepatocytes, such as HCC, are depicted as low-intensity masses. Gd-EOB-DTPA-enhanced MRI may offer a breakthrough for the diagnosis of liver tumours, particularly early HCC [32].

Screening intervals

Since the risk of HCC development does not usually diminish spontaneously in patients who are the typical targets of

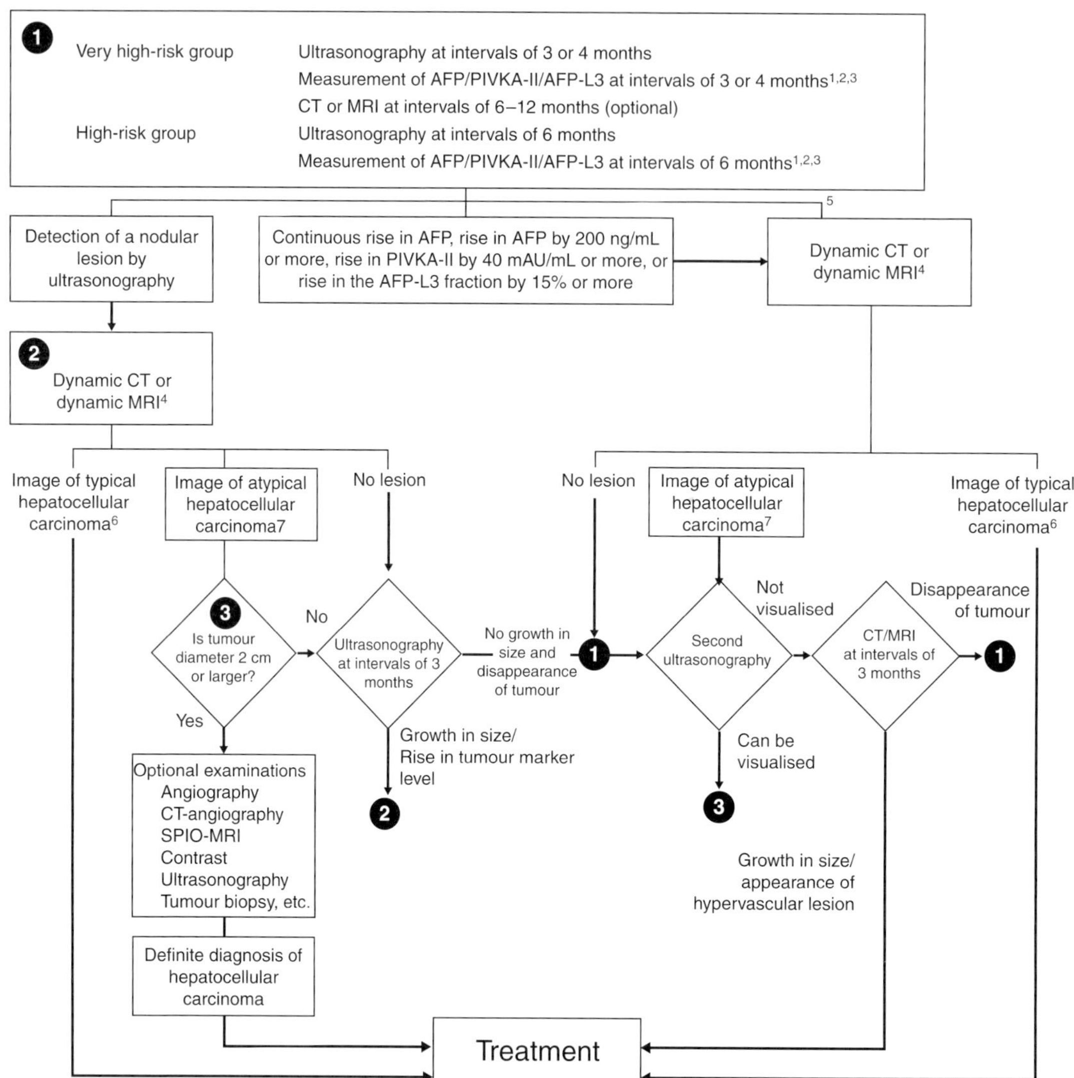

FIG 13.1 Surveillance algorithm for hepatocellular carcinoma in Japan. 1: The current health insurance policy in Japan covers the measurement of AFP or DCP level once per month. 2: AFP L3 can be measured only when patients are suspected of having hepatocellular carcinoma. 3: When AFP is 10 ng/mL or less, the AFP L3 fraction cannot be measured. 4: If patients have renal dysfunction or are suspected of being allergic to iodinated contrast media, dynamic MRI is recommended. 5: CT/MRI at regular intervals. 6: Tumour that is visualised as a high intensity area in the arterial phase and relatively low intensity area in the venous phase. 7: If patients are suspected of having other malignant tumour such as cholangiocellular carcinoma or metastatic liver cancer, they proceed to thorough examination for the underlying disease. AFP, alpha-fetoprotein; DCP, des-gamma carboxyprothrombin; CT, computed tomography; MRI, magnetic resonance imaging.

HCC screening, a surveillance programme for HCC should consist of repeating screenings at determined intervals. Ultrasonography is superior to CT in this setting due to its non-invasiveness and cost-effectiveness. The guidelines of the American Association for the Study of Liver Diseases (AASLD) propose ultrasound surveillance for patients at high risk for HCC at 6-month intervals. The guidelines explicitly indicate that the surveillance interval should depend not on the degree of risk for HCC but exclusively on tumour doubling times to detect cancer nodules while they are small enough to be cured.

In Japan, ultrasound surveillance at a shorter interval of 3–4 months is encouraged for extremely high-risk patients, while a 6-month interval is recommended for those at high risk (Figure 13.1) [33]. In Japanese patients with chronic hepatitis C marked by cirrhosis, the incidence of HCC is 6–8% per year; this group is, therefore, at an extremely high risk of tumour development. While theoretically, shorter surveillance intervals lead to the detection of smaller tumours, whether the potential difference in detected tumour size is large enough to affect prognosis in a cost-effective fashion is not known. Although no prospective comparison of different screening schedules has been performed, both a retrospective study on patients with cirrhosis and a mathematic model applied to HBV carriers suggested that a longer screening interval is just as effective as the 6-month interval in terms of survival.

Opinions also diverge as to whether AFP determination should be included in HCC surveillance programmes. However, if AFP is to be measured, then measurements should be made repeatedly and an abnormal level of AFP must be interpreted not by simple comparison with a given cut-off value, but in the context of a time series of values. An abrupt elevation of serum AFP levels in the absence of exacerbation of hepatitis is suggestive of the development of HCC, even if ultrasonography is apparently negative. In such cases, further evaluation with CT or MRI using contrast enhancement should be considered.

Conclusion

High-risk populations for HCC have been clearly identified in many epidemiological studies and statistical analyses. HCC is a suitable disease for surveillance programmes since it is relatively common, at least in patients with liver disease. The early detection and diagnosis of HCC allow patients to be treated curatively. Nonetheless, whether routine screening and surveillance for HCC actually improve outcome would be best determined by prospective, randomised controlled trials.

References

1. Parkin DM, Bray F, Ferlay J, et al. Estimating the world cancer burden: Globocan 2000. *Int J Cancer* 2001; 94(2):153–156.
2. Bosch FX, Ribes J, Diaz M, et al. Primary liver cancer: worldwide incidence and trends. *Gastroenterology* 2004; 127(5 suppl 1):S5–S16.
3. Capocaccia R, Sant M, Berrino F, et al. Hepatocellular carcinoma: trends of incidence and survival in Europe and the United States at the end of the 20th century. *Am J Gastroenterol* 2007; 102(8):1661–1670; quiz 0, 71.
4. Kiyosawa K, Umemura T, Ichijo T, et al. Hepatocellular carcinoma: recent trends in Japan. *Gastroenterology* 2004; 127(5 suppl 1):S17–S26.
5. El-Serag HB, Davila JA, Petersen NJ, et al. The continuing increase in the incidence of hepatocellular carcinoma in the United States: an update. *Ann Intern Med* 2003; 139(10):817–823.
6. Yoshida H, Shiratori Y, Moriyama M, et al. Interferon therapy reduces the risk for hepatocellular carcinoma: national surveillance program of cirrhotic and noncirrhotic patients with chronic hepatitis C in Japan. IHIT Study Group. Inhibition of hepatocarcinogenesis by interferon therapy. *Ann Intern Med* 1999; 131(3):174–181.
7. Shiratori Y. Different clinicopathological features of hepatitis B- and C-related hepatocellular carcinoma. *J Gastroenterol Hepatol* 1996; 11(10):942–943.
8. Bruix J, Sherman M. Management of hepatocellular carcinoma. *Hepatology* 2005; 42(5):1208–1236.
9. Tanaka K, Hirohata T, Takeshita S, et al. Hepatitis B virus, cigarette smoking and alcohol consumption in the development of hepatocellular carcinoma: a case-control study in Fukuoka, Japan. *Int J Cancer* 1992; 51(4):509–514.
10. Donato F, Tagger A, Gelatti U, et al. Alcohol and hepatocellular carcinoma: the effect of lifetime intake and hepatitis virus infections in men and women. *Am J Epidemiol* 2002; 155(4):323–331.
11. Kuper H, Tzonou A, Kaklamani E, et al. Tobacco smoking, alcohol consumption and their interaction in the causation of hepatocellular carcinoma. *Int J Cancer* 2000; 85(4):498–502.
12. Schoniger-Hekele M, Muller C, Kutilek M, et al. Hepatocellular carcinoma in Austria: aetiological and clinical characteristics at presentation. *Eur J Gastroenterol Hepatol* 2000; 12(8):941–948.
13. El-Serag HB, Mason AC. Risk factors for the rising rates of primary liver cancer in the United States. *Arch Intern Med* 2000; 160(21):3227–3230.
14. Bugianesi E, Leone N, Vanni E, et al., Expanding the natural history of nonalcoholic steatohepatitis: from cryptogenic cirrhosis to hepatocellular carcinoma. *Gastroenterology*, 2002. 123(1):134-40.
15. Shimada M, Hashimoto E, Taniai M, et al. Hepatocellular carcinoma in patients with non-alcoholic steatohepatitis. *J Hepatol* 2002; 37(1):154–160.

16. Castera L, Vergniol J, Foucher J, et al. Prospective comparison of transient elastography, Fibrotest, APRI, and liver biopsy for the assessment of fibrosis in chronic hepatitis C. *Gastroenterology* 2005; 128(2):343–350.
17. Sandrin L, Fourquet B, Hasquenoph JM, et al., Transient elastography: a new noninvasive method for assessment of hepatic fibrosis. *Ultrasound Med Biol* 2003; 29(12):1705–1713.
18. Foucher J, Chanteloup E, Vergniol J, et al. Diagnosis of cirrhosis by transient elastography (FibroScan): a prospective study. *Gut* 2006; 55(3):403–408.
19. Masuzaki R, Tateishi R, Yoshida H, et al. Prospective risk assessment for hepatocellular carcinoma development in patients with chronic hepatitis C by transient elastography. *Hepatology* 2009; 49(6):1954–1961.
20. McMahon BJ, Bulkow L, Harpster A, et al. Screening for hepatocellular carcinoma in Alaska natives infected with chronic hepatitis B: a 16-year population-based study. *Hepatology* 2000; 32(4 Pt 1):842–846.
21. Minami Y, Kudo M, Chung H, et al. Contrast harmonic sonography-guided radiofrequency ablation therapy versus B-mode sonography in hepatocellular carcinoma: prospective randomized controlled trial. *AJR Am J Roentgenol* 2007; 188(2):489–494.
22. Morimoto M, Shirato K, Sugimori K, et al. Contrast-enhanced harmonic gray-scale sonographic-histologic correlation of the therapeutic effects of transcatheter arterial chemoembolization in patients with hepatocellular carcinoma. *AJR Am J Roentgenol* 2003; 181(1):65–69.
23. Horigome H, Nomura T, Saso K, et al. Limitations of imaging diagnosis for small hepatocellular carcinoma: comparison with histological findings. *J Gastroenterol Hepatol* 1999; 14(6):559–565.
24. Sherman M, Peltekian KM, Lee C. Screening for hepatocellular carcinoma in chronic carriers of hepatitis B virus: incidence and prevalence of hepatocellular carcinoma in a North American urban population. *Hepatology* 1995; 22(2):432–438.
25. Pateron D, Ganne N, Trinchet JC, et al. Prospective study of screening for hepatocellular carcinoma in Caucasian patients with cirrhosis. *J Hepatol* 1994; 20(1):65–71.
26. Bolondi L, Sofia S, Siringo S, et al. Surveillance programme of cirrhotic patients for early diagnosis and treatment of hepatocellular carcinoma: a cost effectiveness analysis. *Gut* 2001; 48(2):251–259.
27. Cottone M, Turri M, Caltagirone M, et al. Screening for hepatocellular carcinoma in patients with Child's A cirrhosis: an 8-year prospective study by ultrasound and alphafetoprotein. *J Hepatol* 1994; 21(6):1029–1034.
28. Trevisani F, Cantarini MC, Labate AM, et al. Surveillance for hepatocellular carcinoma in elderly Italian patients with cirrhosis: effects on cancer staging and patient survival. *Am J Gastroenterol* 2004; 99(8):1470–1476.
29. Foley WD, Mallisee TA, Hohenwalter MD, et al. Multiphase hepatic CT with a multirow detector CT scanner. *AJR Am J Roentgenol* 2000; 175(3):679–685.
30. Murakami T, Kim T, Takamura M, et al. Hypervascular hepatocellular carcinoma: detection with double arterial phase multi-detector row helical CT. *Radiology* 2001; 218(3):763–767.
31. Ichikawa T, Kitamura T, Nakajima H et al. Hypervascular hepatocellular carcinoma: can double arterial phase imaging with multidetector CT improve tumor depiction in the cirrhotic liver? *AJR Am J Roentgenol* 2002; 179(3): 751–758.
32. Narita M, Hatano E, Arizono S, et al. Expression of OATP1B3 determines uptake of Gd-EOB-DTPA in hepatocellular carcinoma. *J Gastroenterol* 2009; 44(7):793–798.
33. Makuuchi M, Kokudo N, Arii S, et al. Development of evidence-based clinical guidelines for the diagnosis and treatment of hepatocellular carcinoma in Japan. *Hepatol Res* 2008; 38(1):37–51.

14 What is the value of country-based surveillance programmes?

Peter Ott

Medical Department V (Hepatology and Gastroenterology), Aarhus University Hospital, Aarhus, Denmark

LEARNING POINTS

- Several international societies recommend surveillance for hepatocellular carcinoma (HCC) by ultrasound every 6 months in selected patients with chronic liver disease
- Only few randomised controlled trials (RCTs) address this question and the decision to introduce these costly programmes primarily rest on indirect evidence
- Introduction of country-based surveillance programmes should rest on population-based cohorts, but most often clinic-based cohorts are used. The latter tend to overestimate the risk of HCC and the effect of screening in the populations studied
- The value of ultrasound as a screening test may be lower than generally expected in patients with cirrhosis
- Critical evaluation suggests that the evidence may be insufficient to start country-based surveillance

Introduction

During the last decade, a number of international societies including the American, Japanese, Asia-Pacific, European, British and Spanish professional bodies have recommended introduction of surveillance programmes for selected patients with chronic liver disease to detect HCC. The background is the increased risk of HCC in chronic liver diseases and the availability of potentially effective treatment modalities, such as resection, liver transplantation (LTX) and local ablation. These treatments are most effective when HCC is detected at an early stage and before the tumour becomes symptomatic, which strongly suggest that surveillance could be useful.

Surveillance is applied to a specific group of patients at risk of HCC. It includes the use of a screening tests at regular intervals and structured confirmatory testing when screening raises suspicion of HCC development. As the most well-documented example, it is appropriate to refer to the American Association for the Study of Liver Diseases (AASLD) guidelines [1] that recommend screening by ultrasound every 6 months in the patients listed in Table 14.1.

Implementation of country-based surveillance programmes requires careful evaluation according to the criteria listed in Table 14.2[2]. These aim at securing efficacy and reasonable estimates of the cost–benefit relation before the decision is taken. The efficacy may be expressed by the life years saved (LYS) in the patients under surveillance, as compared with the life expectancy without surveillance. Efficacy is a critical issue; without efficacy, a surveillance programme should be avoided. However, even if a programme has efficacy it may be so expensive that implementation is unreasonable.

National surveillance programmes are costly and should be based on solid evidence. Ideally, they should be supported by large RCTs in which patients were randomised to surveillance or not, showing improved survival in the surveillance group, or at least improved cancer-related mortality. RCTs are especially important in cancer screening, where indirect evidence tends to overestimate the screening effect [2]. In the present case, three RCTs included hepatitis B (HBV) patients with East Asian [3,4] or mainly East Asian background [5]. None were powered to examine the effect of surveillance on overall survival, while the

Clinical Dilemmas in Primary Liver Cancer, First Edition. Edited by Roger Williams and Simon D. Taylor-Robinson.

TABLE 14.1 Patients to be included in surveillance for HCC as recommended by the AASLD HCC guideline [1] and the expected annual incidence of HCC according to these guidelines

Patient group recommended for screening	Expected annual incidence of HCC according to AASLD guidelines
Hepatitis B	
East Asian males > 40 Y	0.4–0.6%
East Asian females > 50 Y	0.3–0.6%
HBV carriers with family history of HCC	Higher than without history
Sub-Saharan African/North American blacks	HCC occur at a younger age
Cirrhotic HBV carriers	3–8%
Hepatitis C and cirrhosis	3–5%
Primary biliary cirrhosis in stage 4	3–5%
Genetic hemochromatosis and cirrhosis	Probably > 1.5%
Alpha-1 antitrypsin deficiency and cirrhosis	Probably > 1.5%
All other types of cirrhosis	Unknown

larger [3] had sufficient power to demonstrate *stage migration* (i.e. HCC detected by surveillance were smaller) and *reduced HCC-related mortality* in the surveillance group. Surprisingly, no RCT has been carried out in the high-risk populations with cirrhosis, where the recommendations rest on indirect evidence with more complex sources of bias. Epidemiologists distinguish between clinic-based and population-based studies. Clinic-based studies include selected patients, typically with more active disease than those in the population. Thus, the decision to implement surveillance on a national scale should rest on data from population, rather than clinic-based cohorts.

In this chapter, the evidence to justify country-based surveillance programmes will be critically reviewed. We will do that by going through the points listed in Table 14.2.

TABLE 14.2 Requirements for a surveillance programme

Effective treatments that require early detection
A well-defined population at risk
A suitable screening test
Screening should improve survival
Acceptable costs per life year gained

Do we have effective treatments?

Most efficient treatments: transplantation, resection and local ablation

LTX, resection and local ablation (such as percutaneous ethanol injection, radiofrequency ablation and others) are regarded as effective treatments when the tumours are small enough. Their assumed efficacy rests on reported 5-year survival rates of 50–75%, which are much higher than 0–10% observed in historical controls. The efficacy depends on careful selection. Extrahepatic HCC always contraindicates local treatment. LTX is generally only used within the Milan Criteria (one lesion smaller than 5 cm or 3 lesions smaller than 3 cm). Resection can be used in patients with relatively good liver function, no portal hypertension and provided that removal of the tumour is technically feasible – again favouring small and single tumours. Local ablation is best when tumours are below 3–5 cm.

Intermediate efficiency: TACE

Transarterial chemoembolisation (TACE) is indicated when neither LTX, resection nor local ablation is possible, provided no extrahepatic spread and less than 50% of the liver is occupied by tumour. The efficacy is supported by seven RCTs [6]. In the largest trial [7], TACE increased median survival from 14 to 28 months. These patients were highly selected and constituted only 10% of the HCC patients that were evaluated for inclusion [7]. In clinical series [8,9], 31–33% of patients with HCC detected in surveillance programmes were offered TACE and results may be inferior to those from the original study [7].

Less efficient therapies: sorafenib

The angiogenesis inhibitor, sorafenib, has shown a statistically significant effect in two RCTs including patients with more advanced cancer and good performance status. The median survival increased from 8 to 11 months in the European study [10] and from 6 to 8 months in the East Asian study [11].

Since only LTX, resection and local ablation potentially provide substantial survival benefits, the efficacy of a surveillance programme will primarily rest on its ability to identify HCC when tumours are less than 3 cm.

Is there a population at risk?

Table 14.1 displays the estimated risk of developing HCC in different patients groups as summarised by the AASLD guidelines [1]. Ideally, these estimates should originate from prospective population-based studies, including large cohorts of unselected patients at risk, but this is not always the case. That is an important dilemma because the use of other (clinic-based) cohorts will tend to overestimate the real risk in a population under surveillance and thus overestimate the efficacy of a nation-wide programme.

Viral hepatitis without cirrhosis

The AASLD guideline recommendation seek to characterise a population of HBV-positive patients (males > 40 years, females > 50) without cirrhosis and a risk of HCC of 0.4–0.6% a year, or at least >0.2% per year, which was considered the threshold for initiation of a screening programme. In two population-based studies of 20,000 [12] and 18,000 [3] HBV-positive patients without cirrhosis, HCC was detected at an annual rate of 0.5% [12] and 0.16% [3], the risk increasing with age and male sex. HBV-positive Caucasians seems less likely to develop HCC, while sub-Saharan Africans or black Americans may develop HCC at a young age, although the rate per year is unknown. Thus, population-based studies exist in HBV, but only in the East Asian population, and suggest an annual risk of HCC from 0.16% to 0.5% per year.

Hepatitis C in patients without cirrhosis carries an increased risk of HCC, but below 0.2% per year [13], and surveillance is not currently recommended in this population [1].

Cirrhosis

The guidelines recommend screening in all patients with cirrhosis of the liver [1]. The expectation is that all types of cirrhosis will carry a risk of >1.5% per year, even though aetiology is known to be of influence.

HBV cirrhosis carries an increased risk of HCC as illustrated by a review of 11 clinic-based studies [14]. The annual rate of HCC ranged from 2.2% in Europe (6 studies, $N = 401$) to 3.2% in China (3 studies, $N = 278$) and 4.3% in Japan (2 studies, $N = 306$), suggesting geographical or racial differences in susceptibility, as has also been seen in viral hepatitis without cirrhosis. Population-based studies are missing and could provide deviating estimates.

HCV cirrhosis is believed to carry the highest risk of HCC with estimates from 3.7% per year in Caucasians to 7.1% per year in Japan [14]. These estimates are based on clinical cohorts that are biased by the accumulation of patients with most active disease and censoring of the milder cases. The largest prospective study was the HALT-C Trail (clinic based, but large scale) [15], where 1050 HCV interferon/ribavirin non-responders with bridging fibrosis or cirrhosis were followed with AFP every 6 months and ultrasound at 6–12 months intervals. The annual rate of HCC was 0.8% among 597 patients with bridging fibrosis and 1.4% among 408 with established cirrhosis. In a prospective clinic-based European study [16] of 312 patients, HCC developed in 1.6% per year. According to the Danish National Registry, the annual rate of HCC was 1.1% in males and 0.6% in females with HCV cirrhosis (P. Jepsen, personal communication). This clearly suggests that clinic-based observations of annual rates of HCC in 3.7–7.1% per year may be much higher than what can be expected in a nationwide surveillance programme where values in the 1–2% range are more likely.

Alcoholic cirrhosis is common in many parts of the world. According to one review [14], the difference between liver clinic-based series (annual rate of HCC 1.7% in Europe, 1.8% in Japan) and population-based series (which may be as low as 0.2% per year) could be larger than with other aetiologies. In a recently described hospital-based cohort of Danish patients with alcoholic cirrhosis [17], the annual rate of HCC was 0.4% per year (P. Jepsen, personal communication).

Other types of cirrhosis were also assumed to carry risks of HCC of >1.5% per year [1], but data are rather limited. Studies in small, highly selected patients suggest a somewhat higher risk in cirrhosis because of genetic haemochromatosis than when primary biliary cirrhosis, autoimmune hepatitis, alpha-1-antitrypsin deficiency or Wilson's disease is the underlying aetiology.

These data illustrate one dilemma for a country-based screening programme. Implementation should rest on expectations for HCC occurrence that are based on population-based studies. Such studies are available for East Asian HBV patients without cirrhosis, but hardly for other populations. Data from HCV and alcoholic cirrhosis strongly suggest that population-based studies estimate lower HCC risks than clinic-based studies. As a result, nationwide surveillance may be less effective and more costly than expected from the clinic-based cohorts.

Is there a suitable screening test?

The perfect screening test with no false positive or negative findings does not exist. In that situation, a screening test that detects all possible HCCs (high sensitivity) will be preferred and a certain rate of false positive tests (suboptimal specificity) accepted. A positive screening test is then followed by confirmatory testing, utilising a method with high specificity.

Alpha-fetoprotein is no longer recommended for screening because of both false-negative and false-positive results [1]. This recommendation rests on studies that primarily included patients with viral hepatitis. It is still a matter of debate whether AFP behaves differently in alcoholic cirrhosis [18].

Abdominal ultrasound is the recommended screening method [1] due to its general availability, patient acceptability, absence of radiation or other side effects and because other imaging modalities such as CT or MR have not proven better for screening purposes. By contrast, multiphase CT, MR and contrast-enhanced ultrasound are superior to ultrasound for confirmatory testing.

The diagnostic performance of ultrasound is usually different in patients with homogenous parenchyma seen in viral hepatitis without cirrhosis, compared with the inhomogeneous parenchyma in cirrhosis. In HBV without cirrhosis, artefacts should be minimal and the most important differential diagnoses for HCC will be benign lesions, such as cysts and haemangiomas that can be differentiated by an experienced ultrasound operator. In the large East Asian RCT [3,19], ultrasound was estimated to have 84% sensitivity and 97% specificity, based on 20,294 ultrasound examinations in 9,373 HBV-positive subjects. In a smaller North American clinic-based study, ultrasound had 79% sensitivity and 94% specificity [5]. So, even in this non-cirrhotic population, ultrasound will overlook 15% of HCCs. A specificity of around 95% is high, but in a population with 0.5% HCC, there would still be 11 false positive diagnoses for each true case.

In cirrhosis, ultrasound is facing additional challenges due to the disrupted architecture of the cirrhotic liver and presence of regenerative nodules [8]. This affects the sensitivity. In one review [20], sensitivity ranged from 35% to 84%. The wide range illustrated the difficulty of finding a suitable 'gold standard'. Another review [21] summarised seven studies, where ultrasound were performed just before LTX and the 'gold standard' was the examination of the explanted liver. In these, the sensitivity ranged from 33% to 66% and specificity from 92% to 98%. The sensitivity depended on tumour size; i.e. in one study, the sensitivities of ultrasound for tumours of >5 cm, 3–5 cm, 2–3 cm, 1–2 cm and <1 cm were 75%, 50%, 20%, 14% and 0%, respectively [22]. As seen, the sensitivity was lowest for the small tumours, where treatment has the greatest impact on survival. This is a dilemma, because the low sensitivity for small tumours could reduce the cost-effectiveness of a surveillance programme.

The operator dependency of ultrasound is an important aspect if country-based surveillance is to be considered. Detecting small HCCs and excluding common benign lesions and regenerative nodules requires specific skills. The latter problem was pointed out by Sherman [5] who expected a larger problem with false positive ultrasound diagnoses if surveillance was taken up by the general health care system.

Will a surveillance programme improve survival?

Even without surveillance, HCC is diagnosed during conventional clinical procedures ('opportunistic screening') [2]. In an ideal world, the addition of a surveillance programme should detect tumours much earlier and with better results. Ideally, a randomised study should demonstrate longer total survival in a group under surveillance, compared with a group following the usual clinical controls. The required sample size for such a study renders it unlikely to be feasible in most settings, and it may acceptable to use HCC-related mortality as the primary endpoint [1].

Chronic HBV infection without cirrhosis has been best studied. Three published RCTs examined surveillance programmes in HBV patients [3–5]. One [4] that used only AFP did not offer efficient treatments to detected HCC and is inappropriate for consideration in this chapter. The two others [3,5] included 18,816 and 1,069 subjects, respectively. The smaller Canadian study [5] was underpowered to study the effects on either total or HCC-related mortality. In the large study from Shanghai [3], subjects with HBV-related hepatitis were randomised to 6 monthly AFP plus ultrasound or no surveillance. In the surveillance group, 86 HCC were detected against 67 in the control group. Five-year HCC-related mortality was lower in the surveillance group (32 deaths, 83 per 100,000 patient years vs. 54 deaths, 131 per 100,000 patient years, $p < 0.05$). That difference was attributed to more HCCs being detected at stage 1 (60% vs. 0%) and more treated by resection (47% vs. 8%). One dilemma is to what extent these data can be generalised to other clinical settings, including other geographical locations and health care systems. The standard of care in the control group was not described [3], so the chances of 'opportunistic screening' cannot be considered and compared with local routine practice. The attendance was low, finally declining to 25–30% [3], which may not apply for other settings. Only resection or TACE were used, and the addition of LTX and local ablation could have changed the results. Finally, the incidence in a selected cohort may have a higher annual incidence of HCC than 0.16% per year as was the case in the study from Zhang and colleagues [3].

It is a real dilemma as to whether these results can be generalised to patients with cirrhosis, where no RCTs have been performed. The somewhat higher incidence of HCC in cirrhosis would tend to favour surveillance. However, a number of factors act in the opposite direction. These include lower sensitivity of ultrasound in the cirrhotic liver, the shorter life expectancy in patients with cirrhosis and the limited possibility to use resection. In addition, these patients will often be followed on a regular basis in specialised clinics and will have ultrasound, CT or MR performed for other reasons than surveillance ('opportunistic screening'). These concerns have different weightings in different aetiologies.

Surveillance in HBV cirrhosis has been scarcely studied, but is probably not much different from HCV cirrhosis. In the absence of RCTs, the rationale for surveillance in this group rests on indirect evidence. Patients with decompensated (Child C) HCV cirrhosis have too short life expectancy to expect any survival effects of surveillance [23]. However, in uncomplicated HCV cirrhosis, HCC is the most common first complication as well as the leading cause of death [24], which should favour the effect of surveillance. In the absence of RCTs, the expectations of effect rest on studies that compare patients with HCC diagnosed in a surveillance programme and patients with HCC diagnosed otherwise ('opportunistic screening'). For example, Bolondi [8] compared 61 patients with surveillance-diagnosed HCC and 104 patients with HCC diagnosed opportunistically. Among surveillance-diagnosed HCC, more were assigned to treatment (69% vs. 59%), a difference accounted for by LXT (26% vs. 13%) and the median survival time was longer (30 vs. 15 months). In a Japanese study [25] of 182 surveillance-diagnosed and 202 'opportunistically' diagnosed HCC patients, the surveillance group had more tumours diagnosed before 30 mm (85% vs. 39%), more patients could be treated with resection or local ablation (76% vs. 46%), and 5-year survival was marginally better (46% vs. 32%) after correction for lead-time bias. Both of these often quoted studies [8,25] suffer from strong *selection bias*, most probably because many HCC patients were not referred to these hospitals, *lead-time bias*, because apparently improved survival may partly be explained by earlier detection, *and length bias*, because HCC detected by screening will preferably be the slower growing and less malignant tumours. All these sources of bias may overestimate the effect of surveillance. This is an illustrative example why experts warn against indirect evidence in support of nationwide surveillance programme to detect cancer [2]. It is quite uncertain whether a proper RCT of surveillance versus conventional standard of care would give similar results.

In alcoholic cirrhosis, surveillance may be less effective than in HCV cirrhosis because the risk of HCC is lower and HCC is not the most common first complication or leading cause of death [17]. In addition, the difference between HCC risk in clinic-based and populations-based studies – 1.7% versus 0.2–0.4% – may be higher in alcoholic cirrhosis than with other aetiologies [14]. Patients with alcoholic cirrhosis have a high non-HCC-related mortality, as exemplified by a 58% 5-year mortality, even in patients with uncomplicated alcoholic cirrhosis [17]. Therefore, the majority of these patients will die from other causes than HCC and even those who develop HCC have a considerable risk to die from non-HCC causes. The lower risk of HCC and the short life expectancy in alcoholic cirrhosis will severely threaten the possible effect of nationwide screening in these patients.

Will the costs be acceptable?

Cost-utility analyses typically estimate the cost per life-year saved (LYS) or the quality-adjusted life year (QALY). It has been suggested that surveillance may be economically acceptable if the costs per LYS are below $50,000 [1,26], but this rather arbitrary limit may apply differently to different socio-economic conditions. In the absence of RCTs, simulations by a Markov model are used to estimate the efficacy and the cost-utility relationship. These analyses can include a large number of factors. They differ in respect to what costs they include (only surveillance or also treatment), and in their assumptions on the attendance to the programme, the annual risk of HCC, the diagnostic values of ultrasound, the available treatment modalities, and the possibility that patients die from other causes than HCC.

The cost benefit relationship of surveillance in non-cirrhotic HBV is poorly studied. The AASLD guideline [1] quotes a Personal Communication as the only evidence that a surveillance programme in non-cirrhotic HBV patients will cost less than $50,000 per LYS. A more recent cost-effectiveness study from Taiwan [27] estimated $15,600 per LYS. However, this estimate is too low because 100% sensitivity and 100% specificity was assumed even for small tumours. Thus, they did not have to include costs of confirmatory testing. In addition, the costs of ultrasound and treatment of HCC were much lower than in most other countries. In the Shanghai Study [3], it took 920 ultrasound examinations and 70 confirmatory testings to prevent one death from HCC, emphasising the economical importance of false positive and false negative screening diagnoses. State of the art cost-utility analyses are clearly needed in this area.

More work has been done to assess the cost-benefit of surveillance programmes in patients with cirrhosis [8,21, 28–33]. Most studies included 6-month interval screening with ultrasound as an option, often in combination with AFP. The estimated cost per QALY gained ranged from $26,000 to $68,800 in simulated patient populations with mixed aetiology [21,29,30,33] and slightly less, $20,800–30,700 in simulations of HCV cirrhosis [28,31,32]. Most of these studies assumed the sensitivity of ultrasound to be 0.85, which is unrealistically high for small tumours in cirrhotic livers and will exaggerate the efficacy of surveillance. Most of these studies did not take available treatments into account, such as LTX [29], local ablation [21,29], TACE [21,29,33] and Sorafenib (all studies). The most comprehensive analysis by Thompson [21] included the lower sensitivity of ultrasound for small tumours and the course of the underlying disease according to aetiology. In the simulated sample of patient with compensated (Child A) cirrhosis of mixed aetiology, surveillance was estimated to increase the life expectancy from diagnosis of cirrhosis to death by 0.110 QALY (from 9.021 to 9.131 QALYs) at an additional cost of $4,800 (from $42,800 to $47,600), corresponding to $43,400 per QALY. The similar estimates were $20,800 per QALY in HBV cirrhosis, $42,900 in HCV cirrhosis, and $57,240 in alcoholic cirrhosis, emphasising the importance of aetiology. The better results for HBV were related to an assumed much younger age at diagnosis (44 years, vs. 53 years in alcoholic and 54 years in HCV cirrhosis). These cost estimates are most probably too low, because the assumed annual rates of HCC (alcoholic 1.7%, HBV 2.2% and HCV 3.7%) were from clinic-based studies, while population-based studies suggest much lower risks (0.4%, unknown, and 1–2%). Also, the assumed annual risks of decompensation (3.3%, 3.3% and 5.3%, respectively) were probably underestimated, at least for alcoholic cirrhosis, where 10–15% is more realistic(17), making death from other complications more likely than death from HCC. Unfortunately, none of the studies included the availability of angiogenesis inhibitors, which is now recommended in advanced HCC [1] and probably the most expensive treatment per LYS at the moment. With all these reservations, the available cost-utility studies suggest that country-based surveillance programmes may not be cost-effective according to the arbitrary $50,000 per LYS threshold, especially when HCV and alcoholic cirrhosis is concerned.

One study [8] indicates that all these simulations may in fact overestimate the cost-utility of surveillance. Bolondi and colleagues [8] compared total treatment costs in patients with HCC diagnosed by screening to other patients referred with HCC diagnosed incidentally. Additional costs per LYS were $113,000, substantially higher than any of the cost-utility analyses quoted above. All together, the cost-efficiency of a surveillance programme in patients with cirrhosis is uncertain and it is a real dilemma whether such programmes should be implemented on a country-based scale without proper RCTs. Again, aetiology matters and the most doubtful case is alcoholic cirrhosis.

Conclusions

The high rate of HCC in chronic liver disease and the availability of effective treatments for small tumours have suggested implementation of country-based surveillance programmes to detect HCC at an early state (Table 14.1).

Ideally, such programmes are supported by large RCTs. This is to some extent the case for the large population of patients with chronic HBV without cirrhosis. Out of three RCTs [5,4,19], only the largest had the power to demonstrate a lower HCC-related mortality in the surveillance group [3]. The value of a national surveillance programme including ultrasound every 6 months will be influenced by geographical variations in the risk of HCC and the local health care systems, including availability of LTX, resection and local ablation. It remains a question as to whether when evidence is sufficient, but a number of large national and international societies now recommend surveillance in selected patients with HBV. While it may be argued that efficacy is documented, the costs are truly uncertain and high-quality cost-utility analyses taking the local conditions into account should be carried out before country-based programmes are launched.

The effect of surveillance in patients with cirrhosis of the liver has never been studied in RCTs. The recommendation rests on generalisations from findings in East Asian HBV patients without cirrhosis [4,5,19], and a large body of indirect evidence. Surveillance in patients with cirrhosis differ in that the incidence is higher, the diagnostic value of ultrasound is poorer and the life expectancy shorter than in patients with non-cirrhotic HBV. Most of the indirect evidence used to justify surveillance in cirrhosis rests on clinic-based cohorts and will most probably overestimate the cost-effectiveness of country-based surveillance. Consequently, it is an open question as whether nationwide programmes will provide a survival benefit and if so, at an acceptable cost. This concern is most prominent with alcoholic cirrhosis. The best answer to this dilemma would be to carry out the relevant RCTs before the decision is taken.

References

1. Bruix J, Sherman M. Management of hepatocellular carcinoma: an update; AASLD management guideline, 2010.
2. Dans LF, Silvestre MA, Dans AL. Trade-off between benefit and harm is crucial in health screening recommendations. Part I: general principles. *J Clin Epidemiol* 2011; 64(5):231–239.
3. Zhang BH, Yang BH, Tang ZY. Randomized controlled trial of screening for hepatocellular carcinoma. *J Cancer Res Clin Oncol* 2004; 130(7):417–422.
4. Chen JG, Parkin DM, Chen QG, et al. Screening for liver cancer: results of a randomised controlled trial in Qidong, China. *J Med Screen* 2003; 10(4):204–209.
5. Sherman M, Peltekian KM, Lee C. Screening for hepatocellular carcinoma in chronic carriers of hepatitis B virus: incidence and prevalence of hepatocellular carcinoma in a North American urban population. *Hepatology* 1995; 22(2):432–438.
6. Llovet JM, Bruix J. Systematic review of randomized trials for unresectable hepatocellular carcinoma: chemoembolization improves survival. *Hepatology* 2003; 37(2):429–442.
7. Llovet JM, Real MI, Montana X, et al. Arterial embolisation or chemoembolisation versus symptomatic treatment in patients with unresectable hepatocellular carcinoma: a randomised controlled trial. *Lancet* 2002; 359(9319): 1734–1739.
8. Bolondi L, Sofia S, Siringo S, et al. Surveillance programme of cirrhotic patients for early diagnosis and treatment of hepatocellular carcinoma: a cost effectiveness analysis. *Gut* 2001; 48(2):251–259.
9. Trevisani F, De NS, Rapaccini G, et al. Semiannual and annual surveillance of cirrhotic patients for hepatocellular carcinoma: effects on cancer stage and patient survival (Italian experience). *Am J Gastroenterol* 2002; 97(3):734–744.
10. Rimassa L, Santoro A. Sorafenib therapy in advanced hepatocellular carcinoma: the SHARP trial. *Expert Rev Anticancer Ther* 2009; 9(6):739–745.
11. Cheng AL, Kang YK, Chen Z, et al. Efficacy and safety of sorafenib in patients in the Asia-Pacific region with advanced hepatocellular carcinoma: a phase III randomised, double-blind, placebo-controlled trial. *Lancet Oncol* 2009; 10(1):25–34.
12. Beasley RP, Hwang LY, Lin CC, Chien CS. Hepatocellular carcinoma and hepatitis B virus. A prospective study of 22 707 men in Taiwan. *Lancet* 1981; 2(8256):1129–1133.
13. Omland LH, Farkas DK, Jepsen P, Obel N, Pedersen L. Hepatitis C virus infection and risk of cancer: a population-based cohort study. *Clin Epidemiol* 2010; 2:179–186.
14. Fattovich G, Stroffolini T, Zagni I, Donato F. Hepatocellular carcinoma in cirrhosis: incidence and risk factors. *Gastroenterology* 2004; 127(5 suppl 1):S35–S50.
15. Lok AS, Seeff LB, Morgan TR, et al. Incidence of hepatocellular carcinoma and associated risk factors in hepatitis C-related advanced liver disease. *Gastroenterology* 2009; 136(1):138–148.
16. Benvegnu L, Gios M, Boccato S, Alberti A. Natural history of compensated viral cirrhosis: a prospective study on the incidence and hierarchy of major complications. *Gut* 2004; 53(5):744–749.
17. Jepsen P, Ott P, Andersen PK, Sorensen HT, Vilstrup H. Clinical course of alcoholic liver cirrhosis: a Danish population-based cohort study. *Hepatology* 2010; 51(5):1675–1682.
18. Trevisani F, D'Intino PE, Morselli-Labate AM, et al. Serum alpha-fetoprotein for diagnosis of hepatocellular carcinoma in patients with chronic liver disease: influence of HBsAg and anti-HCV status. *J Hepatol* 2001; 34(4):570–575.
19. Zhang B, Yang B. Combined alpha fetoprotein testing and ultrasonography as a screening test for primary liver cancer. *J Med Screen* 1999; 6(2):108–110.
20. Peterson MS, Baron RL. Radiologic diagnosis of hepatocellular carcinoma. *Clin Liver Dis* 2001; 5(1):123–144.
21. Thompson CJ, Rogers G, Hewson P, et al. Surveillance of cirrhosis for hepatocellular carcinoma: systematic review and economic analysis. *Health Technol Assess* 2007; 11(34): 1–206.
22. Bennett GL, Krinsky GA, Abitbol RJ, Kim SY, Theise ND, Teperman LW. Sonographic detection of hepatocellular carcinoma and dysplastic nodules in cirrhosis: correlation of pretransplantation sonography and liver explant pathol-

ogy in 200 patients. *AJR Am J Roentgenol* 2002; 179(1): 75–80.

23. Trevisani F, Santi V, Gramenzi A, et al. Surveillance for early diagnosis of hepatocellular carcinoma: is it effective in intermediate/advanced cirrhosis? *Am J Gastroenterol* 2007; 102(11):2448–2457.
24. Sangiovanni A, Prati GM, Fasani P, et al. The natural history of compensated cirrhosis due to hepatitis C virus: A 17-year cohort study of 214 patients. *Hepatology* 2006; 43(6):1303–1310.
25. Tanaka H, Nouso K, Kobashi H, et al. Surveillance of hepatocellular carcinoma in patients with hepatitis C virus infection may improve patient survival. *Liver Int* 2006; 26(5): 543–551.
26. Naimark D, Naglie G, Detsky AS. The meaning of life expectancy: what is a clinically significant gain? *J Gen Intern Med* 1994; 9(12):702–707.
27. Shih ST, Crowley S, Sheu JC. Cost-effectiveness analysis of a two-stage screening intervention for hepatocellular carcinoma in Taiwan. *J Formos Med Assoc* 2010; 109(1):39–55.
28. Patel D, Terrault NA, Yao FY, Bass NM, Ladabaum U. Cost-effectiveness of hepatocellular carcinoma surveillance in patients with hepatitis C virus-related cirrhosis. *Clin Gastroenterol Hepatol* 2005; 3(1):75–84.
29. Sarasin FP, Giostra E, Hadengue A. Cost-effectiveness of screening for detection of small hepatocellular carcinoma in western patients with Child-Pugh class A cirrhosis. *Am J Med* 1996; 101(4):422–434.
30. Nouso K, Tanaka H, Uematsu S, et al. Cost-effectiveness of the surveillance program of hepatocellular carcinoma depends on the medical circumstances. *J Gastroenterol Hepatol* 2008; 23(3):437–444.
31. Lin OS, Keeffe EB, Sanders GD, Owens DK. Cost-effectiveness of screening for hepatocellular carcinoma in patients with cirrhosis due to chronic hepatitis C. *Aliment Pharmacol Ther* 2004; 19(11):1159–1172.
32. Arguedas MR, Chen VK, Eloubeidi MA, Fallon MB. Screening for hepatocellular carcinoma in patients with hepatitis C cirrhosis: a cost-utility analysis. *Am J Gastroenterol* 2003; 98(3):679–690.
33. Andersson KL, Salomon JA, Goldie SJ, Chung RT. Cost effectiveness of alternative surveillance strategies for hepatocellular carcinoma in patients with cirrhosis. *Clin Gastroenterol Hepatol* 2008; 6(12):1418–1424.

PART 4

Choice of Radiological Diagnostic Technique

15 Computed tomography or magnetic resonance imaging for the diagnosis of hepatocellular carcinoma

Wladyslaw Gedroyc
MRI Unit, St. Mary's Hospital, Imperial College Health Care Trust, London, UK

LEARNING POINTS

- The nature of the new technologies that have improved computed tomography (CT) and magnetic resonance imaging (MRI) in the last 5 years
- Advantages and disadvantages of CT and MRI in the liver
- Relative performance of CT and MRI in the diagnosis of small hepatocellular carcinoma (smaller than 2 cm)
- Utility of new hepatocyte specific MR contrast agents and how to use them

MRI and computed X-ray tomography have completely changed the understanding and investigation of hepatic masses over the last 25 years. Both these techniques allow detailed cross-sectional images of the body to be obtained with good soft tissue contrast, completely independent of the operator. These two techniques, of course, have themselves changed radically since they were first introduced into clinical practice, and this chapter attempts to describe the role of the newer developments in these technologies and places these two modalities in their appropriate context in terms of the diagnosis of hepatocellular carcinoma (HCC).

New developments

Both CT and MR have undergone important technological improvements in the last 5 years, which have significantly improved the ability to detect and diagnose hepatic abnormalities. The current crop of CT and MR scanners are consistently able to visualise liver masses below 1 cm in diameter and their role in this area will be discussed specifically.

The most important change in CT has been the widespread adoption of multidetector (MD) technology. The implementation of this new development allows extremely rapid acquisition of large volumes of tissue simultaneously, in an isotropic manner, using only a few breath holds. These volumes can be rapidly repeated so that they can detect multiple sequential phases of vascularity after intravenous contrast administration and can, therefore, clearly show a lesion's behaviour in terms of its enhancement. The imaging volumes that are acquired using this technology produce isotropic voxels that are the same size in all directions, which means that multiplanar reconstruction can be easily carried out, producing good-quality multiplanar images, despite the inevitable axial plane of acquisition. MD technology allows multiple slices to be acquired simultaneously and the amount of slices that can be acquired in this manner varies from 16 slices up to 256 slices, depending on the individual CT machine. The improvement in visualisation of liver masses using these techniques is significant, but the physical principles of lesion appreciation using CT are not altered in any way. Lesion depiction still relies on differences in X-ray attenuation between pathological areas and abnormal areas and their pattern of enhancement after substantial volumes of contrast.

MRI continues to expand technologically with new hardware and new sequences continuously emerging, which improves the ability to image abnormal tissue. Over the last 5 years, parallel acquisition and reconstruction

Clinical Dilemmas in Primary Liver Cancer, First Edition. Edited by Roger Williams and Simon D. Taylor-Robinson.

techniques using multi-element coils have become commonplace, allowing a substantial improvement in spatial resolution and speed of imaging, which have been especially valuable in imaging the liver and thus facilitating multiple phases post-contrast to be easily acquired. The whole volume of the liver can be acquired using gradient echo T_1-weighted fat saturated sequences, which are extremely sensitive to contrast enhancement and can cover the whole liver in approximately 25 seconds with slice thicknesses of between 3 and 5 mm at 1.5 T. Similar volumes with similar sequences, but with much higher resolution can be acquired in 12 seconds at 3 T, using current state-of-the-art machinery.

Over the last 5 years, diffusion-weighted imaging has also begun to have a huge impact in the liver [1,2]. This type of sequence assesses water mobility in tissues (Brownian motion). In areas of significant hypercellularity, such as in tumours, water is bound tightly and much more avidly than in normal tissues, where it is loosely bound. Using sequences that measure the ability of water to move freely allows areas of diffusion restriction, as in areas of hypercellularity (tumours), to be easily distinguished from normal tissue [3]. Diffusion imaging has become an excellent modality for visualising small hepatic metastasis [4,5]. It is equally very effective at demonstrating HCCs, but is perhaps slightly less reliable in differentiating small HCCs from surrounding tissue in cirrhotic livers [6–8] and in particular, it is quite difficult to differentiate well-differentiated HCCs from surrounding dysplastic nodules and uninvolved cirrhotic tissue. Several types of liver-specific MR contrast agents are also now available. The most recent hepatocyte-specific contrast medium to emerge is gadolinium ethoxy-benzoic acid (Gd EOB), commercially marketed as Primovist™ (Bayer AG Leverkusen Germany), which is a dual action agent [9]. This compound will act as a conventional extracellular fluid (ECF) gadolinium agent in its first pass through the liver, demonstrating areas of hypervascularity in the same way that conventional ECF agents do. Subsequently, 50% of this agent is taken up and excreted by hepatocytes. Therefore, approximately 20 minutes after an intravenous injection of this compound, there is a strong hepatocyte-enhanced phase, often termed the hepatobiliary phase and this allows the parenchyma to be imaged effectively, and, therefore, tumours or other abnormalities that do not contain functioning hepatocytes are visualised as filling defects within this hepatobiliary-enhanced phase.

3-T MR machines have also improved substantially over the last 2 years. The current crop of high-field scanners can now produce high-resolution images more rapidly and with almost no artefacts in comparison to 3-T scanners from several years ago, which produced images of the liver with extensive artefacts. The ability to effectively utilise the greatly increased signal available at 3T is a huge step forward for MRI of the liver. It seems very likely that 3-T MR scanners will become the standard clinical work horses over the next 5 years, slowly replacing the existing 1.5-T scanners.

Disadvantages of CT and MRI

Despite its increased speed, CT still requires a substantial ionising radiation dose to obtain images. This may increase even further with the use of MD technology, because this allows multiple large tissue volumes to be acquired in a very short space of time and because each pass through the area in question is so quick, acquisitions are commonly repeated. However, each acquisition has the full radiation dose of a standard whole CT abdominal examination, so it is common for increased doses of radiation to be encountered in modern CT liver imaging. Significant volumes of iodinated contrast media must also be utilised, and these agents have multiple well-known problems that are inherent including allergic phenomena.

MRI for all its improvements in speed of acquisition is still affected by significant patient movement and by breathing artefact. It is much more susceptible than CT to this problem. MR images still have lower spatial resolution than standard CT acquisitions. The new breed of MR scanners now available are much shorter physically than previous large MR machines and the newest scanners also have a much wider bore, so that whereas previously the standard width of the MRI bore in which the patient lies was 55 cm, newer machines have a bore of between 70 and 75 cm, which is a great improvement for patient comfort and decreases the incidence of failed scans from claustrophobia.

Advantages of MRI and CT

The speed of acquisition and the high spatial resolution of CT, in addition to its ready availability in most radiology departments across the world are its unequivocal advantages. MRI, in comparison, has much greater soft tissue contrast and more importantly, it uses measurements of multiple different physical parameters to visualise and display lesions. MR is sensitive to proton relaxation factors, temperature of tissues, diffusion coefficients of tissue, vascular flow, mineral content and other related aspects. Also the sensitivity of T_1-weighted fat saturated MRI sequences to very small amounts of gadolinium-based contrast is much greater than the sensitivity of CT to small changes in attenuation induced by the presence of iodinated intravenous contrast. This aspect means that very slight areas of tissue contrast enhancement are likely to be much more easily detected by MRI than CT. It is also much easier to make more tissue-specific diagnoses in liver tumours and other soft tissue areas by using the information available from the multiple different sequences that are carried out in MRI (which examine some of the different physical tissue properties described in the preceding text). However, access to MRI is always more difficult than it is to CT, simply because there are fewer MR scanners available than CT scanners.

Detection of small lesions using MRI and CT

Detection of small lesions and their accurate diagnosis is a particular problem in the cirrhotic liver, where there are a large variety of nodules and distortions that may be visualised by different modalities and many of these lesions will have uncertain or no malignant potential and must be differentiated from the much more important small HCCs, which have immense relevance for subsequent treatment [10]. The use of ablative percutaneous technologies, such as radiofrquency ablation, laser ablation or microwave ablation, in the treatment of HCC has also become more sophisticated, and in many instances, simplified treatment strategies away from ineffective chemotherapy and larger surgical resections. This type of technology allows equivalent survival to be obtained, comparable to surgical resection [11], but it is clear that the smaller the HCC lesion at the time of ablation, the better the long-term results following the ablation. Therefore, if this type of percutaneous technology is to be utilised for the treatment of HCCs, the diagnosis of HCC must be as accurate as possible and the technology must be able to detect these lesions at an early stage when they are as small as possible. This also pertains to any subsequent technological successors that will evolve in the next 5 years.

The detection and diagnosis of HCC in the liver has predominantly been based on demonstrating abnormal, very early arterial enhancement within suspicious lesions after intravenous contrast. This applies equally to CT using iodinated contrast media or MRI using gadolinium agents. Current MD CT technology is equivalent to MRI and all other modalities in the detection of liver lesions, greater than 2 cm in diameter. The diagnosis is less specific in this tumour size range using CT rather than MRI, but most lesions detected within this size range can usually be visualised currently by all available modalities of imaging including ultrasound when used optimally, which can usually effect lesion detection of hepatic tumours of 2 cm or greater in non-cirrhotic livers.

However, mass lesions less than 2 cm diameter in cirrhotic livers are a completely different proposition. The differential diagnosis of a potential hepatic mass under these circumstances is much wider. Fibrosis, regenerative nodules, siderotic nodules and various grades of dysplastic nodules and arterial portal shunting, as well as HCCs, all have to be considered in this differential. CT as described in the preceding text (Figure 15.1A) relies on arterial enhancement using contrast to visualise HCC, but if this is not evident or is ambivalent in some way, then CT diagnosis immediately becomes problematic. At what stage does an evolving HCCs start to display neo-angiogenesis that can be picked up by CT [12,13]? The answer to this question is immensely variable between patients and between different areas within the same liver and no real consensus exists.

MR conventionally also relies heavily on arterial enhancement visualised after intravenous contrast administration for the positive diagnosis of HCC. The other physical factors mentioned in the preceding text and the high soft tissue contrast available to MR means that in many instances a positive diagnosis of one of the other causes of small nodules in cirrhotic livers can be made. Siderotic nodules usually show typical low signal susceptibility changes on all sequences, allowing a confident positive diagnosis. Areas of fibrosis show low signal without susceptibility changes on T_1-weighted and T_2-weighted sequences and regenerative nodules frequently, although not invariably, show mild hypertensity on T_1-weighted sequences without any enhancement being visible subsequently. Diffusion is usually not altered under these circumstances. The spectrum of changes that are seen in dysplastic nodules on their way to becoming frank HCCs [14] are rarely visible on imaging criteria alone and may even be very hard to

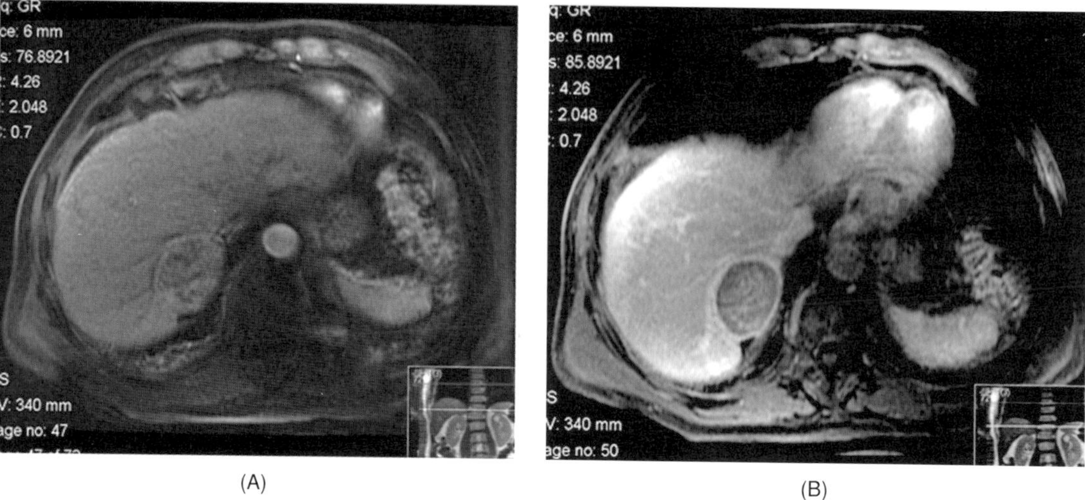

(A) (B)

FIG 15.1 (A) Arterial phase post-intravenous contrast using Gd EOB. Large mass lesion in posterior aspect of segment 7 is visible, which shows early but mild arterial enhancement in this first pass image. (B) Hepatobiliary phase of post Gd EOB examination. This image was taken 20 minutes post-contrast administration. *Note*: substantial liver parenchymal enhancement, but decreased uptake at the site of the mass in segment 7.

detect pathologically. Commonly, it is believed that arterial neo-angiogenesis does not occur until a dysplastic nodule has become a frank HCC and it is this finding that imaging visualises on arterial enhancement [15]. Since MR is so much more sensitive to small amounts of contrast than CT, MR does visualise such very early lesions before they can be seen with CT. Well-differentiated HCCs are a more difficult problem [16]. These lesions may not have much arterial enhancement in the early post-contrast phases and may potentially have some residual hepatocyte function to make visualisation and differential diagnosis extremely problematic. There are recent suggestions that the use of Gd EOB (Primovist) may depict such lesions in the delayed hepatobiliary phase (20-minute post-administration) as an area of non-enhancement [17]. Over the past 8 years, superparamagnetic iron oxide particles (SPIO) that are specific reticuloendothelial agents have been quite widely investigated as a method of diagnosing HCC [18–20]. More recently, these agents have also been combined with conventional MR gadolinium contrast agents that have an ECF distribution as a dual contrast administration study [21]. The principle here is that the SPIO agent blackens normal liver parenchyma by susceptibility effects and areas that do not contain normal Kupffer cells, such as tumours, are highlighted as bright areas on a normal dark liver background (Figure 15.1B). SPIO agents used on their own have been shown to be less sensitive for the diagnosis of small HCCs than conventional ECF gadolinium agents alone (which show more small lesions just by using early arterial enhancement). Therefore, some groups have combined these two agents with the belief that reducing the liver signal will highlight areas of gadolinium arterial enhancement, thus showing more small HCCs than either agent can achieve alone. These dual contrast studies have been reasonably successful in this and are an improvement on just using SPIO particles alone [21].

The widespread introduction of a new biphasic hepatocyte specific gadolinium contrast agent (Gd EOB) has changed the balance of MR liver-specific contrast agent utilisation. Fifty per cent of this agent is excreted by the liver after hepatocyte uptake, so that at 20-minute post-intravenous administration, the liver parenchyma is strongly enhanced with areas of functioning hepatocytes appearing brighter in this hepatobiliary phase. On the first pass, post-intravenous injection, this agent also acts like a conventional ECF gadolinium contrast agent, demonstrating vascularity and arterial and venous enhancement. Initially, there was a concern that this agent would be very poor in the early arterial phase, because the total gadolinium dose used in this compound, in comparison to conventional ECF gadolinium preparations, is four times lower. However, the T_1 relaxivity of Gd EOB is at least double that of other gadolinium compounds [17], and widespread use and assessment of the arterial phase of HCCs has not resulted in any change in visualisation of small lesions in the early arterial phase using Gd EOB. Decreased intensity on the delayed hepatobiliary phase is indicative of a lack of hepatocyte function in the area in question. This is usually believed to indicate an HCC in a cirrhotic liver. Kim et al. [17] described finding four hypointense areas in the hepatobiliary delayed phase post-Gd EOB, which were not visualised as areas of abnormality on any other sequences. Three of these lesions proved to be well-differentiated HCCs, but the remaining lesion turned out to be a dysplastic nodule. The conclusion from this seems to be that the hepatobiliary phase can take the problematic differential diagnosis of small HCCs much further than using the simple post-contrast sequences alone, but the problems of differentiating dysplastic nodules and other benign nodules from small HCCs still unsurprisingly remain.

The last 2 years have seen multiple studies examining the performances of Gd EOB-enhanced MRI sequences in comparison to CT MD scans and other MR contrast studies in the detection of small HCCs. Ichikawa et al. [22] examined 178 patients with hepatic masses using Gd EOB and compared their results to MD CT (64 slice scanner) in the same patients in a large multi-institutional study in Japan. MRI showed a significantly greater amount of all lesions (67.5–79.5%) than CT (61–73%). Lesions below 2 cm in diameter also showed significant further differences. Lesions 10–20 mm in diameter showed 71–87% detection with MR and 65.7–78.7% detection for CT. In the case of lesions below 10 mm in diameter, the results are 38–55% detection for MRI and 26–47% detection for CT.

Di Martino et al. [23] examined 87 HCCs using Gd EOB MRI and 64 slice MD CT. Their results show sensitivity for lesion detection of 85% for MRI and only 69% for CT (a significant difference) for all lesions in their study. In the subgroup of lesions smaller than 2 cm diameter, these auhors also found significantly more lesions detected with MR than with equivalent CT. Hammerstingl et al. [9] in an earlier multi-institutional study also noted that Gd EOB was significantly superior for the detection of small HCCs. In this study MR had a detection rate of 82% of lesions, as opposed to 71% for equivalent CT, and interestingly this group commented that the extra information available from MRI changed the surgical therapy in their group in 19/131 cases.

Several studies have also compared Gd EOB MRI with SPIO-enhanced liver imaging. Kim et al. [24] examined the direct comparison with SPIO alone and in a subsequent paper [17] made a comparison with a dual contrast administration technique using SPIO and Gd ECF agents as described above. In the first paper GD EOB imaging was significantly more sensitive than SPIO particles alone, 91% as opposed to 84.7%, respectively. In the case of the dual contrast technique, the sensitivities of the two examinations were completely equivalent suggesting that the very simple Gd EOB examination could replace the much more awkward and expensive dual contrast technique.

Conclusions

CT has long been regarded as the imaging work horse in the abdomen with its ready availability and ease-of-use. These advantages have readily overcome its main problems of high radiation dose and relative diagnostic non-specificity in terms of its results (Table 15.1). MD technology has improved CT usability immensely and has introduced much better quality multiplanar reconstructions and thinner axial sections both of which add substantially to disease assessment. CT remains limited by its physical nature, which requires the use of large radiation doses and relatively large doses of iodinated contrast, if significant tissue discrimination is to be achieved for proper diagnosis. MRI used to be viewed as a diagnostic problem solver in the abdomen with artefacts due to motion from breathing and pulsation limiting its application. Continuous improvements in movement suppression have addressed many of these concerns. The variety of different physical parameters that MR can measure in the body allows much more information to be acquired about a target tissue, leading to a much more specific diagnosis than is possible with CT. This allows MR images to advance the differential diagnosis of small lesions on a background of cirrhosis much further than is conventionally achieved by CT. The addition of more hepatocyte-specific contrast media has also had a great impact in this field. Gd EOB images have allowed MR to consistently outperform current state-of-the-art CT in the depiction of small HCCs, overcoming the higher spatial resolution inherent to CT. MR diffusion imaging has also become an important extra strand in imaging of the liver, improving the diagnostic confidence in many focal

TABLE 15.1 The advantages and disadvantages of CT and MRI in the context of diagnosing small hepatocellular carcinomas in cirrhosis

	Advantages	Disadvantages
CT	Quick High spatial resolution Resistant to movement Readily available everywhere	High radiation dose Needs large doses iodinated contrast to differentiate between tissues Poor soft tissue contrast Only moderately sensitive to enhancement Less sensitive to small HCCs in cirrhosis Less specific diagnostically
MRI	High soft tissue resolution No ionising radiation used Very sensitive to small amount contrast Hepatocyte-specific contrast available Multiple physical factors measured to produce image Very specific diagnostically Better at diagnosing small HCC on cirrhotic background Differentiates between benign cirrhotic change and malignancy	Susceptible to motion artefacts Lower spatial resolution Fewer machines available More claustrophobic

liver masses. Perhaps its most important role in cirrhosis is in increasing diagnostic confidence when a normal scan is assessed.

Therefore, it is clear that good quality MR should be the primary diagnostic modality for the assessment of focal liver masses in the cirrhotic liver at this time. Current scanners coupled with new hepatocyte specific contrast agents when used effectively can provide a much more complete assessment of the liver and advance the differential diagnosis of small HCCs much further than is possible with CT alone with a much greater potential impact on subsequent therapy. Many more advances in MRI in terms of hardware and software will be seen in the near future, which will accentuate the advantages of MR further, particularly when 3 T scanners start to become used routinely in this field.

References

1. Kele PG, van der Jagt EJ. Diffusion weighted imaging in the liver. *World J Gastroenterol* 2010; 16(13):1567–1576.
2. Pauls S, Schmidt SA, Juchems MS, et al. Diffusion-weighted MR imaging in comparison to integrated [(18)F]-FDG PET/CT for N-staging in patients with lung cancer. *Eur J Radiol* 2010 (in press).
3. Sandrasegaran K, Akisik FM, Lin C, et al. Value of diffusion-weighted MRI for assessing liver fibrosis and cirrhosis. *AJR Am J Roentgenol* 2009; 193(6):1556–1560.
4. Demir OI, Obuz F, Sağol O, Dicle O. Contribution of diffusion-weighted MRI to the differential diagnosis of hepatic masses. *Diagn Interv Radiol* 2007; 13(2):81–86.
5. Lichy MP, Aschoff P, Plathow C, et al. Tumor detection by diffusion-weighted MRI and ADC-mapping – initial clinical experiences in comparison to PET-CT. *Invest Radiol* 2007; 42(9):605–613.
6. Xu H, Li X, Xie JX, Yang ZH, Wang B. Diffusion-weighted magnetic resonance imaging of focal hepatic nodules in an experimental hepatocellular carcinoma rat model. *Acad Radiol* 2007; 14(3):279–286.
7. Zech CJ, Reiser MF, Herrmann KA. Imaging of hepatocellular carcinoma by computed tomography and magnetic resonance imaging: state of the art. *Dig Dis* 2009; 27(2):114–124.
8. Parikh T, Drew SJ, Lee VS, et al. Focal liver lesion detection and characterization with diffusion-weighted MR imaging: comparison with standard breath-hold T2-weighted imaging. *Radiology* 2008; 246(3):812–822.
9. Hammerstingl R, Huppertz A, Breuer J, et al. European EOB-study group. Diagnostic efficacy of gadoxetic acid (Primovist)-enhanced MRI and spiral CT for a therapeutic strategy: comparison with intraoperative and histopathologic findings in focal liver lesions. *Eur Radiol* 2008; 18(3):457–467.
10. Mita K, Kim SR, Kudo M, et al. Diagnostic sensitivity of imaging modalities for hepatocellular carcinoma smaller than 2 cm. *World J Gastroenterol* 2010; 16(33):4187–4192.
11. Chen M, Li J, Zheng Y. Surgical resection versus percutaneous thermal ablation for early-stage hepatocellular carcinoma: a

randomized controlled trial. *Annals of Surgery* 2006; 243: 321–328.

12. Hayashi M, Matsui O, Ueda K, Kawamori Y, Gabata T, Kadoya M. Progression to hypervascular hepatocellular carcinoma: correlation with intranodular blood supply evaluated with CT during intraarterial injection of contrast material. *Radiology* 2002; 225(1):143–149.
13. Tajima T, Honda H, Taguchi K, et al. Sequential hemodynamic change in hepatocellular carcinoma and dysplastic nodules: CT angiography and pathologic correlation. *AJR Am J Roentgenol* 2002; 178(4):885–897.
14. Theise ND, Schwartz M, Miller C, Thung SN. Macroregenerative nodules and hepatocellular carcinoma in forty-four sequential adult liver explants with cirrhosis. *Hepatology* 1992; 16(4):949–955.
15. Mion F, Grozel L, Boillot O, Paliard P, Berger F. Adult cirrhotic liver explants: precancerous lesions and undetected small hepatocellular carcinomas. *Gastroenterology* 1996; 111(6):1587–1592.
16. Kogita S, Imai Y, Okada M, et al. Gd-EOB-DTPA-enhanced magnetic resonance images of hepatocellular carcinoma: correlation with histological grading and portal blood flow. *Eur Radiol* 2010; 20(10):2405–2413.
17. Kim YK, Kim CS, Han YM, Park G. Detection of small hepatocellular carcinoma: can gadoxetic acid-enhanced magnetic resonance imaging replace combining gadopentetate dimeglumine-enhanced and superparamagnetic iron oxide-enhanced magnetic resonance imaging? *Invest Radiol* 2010; 45(11):740–746.
18. Choi D, Kim S, Lim J, Lee W, Jang H, Lee S, Lim H. Preoperative detection of hepatocellular carcinoma: ferumoxides-enhanced mr imaging versus combined helical CT during arterial portography and CT hepatic arteriography. *AJR Am J Roentgenol* 2001; 176(2):475–482.
19. Kim SK, Kim SH, Lee WJ, et al. Preoperative detection of hepatocellular carcinoma: ferumoxides-enhanced versus mangafodipir trisodium-enhanced MR imaging. *AJR Am J Roentgenol* 2002; 179(3):741–750.
20. Raman SS, Lu DS, Chen SC, Sayre J, Eilber F, Economou J. Hepatic MR imaging using ferumoxides: prospective evaluation with surgical and intraoperative sonographic confirmation in 25 cases. *AJR Am J Roentgenol* 2001; 177(4):807–812.
21. Ward J, Guthrie JA, Scott DJ, et al. Hepatocellular carcinoma in the cirrhotic liver: double-contrast MR imaging for diagnosis. *Radiology* 2000; 216(1):154–162.
22. Ichikawa T, Saito K, Yoshioka N, et al. Detection and characterization of focal liver lesions: a Japanese phase III, multicenter comparison between gadoxetic acid disodium-enhanced magnetic resonance imaging and contrast-enhanced computed tomography predominantly in patients with hepatocellular carcinoma and chronic liver disease. *Invest Radiol* 2010; 45(3):133–141.
23. Di Martino M, Marin D, Guerrisi A, et al. Intraindividual comparison of gadoxetate disodium-enhanced MR imaging and 64-section multidetector CT in the Detection of hepatocellular carcinoma in patients with cirrhosis. *Radiology* 2010; 256(3):806–816.
24. Kim YK, Kim CS, Han YM, Park G, Hwang SB, Yu HC. Comparison of gadoxetic acid-enhanced MRI and superparamagnetic iron oxide-enhanced MRI for the detection of hepatocellular carcinoma. *Clin Radiol* 2010; 65(5):358–365.

16 Is microbubble ultrasound useful?

Adrian Lim

Imperial College Health Care NHS Trust, Charing Cross Hospital, London, UK

LEARNING POINTS

- Hepatocellular carcinomas (HCCs) are hypervascular in the arterial phase and the majority washout in the portal and late phases. Those that do not demonstrate significant washout are commonly associated with a lower grade tumour
- Microbubble contrast-enhanced ultrasound (CEUS) improves liver lesion detection, but is yet to be proven for screening HCCs in multicentre studies
- The advantage of CEUS is its real-time capability in comparison to computed tomography (CT) or magnetic resonance imaging (MRI), where sometimes the timing of scan acquisition may miss key characteristics
- CEUS is cheaper and more widely available than CT or MRI, but it has the disadvantages of ultrasound where penetration can be a problem in hepatic steatosis and in larger patients
- The hepatic vein transit time (HVTT) of microbubbles has been shown to be able to stage chronic liver disease

Ultrasound remains the first-line imaging modality of choice in HCC surveillance owing to its accessibility and relatively low cost. On a background of cirrhosis where there are multiple regenerative and dysplastic nodules, conventional ultrasound has difficulty in distinguishing these benign nodules from malignancy. The grey-scale appearances are similar where the nodules and HCCs are typically hypoechoic, although HCCs may sometimes demonstrate variable echotexture and necrosis. HCCs are also typically more vascular, but even with Doppler ultrasound, the accuracy of conventional ultrasound in determining HCCs from regenerative nodules, dysplastic nodules or other coincidental focal liver lesions (such as haemangiomata and focal nodular hyperplasia (FNH)) remains low.

In the last 15 years, the advent of contrast agents for ultrasound (microbubbles) has allowed real-time characterisation of focal liver lesions, where grey-scale imaging is typically unhelpful. Microbubbles have been shown to play an important imaging role in characterising focal liver lesions [1,2].

Many studies corroborate that the neo-angiogenic properties of HCC are key to its diagnosis with CEUS [2–4]. HCCs are typically hypervascular in the arterial phase with a reticular network of angiogenic vessels in a 'basket weave' pattern and enhancement in a haphazard way, predominantly from the periphery inwards (Plate 16.1). The contrast then begins to wash out in the portal phase, in comparison to the enhancing adjacent liver and, in the late phase (more than 2-minute post-injection), HCCs typically appear as signal defects within the enhanced liver parenchyma (Plate 16.2).

HCCs are predominantly hypervascular in the arterial phase, but in a very small proportion, they can be hypovascular or isovascular in the arterial phase, and therefore, interpretation with the portal and late phases are key. The majority of these lesions washout in the late phase and it is this washout phase that has high accuracy of over 95% for detecting malignancy in CEUS, as demonstrated in a previous multicentre study [1]. While the latter is true for all metastases, the washout can be variable with HCCs [3,6–8] and has been to shown to be associated with the grade of tumour, where the well-differentiated HCCs tend to have less washout in the late phases at 5 minutes and 10 minutes

Clinical Dilemmas in Primary Liver Cancer, First Edition. Edited by Roger Williams and Simon D. Taylor-Robinson.

post-injection. Of note, in a recent study, only 10 out of 26 well-differentiated HCCs demonstrated washout in contrast to 44 out of 51 moderately- and poorly differentiated HCCs [3].

These microbubble enhancement characteristics, although similar to that seen on CT or MRI, have certain advantages. The key is the real-time CEUS property that allows the early hypervascularity of a lesion to be visualised and this can sometimes be missed depending on the timing of the dynamic scans on CT and MRI. In addition, the ability to watch the lesion enhance centrifugally or centripetally allows the distinction of a HCC from other hypervascular lesions, in particular FNH with high accuracy [4–6]. In addition, the higher resolution of ultrasound allows smaller lesions (less than 10 mm) to be characterised with confidence.

In recent studies [3,6–8], the use of microbubbles have been shown to detect the hypervascularity of HCCs where they were hypoenhancing lesions on CT or MRI on a background of chronic liver disease. This again may have been due to the phase and timing of the CT/MRI scan and enforces the key advantage of real-time capability of CEUS in comparison to the other two modalities.

A multicentre study that compared microbubble utlrasound with CT and MRI showed that CEUS was the most sensitive, most specific and thus most accurate imaging modality for the characterisation of focal liver lesions [5].

Another benefit for this technique in comparison to other imaging modalities is the widespread availability of relative high-end ultrasound equipment, unlike state-of-the-art CT or MRI scanners, particularly in developing countries, where they can be limited to major teaching hospitals. The cost of a CEUS in comparison to these other two techniques is substantially less, and one study estimated a CEUS-related cost saving of approximately 13%, compared with CT, and approximately 33% when compared with MRI when these techniques were used as first-line diagnosis for characterisation of focal liver lesions [9]. A cost analysis study by Piscaglia and colleagues [10] also showed that the least expensive recall strategy in patients with cirrhosis and a screen-detected nodule of 10–19 mm on grey-scale ultrasound would be CEUS initially and CT to confirm the hypervascularity of the lesion in accordance with European Association for the Study of the Liver (EASL) guidelines [11]. In patients with single 20–30 mm nodules, the least expensive strategy is to start with CT and to use contrast-enhanced ultrasound as a second step technique [12]. The use of CEUS would obviate the need for MRI as a second technique for staging and liver lesion characterisation.

There has also been much work in utilising microbubbles as a tracer and measuring the HVTT of these microbubbles through the liver in patients with chronic liver disease. It would appear that, with increasing damage and fibrosis, the HVTT is shortened owing to the arteriovenous shunts that develop. Studies have shown that an HVTT of less than 24 seconds using the microbubble agent, Levovist™ (Schering AG, Berlin, Germany) as a tracer or less than 12 seconds with the agent, SonoVue™ (Bracco, Milan, Italy) can reliably diagnose cirrhosis [13,14]. Importantly, in a histologically stratified group of patient with hepatitis C virus (HCV)-related liver disease, the HVTT appeared able to separate mild hepatitis from moderate/severe hepatitis and cirrhosis [15]. These findings suggest that microbubbles can be a useful and non-invasive technique for staging chronic liver disease, in addition to characterising focal lesions within these damaged livers [15,16].

Although the modality used for screening is variable, conventional ultrasound performed at 6-month intervals is most common and current practice as recommended by the British Society of Gastroenterology guidelines [17]. In the experience reported from the world literature, CEUS is invaluable for its contribution to characterisation of nodules detected in a cirrhotic liver. However, detection of HCC, especially in a cirrhotic liver, presents more of a challenge, particularly because of the heterogeneous behaviour of HCC in the portal phase. In addition, the small end-stage cirrhotic liver and the chronic liver with substantial fat deposition may be much more difficult to image with sonography than a normal liver and one of the main limitations of CEUS is the poor penetration at depths greater than 10 cm and sometimes substantially less in a very fatty liver. Our unpublished database from Imperial College Health Care Trust, London, on over 100 patients with biopsy-proven hepatitis C-related chronic liver disease and 35 patients with cirrhosis provided information over a period of 3 years with 6 monthly interval ultrasound, includes CEUS. In this screening cohort, only two HCCs were detected and these were seen on grey-scale ultrasound without microbubbles, although the latter provided lesion characterisation and confirmatory evidence that the lesion was a HCC. Detection of HCC in a cirrhotic liver is predominantly dependant on visualising the hypervascularity of the lesion in the arterial phase and in most cases, washout in the portal and late phases. With CEUS, it can be difficult to completely assess the whole liver within the limited arterial phase period and as washout in the late phase is variable, lesions can be missed. Therefore, the use of CEUS as part of screening and detection is still controversial and requires large multicentre trials for validation.

It may be that with the development of targeted and more liver-specific microbubble agents, such as Sonazoid™ (GE Healthcare, Amersham, Buckinghamshire, UK), the detection of HCCs and differentiation of dysplastic nodules from HCCs may be improved. This newer agent has been shown to have detection capability, even for small well-differentiated HCCs, to rival that of liver-specific superparamagnetic iron oxide (SPIO) MRI scans and has improved sensitivity over triple-phase multislice CT [18–20].

Overall, microbubble (contrast-enhanced ultrasound) is a relatively inexpensive and widely accessible imaging modality with high accuracy for characterising focal liver lesions in patients with chronic liver disease and liver cirrhosis comparable to that of CT and MRI. It has potential for assessing the severity of fibrosis non-invasively in chronic liver disease and may aid detection of HCCs, although the latter has yet to be proven in large-scale studies. The development of targeted and more liver-specific microbubbles has allowed the sensitivity and specificity of this technique to rival that of SPIO MRI scans. CEUS is proving an invaluable technique in the imaging armamentarium for problem solving difficult lesions in the diseased/cirrhotic liver.

References

1. Bryant TH, Blomley MJ, Albrecht T, et al. Improved characterization of liver lesions with liver-phase uptake of liver-specific microbubbles: prospective multicenter study. *Radiology* 2004; 232(3):799–809.
2. Claudon M, Cosgrove D, Albrecht T, et al. Guidelines and good clinical practice recommendations for contrast enhanced ultrasound (CEUS) - update 2008. *Ultraschall Med* 2008; 29(1):28–44.
3. Jang HJ, Kim TK, Burns PN, Wilson SR. Enhancement patterns of hepatocellular carcinoma at contrast enhanced US: Comparison with histologic differentiation. *Radiology* 2007; 244(3):898–906.
4. Morin SH, Lim AK, Cobbold JF, Taylor-Robinson SD. Use of second generation contrast-enhanced ultrasound in the assessment of focal liver lesions. *World J Gastroenterol* 2007; 13(45):5963–5970.
5. Trillaud H, Bruel JM, Valette PJ, et al. Characterization of focal liver lesions with SonoVue-enhanced sonography: international multicenter-study in comparison to CT and MRI. *World J Gastroenterol* 200914; 15(30):3748–3756.
6. Wang WP, Wu Y, Luo Y, et al. Clinical value of contrast-enhanced ultrasonography in the characterization of focal liver lesions: a prospective multicenter trial. *Hepatobiliary Pancreat Dis Int* 2009; 8(4):370–376.
7. Numata K, Luo W, Morimoto M, et al. Contrast enhanced ultrasound of hepatocellular carcinoma. *World J Radiol* 2010; 2(2):68–82.
8. Takahashi M, Maruyama H, Ishibashi H, Yoshikawa M, Yokosuka O. Contrast-enhanced ultrasound with perflubutane microbubble agent: evaluation of differentiation of hepatocellular carcinoma. *AJR Am J Roentgenol* 2011; 196(2):W123–31.
9. Sirli R, Sporea I, Martie A, Popescu A, Dănilă M. Contrast enhanced ultrasound in focal liver lesions–a cost efficiency study. *Med Ultrason* 2010; 12(4):280–285.
10. Piscaglia F, Leoni S, Cabibbo G, et al. Cost analysis of recall strategies for non-invasive diagnosis of small hepatocellular carcinoma. *Dig Liver Dis* 2010; 42(10):729–734.
11. Bruix J, Sherman M, Llovet JM, et al. EASL Panel of Experts on HCC. Clinical management of hepatocellular carcinoma. Conclusions of the Barcelona-2000 EASL conference. European Association for the Study of the Liver. *J Hepatol* 2001; 35(3):421–430.
12. Giesel FL, Delorme S, Sibbel R, Kauczor HU, Krix M. Contrast-enhanced ultrasound for the characterization of incidental liver lesions – an economical evaluation in comparison with multi-phase computed tomography. *Ultraschall Med* 2009; 30:259–268.
13. Albrecht T, Blomley MJ, Cosgrove DO, et al. Non-invasive diagnosis of hepatic cirrhosis by transit-time analysis of an ultrasound contrast agent. *Lancet* 1999; 353(9164): 1579–1583.
14. Lim AK, Patel N, Eckersley RJ, et al. Hepatic vein transit time of SonoVue: a comparative study with Levovist. *Radiology* 2006; 240(1):130–135.
15. Lim AK, Taylor-Robinson SD, Patel N, et al. Hepatic vein transit times using a microbubble agent can predict disease severity non-invasively in patients with hepatitis C. *Gut* 2005; 54(1):128–133.
16. Blomley MJ, Lim AK, Harvey CJ, et al. Liver microbubble transit time compared with histology and Child-Pugh score in diffuse liver disease: a cross sectional study. *Gut* 2003; 52(8):1188–1193.
17. Ryder SD. Guidelines for the diagnosis and treatment of hepatocellular carcinoma (HCC) in adults. *Gut* 2003; 52(suppl 3):iii1–8.

18. Kawada N, Ohkawa K, Tanaka S, et al. Improved diagnosis of well-differentiated hepatocellular carcinoma with gadolinium ethoxybenzyl diethylene triamine pentaacetic acid-enhanced magnetic resonance imaging and Sonazoid contrast-enhanced ultrasonography. *Hepatol Res* 2010; 40(9):930–936.
19. Korenaga K, Korenaga M, Furukawa M, Yamasaki T, Sakaida I. Usefulness of Sonazoid contrast-enhanced ultrasonography for hepatocellular carcinoma: comparison with pathological diagnosis and superparamagnetic iron oxide magnetic resonance images. *J Gastroenterol* 2009; 44(7):733–741.
20. Liu F, Wang X, Yang L, Jiang B. A novel method for preparing microbubbles targeting hepatocellular carcinoma. *Hepatogastroenterology* 2009; 56(93):1163–1168

17 Value of PET scanning

Tara D. Barwick, Imene Zerizer, Adil Al-Nahhas

Imperial College Health Care NHS Trust, London, UK

LEARNING POINTS

- FDG-PET has limited role in the detection of hepatocellular carcinoma (HCC), as it may not identify small lesions and well-differentiated HCC in particular.
- FDG-PET is a non-invasive biomarker of tumour differentiation, prognostic indicator and may detect extrahepatic metastases, thereby aiding selection of appropriate therapy.
- Dual tracer imaging with FDG-PET and tracers targeting tumour cell proliferation, cell membrane activity and amino acid transport may improve detection of HCC.

Introduction

Positron emission tomography (PET) imaging involves the intravenous administration of a small amount of short-lived radioactive tracers that emit positrons (positively charged electrons) from a parent nucleus. The tracers are bound to molecules that target different biological processes. The most widely used tracer is F-18-2-fluoro-2-deoxy-D-glucose (F-18 FDG), a glucose analogue, which is actively transported into cells via glucose transporter (GLUT) membrane receptors. FDG is phosphorylated by hexokinase to FDG-glucose-6-phophate, which has a much slower rate of dephosphorylation, compared with glucose-6-phosphate, thus it is progressively trapped within metabolically active cells (Plate 17.1). Cellular uptake of F-18 FDG is related to expression of GLUT membrane transporters and hexokinase activity, which are increased in a number of malignant processes. The distribution of tracer within the body is detected by a PET camera. Recently introduced combined PET/CT cameras permit functional PET images to be fused to a computed tomography (CT) study, acquired in the same sitting.

To date, FDG-PET has been shown to be beneficial for the staging, monitoring response to therapy and detection of recurrent disease in a variety of cancers. The role of FDG-PET in the management of HCC patients is controversial and has not been fully established. This chapter covers the current evidence for the use of FDG-PET in detection and staging of HCC, selection of patients for liver transplant, response to therapy and detection of recurrent disease. The use of new tracers and dual tracer imaging is also discussed.

FDG-PET and HCC

Diagnosis and staging of HCC

Diagnostic confirmation and accurate assessment of the extent of disease are paramount for the selection of appropriate management for patients with HCC. Currently, dynamic CT and magnetic resonance imaging (MRI), which are discussed in the preceding chapters, are widely accepted in this regard.

There are variable reports of the sensitivity of FDG-PET for the detection of primary untreated HCC above background liver levels, ranging from 50% to 70% in early case cohorts performed on PET only scanners [1–3]. Trojan and colleagues assessed 14 patients with HCC of which 7/14 (50%) demonstrated increased tracer uptake [2]. Extrahepatic disease was detected in 3/7. Khan and co-workers reported a sensitivity of 55% (11/20), compared with 90% detected by dynamic contrast-enhanced CT. However, 5%

Clinical Dilemmas in Primary Liver Cancer, First Edition. Edited by Roger Williams and Simon D. Taylor-Robinson.

of tumours and extrahepatic metastases in three patients were visualised on PET and not CT [1]. Delbeke and coworkers assessed uptake of FDG in 120 patients with a variety of liver lesions (all greater than 1 cm), 23 of which had proven HCC. Of these, 16/23 (70%) had increased tracer uptake above background liver [3]. The higher detection rate in this series may relate in part to the lesions all being greater than 1 cm and the degree of tumour differentiation.

A recent study using PET/CT reported sensitivity for detection of primary HCC in 90 patients of 60.9% and, in relation to tumour differentiation and size of lesion, 27.2%, 47.8% and 92.8% in index lesions sized 1–2 cm, 2–5 cm and >5 cm, respectively [4].

Limited detection of small lesions is a known technical limitation of PET, related to spatial resolution of the camera, partial volume effects and respiratory motion, as mentioned later in the pitfalls section. However, the size limitation means PET is not reliable for the morphological distinction between small HCCs, regenerative nodules and pre-malignant dysplastic nodules.

The differences in FDG avidity may be explained by levels of glucose-6-phosphatase, which converts FDG-6-P to FDG (Plate 17.1). In general, high levels of glucose-6-phosphatase are present in normal liver and low levels in metastatic liver lesions, leading to increased FDG-6-phosphate accumulation in metastatic liver lesions, compared with background normal liver.

However, the activity of glucose-6-phosphatase within HCCs is variable and related to the degree of differentiation. Well-differentiated HCCs have high levels of glucose-6-phosphatase, leading to dephosphorylation of F-18 FDG and thus low FDG avidity escaping detection, compared with poorly differentiated HCCs that have low levels of glucose-6-phosphatase and tend to be FDG avid [1]. The level of FDG tracer uptake has been shown to relate to degree of tumour differentiation with poorly differentiated aggressive HCC taking up FDG more avidly [5].

Detection of extrahepatic metastases

One of the main advantages of PET over other imaging modalities is that it provides whole body imaging, allowing the detection of multifocal and extrahepatic disease. Although extrahepatic disease is relatively uncommon, especially for well-differentiated tumours, its detection can significantly change management. Several of the studies assessing FDG-PET for diagnosis and staging of HCC have reported unexpected extrahepatic metastases [1–3]. In a study of 19 patients suspected of having extrahepatic disease (14 patients by conventional CT, MRI or ultrasound; 5 patients by raised tumour markers, conventional studies negative), the detection rate of FDG-PET was 83% (24 out of 29) for metastases with lesions greater than 1 cm [6]. Nagaoka and colleagues also reported that PET alone detected 52 of 58 (89.6%) extrahepatic metastases [7]. A recent study by Kawaoka and colleagues compared the efficacy of PET/CT with multidetector CT (MDCT) for the detection of lung, lymph node and bone metastases in 34 consecutive HCC patients diagnosed with extrahepatic metastases [8]. MDCT was more sensitive than PET/CT for the detection of lung metastases; both performed equally well for nodal metastases, but bone metastases were more accurately detected by PET/CT [8]. Of note, the three false negative lung metastases were <8 mm in size. HCC bone metastases are typically osteolytic and it has been documented in breast and lung cancer that FDG-PET is more sensitive than bone scintigraphy for detection of osteolytic metastases.

Wudel and colleagues reported that FDG-PET lead to a change in management in 26 of 91 (28%) HCC patients, including detection of unsuspected metastatic disease and monitoring response to hepatic-directed therapy [9]. Their population included both staging and suspected recurrence patients.

Dual time point imaging (at the normal 60–90 minutes post-tracer injection and delayed at 3 hours) has been reported to improve detection of malignant solitary pulmonary nodules, as malignant lesions tend to accumulate FDG over time. This method could potentially improve sensitivity.

FDG-PET as a prognostic indicator

In post-operative HCC patients various factors based on pathological evaluation such as the presence of microvascular invasion, poor histological differentiation and satellite lesions may predict tumour recurrence [10]. However, there is a need for a non-invasive indicator of tumour viability and predictor of prognosis, especially in patients after non-operative therapy. Pre-operative FDG-PET has been shown to predict tumour differentiation and outcome after liver resection [11,12].

Pre-operative FDG-PET in 120 patients was predictive of tumour differentiation, p-glycoprotein expression (a marker of chemoresistance) and outcome post-surgery [5]. The level of metabolic activity, using the semi-quantitative measure, standardised uptake value (SUV), was significantly higher in poorly differentiated HCCs (10.1 ± 6.5) than in well-differentiated HCCs (3.4 ± 1.4; $p = 0.001$) or moderately differentiated HCCs (4.5 ± 1.8; $p < 0.0001$). The outcomes of patients with a high SUV and a high tumour to non-tumour SUV ratio (TNR) were worse than those with a low SUV and a low TNR.

A further study in 31 patients who underwent pre-operative FDG-PET reported SUV ratio to relate to disease-related death [11]. The overall survival was significantly longer in the lower SUV ratio group than in the higher SUV ratio group (5-year survival rate: 63% vs. 29%; $p = 0.006$). PET could potentially stratify patients for closer post-operative surveillance or adjuvant treatment.

Pre-liver transplant

HCC is a major indication for liver transplantation and appropriate selection of patients can be challenging. Recently, in a retrospective single centre study of 43 patients, a positive PET pre-transplant was predictive of microvascular invasion and tumour recurrence post-liver transplantation: HCC recurrence rate was 50% in PET +ve versus 3.8% in PET −ve [13]. Furthermore, patients with tumours beyond the Milan criteria and negative pre-operative PET had a 3-year recurrence free survival (80%), comparable to tumours meeting the Milan criteria (94%) and significantly better than tumours beyond Milan criteria with a positive PET (35%) [13]. This suggests a subset of patients with advanced HCC may benefit from liver transplantation because of biological low aggression behaviour of the tumour, which may be identified by PET. As such, PET may act as a non-invasive biomarker of tumour aggressiveness and potentially may optimise selection of patients for liver transplant.

Response to therapy of HCC

Treatment modalities are discussed in detail in Part V of the book. In general, tumour resection and liver transplantation achieve the best outcomes in well-selected candidates. In non-operative patients, therapies include transcatheter arterial chemoembolisation (TACE), selective internal radiation therapy with yttrium-90 microspheres and transcatheter arterial infusion (TAI) chemotherapy for relatively large/advanced HCC, radiofrequency ablation (RFA) and percutaneous ethanol injection for small HCC. For patients with distant metastases, systemic chemotherapy and novel targeted therapy such as sorafenib, a multitargeted tyrosine kinase inhibitor may be employed. Traditionally, radiological response assessment post-therapy has relied on the Response Evaluation Criteria in Solid tumours (RECIST), which is primarily based on changes in tumour size (CT, MRI and contrast ultrasound discussed in Chapters 14 and 15). Recently, tumour enhancement quantified with Hounsfield units (HU) on CT has also been proposed as a means of assessing response following vascular interventional therapies and RFA.

In a comparative study in 30 patients of FDG-PET post-TACE and histopathology, increased or similar uptake relative to normal liver post-chemoembolisation was suggestive of residual viable tumour, while decreased or absent FDG uptake indicated more than 90% necrosis [14]. Thus PET may predict tumour viability post-interventional therapy.

A study of 33 lesions in 24 patients comparing FDG-PET to contrast-enhanced CT for detection of tumour recurrence post-RFA reported earlier detection with PET and a higher overall detection rate (92% for FDG-PET vs. 75% for CT) [15]. However, the optimal timing of PET post-local interventions, such as RFA, has not been established as post-treatment inflammatory response can mimic residual disease.

New functional techniques, such as elastography and contrast-enhanced ultrasound, perfusion imaging and diffusion-weighted MRI, are developing in parallel to PET/CT and the role of these in the detection and characterisation of small tumours in particular shall be evaluated in future.

Non-FDG-PET tracers

The above discussion highlights the fact that metabolic imaging with F-18 FDG is not ideal for routine diagnosis and management of patients with HCC. This is due to the fact that increased glycolysis is not the preferred kinetic pathway for this tumour, which may demonstrate a rate of glycolysis that is similar or even less than surrounding liver tissue [1]. Therefore, the search has continued to find an ideal PET radiopharmaceutical that specifically targets HCC cells and can be routinely used for diagnosis as well as staging and monitoring response to therapy.

Other F-18 labelled tracers were used to evaluate HCC. F-18 fluorthymidine (FLT) is well established in oncology to target proliferative components of tumours rather than detecting increased glycolysis. Eckel and colleagues examined the utility of F-18 FLT in a group of 16 patients with

HCC and reported a sensitivity of 69%. They also suggested a prognostic value in that high initial uptake of F-18 FLT was associated with reduced overall survival but the small sample number rendered this as statistically insignificant [16].

Carbon-11 radiopharmaceuticals

Carbon-11 (C-11) is another positron emitter that has been used in oncological imaging. Despite its short half-life of 20 minutes (necessitating the presence of an on-site cyclotron), it has excellent radiochemical characteristics in being easily labelled with a number of compounds and amino acids that reflect tumour activity including acetate, choline and methionine.

C-11 acetate has been used in the diagnosis of urological tumours, such as prostate cancer. It enters the Krebs cycle as a substrate for β-oxidation in fatty acid and cholesterol synthesis, and the former is thought to be the main factor affecting its uptake by HCC (Plate 17.2). The first attempt to use C-11 acetate in the evaluation of HCC was done by Ho and colleagues [17]. These authors described their findings in 57 patients with liver masses, including 39 HCC, 3 cholangiocarcinoma, 10 liver metastases and 5 benign masses. All patients underwent PET imaging with F-18 FDG and C-11 acetate and the results of both imaging tests were compared with histology. Patients who had three or less HCC lesions were detected with a high sensitivity of 87.3% by C-11 acetate, compared with 47.3% for F-18 FDG. All HCC tumours were detected by the combined use of both tracers, suggesting that they are complementary to each other. As anticipated, histopathological correlation suggested that well-differentiated HCC were better detected by C-11 acetate and poorly differentiated HCC by F-18 FDG. Interestingly, non-HCC tumours and benign lesions were not detected by C-11 acetate. However, another group documented the finding of one false positive case amongst 18 patients with HCC (5.5%), but confirmed a good sensitivity of 78% in detecting true lesions [18].

In another study by the former group [19], with the improved technique of PET/CT, the value of both tracers in detecting extrahepatic metastases was tested in 121 patients. The results showed that ^{18}F-FDG was better in detecting extrahepatic metastases. Dual tracer imaging was very effective in identifying candidates for curative therapy with a negative predictive value of 90% (19/21). The false negative cases with dual tracer imaging were in very small lung lesions and sub-centimetre mediastinal lymph nodes. A similarly designed PET/CT study, involving 99 patients with HCC, confirmed a better sensitivity of F-18 FDG to detect extrahepatic metastases with a tendency for both tracers to miss small lesions [4].

C-11 choline is another C-11 labelled radiopharmaceutical that has been tried in this respect. Choline is a water-soluble nutrient related to the B-complex vitamins that is incorporated into cell membrane phospholipids. Tumours with increased metabolism of cell membrane components can demonstrate increased choline uptake and this is the basis for its use in HCC. In a comparative animal model PET study, Salem and colleagues used F-18 FDG, C-11 acetate and C-11 choline and found that C-11 choline was positive in 5/5 HCC lesions that were well differentiated [20]. Yamamoto and colleagues [21] studied the utility of C-11 choline PET in 12 patients with HCC and compared the results with F-18 FDG PET. The sensitivity of C-11 choline was slightly better than that of F-18 FDG (63% vs. 50%). They confirmed the tendency of C-11 choline to detect moderately differentiated tumours, compared with poorly differentiated types (75% vs. 25%) in contrast with F-18 FDG (42% vs. 75%). Their conclusion was that both tracers should be used together to achieve better results.

C-11 methionine, an essential amino acid that reflects increased amino acid transport and protein synthesis, can be utilised as a tumour marker. Zhao and colleagues examined its usefulness to differentiate HCC from granulomas, induced in a rat model, and compared the findings with those obtained with F-18 FDG and F-18 FLT PET. They found that uptake of C-11 methionine was significantly reduced in granulomas, compared with HCC, unlike uptake of F-18 FDG and F-18 FLT, which were unable to differentiate between the two [22].

As mentioned above, the clinical use of C-11 labelled radiopharmaceuticals has been limited by its short half-life and reduced routine availability, compared with F-18 products, and efforts to replace the latter with the former have been achieved lately with the labelling of choline.

F-18 choline was evaluated by Talbot and colleagues in 34 patients with HCC and was shown to have significantly higher site-based sensitivity of 94%, compared with 59% for F-18 FDG at detecting HCC, particularly in well-differentiated forms [23]. This combination of a suitable positron emitter and HCC-specific ligand is likely to be pursued (Figure 17.1) as the ideal imaging approach, but further studies are still awaited.

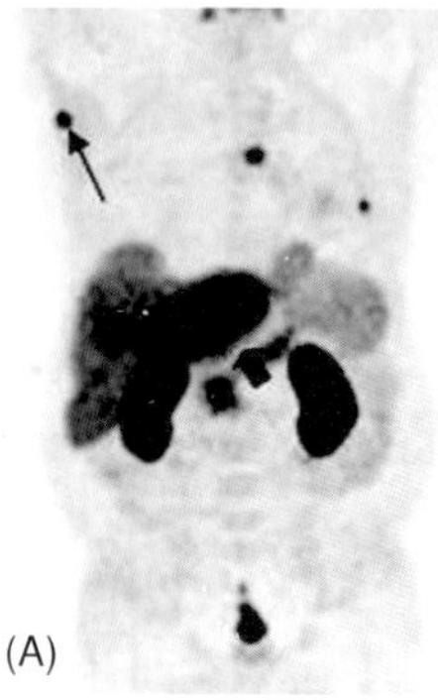
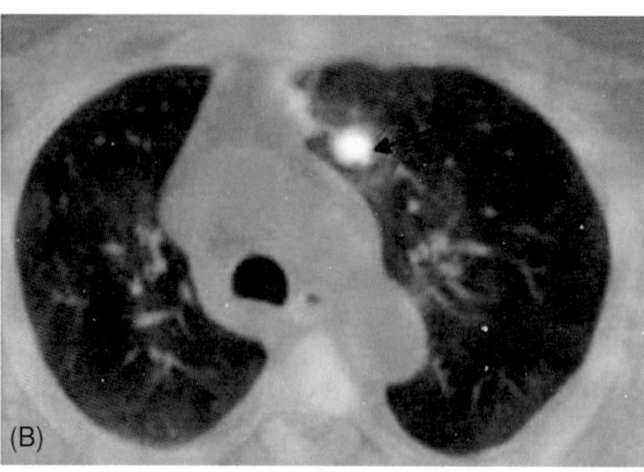

FIG 17.1 F-18 choline PET/CT study of a patient previously treated for HCC. (A) Coronal PET image demonstrates disease in axillary lymph nodes (arrow) and pulmonary metastases. Note the increased tracer uptake in the primary lesion in the left lobe of the liver (arrow). (B) Fused PET/CT image of the active pulmonary nodule in the anterior segment of the left upper lobe (arrow). (Image courtesy of Dr. D. Rubello.)

Angiogenesis tracers are under development, which have yet to be evaluated in HCC, but may be beneficial given the neo-angiogenesis, which is associated with HCCs, particularly if dynamic imaging is employed.

Pitfalls

All PET tracers have reduced sensitivity for detection of small lesions (<8–10 mm), because of the limited spatial resolution of the camera. Furthermore, because the PET acquisition takes approximately 2–4 minutes per bed position (approximately 20 minutes per scan), compared with the CT scan, which is acquired in a matter of seconds, PET is subject to artefacts, secondary to patient movement and respiratory motion. Respiratory motion can be particularly problematic close to the hemi-diaphragm and limits the sensitivity for small liver lesions, especially close to the dome of the liver. Both the CT scan and PET are generally acquired during free respiration to reduce fusion artefacts. In future, advances in PET technology that permit quicker imaging and respiratory gating methods may reduce motion artefacts. A further pitfall for FDG-PET is that FDG is non-specific for malignancy and increased glucose metabolism in inflammatory conditions can cause false positive findings.

Summary

The sensitivity of FDG-PET for HCC is insufficient for accurate detection and staging, but it may act as an adjunct to anatomical methods as a non-invasive biomarker of tumour differentiation, prognostic indicator and in the detection of extrahepatic metastases. In FDG avid tumours, PET imaging may have a role in response assessment after treatment with TACE or RFA.

Other F-18 and C-11 PET radiopharmaceuticals have been used in the assessment of HCC. C-11 is easily labelled with ligands that highlight tumour cell proliferation, cell membrane activity and amino acid transport, such as acetate, choline and methionine with better results compared with F-18 FDG. Furthermore, dual tracer imaging with F-18 FDG appears to be complimentary. However, the routine use of C-11 is logistically limited, and the recent success in labelling choline with F-18 may pave the way for better imaging of HCC that, in addition to diagnostic value, may aid in staging and assessing response to therapy.

References

1. Khan MA, Combs CS, Brunt EM, et al. Positron emission tomography scanning in the evaluation of hepatocellular carcinoma. *J Hepatol* 2000; 32(5):792–797.
2. Trojan J, Schroeder O, Raedle J, et al. Fluorine-18 FDG positron emission tomography for imaging of hepatocellular carcinoma. *Am J Gastroenterol* 1999; 94(11):3314–3319.
3. Delbeke D, Martin WH, Sandler MP, Chapman WC, Wright JK, Jr., Pinson CW. Evaluation of benign vs malignant hepatic lesions with positron emission tomography. *Arch Surg* 1998; 133(5):510–515.
4. Park JW, Kim JH, Kim SK, et al. A prospective evaluation of 18F-FDG and 11C-acetate PET/CT for detection of primary and metastatic hepatocellular carcinoma. *J Nucl Med* 2008; 49(12):1912–1921.
5. Seo S, Hatano E, Higashi T, et al. Fluorine-18 fluorodeoxyglucose positron emission tomography predicts tumor differentiation, P-glycoprotein expression, and outcome after resection in hepatocellular carcinoma. *Clin Cancer Res* 2007; 13(2 Pt 1):427–433.

6. Sugiyama M, Sakahara H, Torizuka T, et al. 18F-FDG PET in the detection of extrahepatic metastases from hepatocellular carcinoma. *J Gastroenterol* 2004; 39(10):961–968.
7. Nagaoka S, Itano S, Ishibashi M, et al. Value of fusing PET plus CT images in hepatocellular carcinoma and combined hepatocellular and cholangiocarcinoma patients with extrahepatic metastases: preliminary findings. *Liver Int* 2006; 26(7):781–788.
8. Kawaoka T, Aikata H, Takaki S, et al. FDG positron emission tomography/computed tomography for the detection of extrahepatic metastases from hepatocellular carcinoma. *Hepatol Res* 2009; 39(2):134–142.
9. Wudel LJ, Jr., Delbeke D, Morris D, et al. The role of [18F]fluorodeoxyglucose positron emission tomography imaging in the evaluation of hepatocellular carcinoma. *Am Surg* 2003; 69(2):117–124.
10. Higashi T, Hatano E, Ikai I, et al. FDG PET as a prognostic predictor in the early post-therapeutic evaluation for unresectable hepatocellular carcinoma. *Eur J Nucl Med Mol Imaging* 2010; 37(3):468–482.
11. Hatano E, Ikai I, Higashi T, et al. Preoperative positron emission tomography with fluorine-18-fluorodeoxyglucose is predictive of prognosis in patients with hepatocellular carcinoma after resection. *World J Surg* 2006; 30(9):1736–1741.
12. Seo S, Hatano E, Higashi T, et al. Fluorine-18 fluorodeoxyglucose positron emission tomography predicts tumor differentiation, P-glycoprotein expression, and outcome after resection in hepatocellular carcinoma. *Clin Cancer Res* 2007; 13(2 Pt 1):427–433.
13. Kornberg A, Freesmeyer M, Barthel E, et al. 18F-FDG-uptake of hepatocellular carcinoma on PET predicts microvascular tumor invasion in liver transplant patients. *Am J Transplant* 2009; 9(3):592–600.
14. Torizuka T, Tamaki N, Inokuma T, et al. Value of fluorine-18-FDG-PET to monitor hepatocellular carcinoma after interventional therapy. *J Nucl Med* 1994; 35(12):1965–1969.
15. Paudyal B, Oriuchi N, Paudyal P, et al. Early diagnosis of recurrent hepatocellular carcinoma with 18F-FDG PET after radiofrequency ablation therapy. *Oncol Rep* 2007; 18(6):1469–1473.
16. Eckel F, Herrmann K, Schmidt S, et al. Imaging of proliferation in hepatocellular carcinoma with the in vivo marker 18F-fluorothymidine. *J Nucl Med* 2009; 50(9):1441–1447.
17. Ho CL, Yu SC, Yeung DW. 11C-acetate PET imaging in hepatocellular carcinoma and other liver masses. *J Nucl Med* 2003; 44(2):213–221.
18. Li S, Beheshti M, Peck-Radosavljevic M, et al. Comparison of (11)C-acetate positron emission tomography and (67)Gallium citrate scintigraphy in patients with hepatocellular carcinoma. *Liver Int* 2006; 26(8):920–927.
19. Ho CL, Chen S, Yeung DW, Cheng TK. Dual-tracer PET/CT imaging in evaluation of metastatic hepatocellular carcinoma. *J Nucl Med* 2007; 48(6):902–909.
20. Salem N, Kuang Y, Wang F, Maclennan GT, Lee Z. PET imaging of hepatocellular carcinoma with 2-deoxy-2[18F]fluoro-D-glucose, 6-deoxy-6[18F] fluoro-D-glucose, [1-11C]-acetate and [N-methyl-11C]-choline. *Q J Nucl Med Mol Imaging* 2009; 53(2):144–156.
21. Yamamoto Y, Nishiyama Y, Kameyama R, et al. Detection of hepatocellular carcinoma using 11C-choline PET: comparison with 18F-FDG PET. *J Nucl Med* 2008; 49(8):1245–1248.
22. Zhao S, Kuge Y, Kohanawa M, et al. Usefulness of 11C-methionine for differentiating tumors from granulomas in experimental rat models: a comparison with 18F-FDG and 18F-FLT. *J Nucl Med* 2008; 49(1):135–141.
23. Talbot JN, Fartoux L, Balogova S, et al. Detection of hepatocellular carcinoma with PET/CT: a prospective comparison of 18F-fluorocholine and 18F-FDG in patients with cirrhosis or chronic liver disease. *J Nucl Med* 2010; 51(11):1699–1706.

PART 5
Can Treatment be Tailored to the Patient?

18 Who could benefit from chemoembolisation?

Gisèle N'Kontchou[1], Olivier Seror[1,2], Michel Beaugrand[1,2]

[1]Hôpital Jean Verdier, Bondy, France
[2]Université Paris XIII, France

LEARNING POINTS

- Chemoembolisation is a widely used palliative treatment of hepatocellular carcinoma (HCC) that associates intra-arterial injection of cytotoxic drugs with Lipiodol followed by embolisation using Gelfoam particles
- The proper role of cytotoxic agents in this setting has never been demonstrated. Ischaemia of the tumour due to embolisation by Gelfoam particles and Lipiodol is likely to be the main mechanism of tumoural response
- Several small-sized randomised studies have shown that the procedure induces tumoural necrosis and delays portal vein invasion. The effect on tumoural growth seems particularly clear in well-circumscribed hypervascularised tumours of medium size and when a selective or hyperselective approach is used
- The main contraindications to chemoembolisation are inadequate portal flow particularly portal vein thrombosis and liver failure
- Chemoembolisation has numerous side effects and complications. In patients with cirrhosis it may lead to decompensation and liver failure with progressive liver atrophy when the procedures are repeated
- The overall influence of chemoembolisation on survival is still controversial as results are different from one study to another. As a whole the benefit seems more important in Asia in patients with HBV liver disease. Studies including a majority of patients with alcoholic cirrhosis have provided disparate results
- New promising related techniques have been reported, mainly embolisation by doxorubicin-eluding beads and internal radiotherapy with yttrium-90. These techniques have been credited of lesser secondary effects and could achieve more complete responses. Both are costly and failed up to now to demonstrate a survival benefit in comparison to chemoembolisation

Introduction

Chemoembolisation is the most widely used treatment in patients with HCC. Millions of procedures, particularly in Asia, have been performed since it was introduced more than 20 years ago. Therefore, it is paradoxical that the benefits of this treatment, in terms of survival, are still uncertain and that patients who could benefit from this procedure are difficult to define. At first glance, several reasons could be advocated to explain this unsustainable failure: the heterogeneity of techniques used and, mostly, the heterogeneity of the patients, who differ not only in their tumour's characteristics and behaviour, but also in the nature and severity of the underlying liver disease, which can influence sensitivity to ischaemia of the non-tumorous liver and, more hypothetically, of the tumour itself. Further, chemoembolisation is performed in countries, where the main causes of HCC are markedly different. Not surprisingly, results differ according to the different countries. If one considers that only a few randomised trials have been published and that no meta-analysis has been performed that takes into account all the individual data, one can see why the answer to this question remains largely empirical.

Clinical Dilemmas in Primary Liver Cancer, First Edition. Edited by Roger Williams and Simon D. Taylor-Robinson.

Rational basis, limitations and potential deleterious effects of chemoembolisation

The most common procedure for transarterial chemoembolisation (TACE) is the injection of an anticancer drug, mixed with Lipiodol into the hepatic artery or one of its branches, followed by arterial embolisation using Gelfoam particles or powder. The rationale for embolisation is to induce selective tumoural ischaemia because as the tumour grows in size, the HCC nodule shifts its blood supply from the portal vein to the hepatic-artery vessels. Lipiodol is an oily contrast medium, which contributes to the embolisation of arterial vessels inside the tumour, and helps retain the cytotoxic drugs [1]. The most commonly used anticancer drugs in this setting are Adriamycin and cisplatin, which are delivered via the hepatic artery to enhance their concentration in the tumour and obviate systemic effects. They are also supposed, when mixed with Lipiodol, to form a stable mixture that stay in close contact with the tumoural cells for days or weeks. The limitations to this ideal scenario are the following: (a) some HCCs, and particularly the most malignant, are insensitive to ischaemia, (b) most HCCs are resistant to doxorubicin and cisplatin, as well as to other cytotoxic drugs, and (c) the mixture of Lipiodol with amphiphilic drugs is unstable, and they are released very rapidly to the general circulation, inducing systemic toxicity (d) the procedure of embolisation leads to increased serum growth and angiogenic factors that may accelerate tumoural growth [2], (e) spread of tumoural cells into the general circulation may occur [3], and increase the rate of metastasis (f) the non-tumorous liver, particularly in cases of cirrhosis, is not insensitive to arterial ischaemia, and embolisation can lead to decompensation and liver failure [4].

What is consensual concerning chemoembolisation?

TACE can induce partial or, rarely, macroscopically complete tumour necrosis, as assessed by examination of resected liver specimens [5]. However, complete necrosis at histology is exceptional, and when results are evaluated by a computed tomography (CT)-scan, there is often overestimation of the extent of necrosis [5]. The 'capture' of Lipiodol by the tumour, which is associated with a good response, precludes using CT to evaluate the active remnants characterised by persistent vascularity, as it is masked by Lipiodol. Magnetic resonance imaging (MRI) is certainly more reliable in this setting [6], but is still rarely performed. Randomised studies have brought some objective data: the French cooperative trial showed that a significant decrease in active tumoural mass was observed in 50% of treated patients and an increase in 9% versus 50% in control subjects. In the same trial, a decrease in incidence of portal obstruction was also demonstrated, occurring in 7% of treated patients versus 27% of controls [4]. Overall, therefore, there is no doubt regarding the reality of an antitumour effect.

The second point of consensus is that TACE can be detrimental to liver function, particularly in cases of cirrhosis, and may lead to severe decompensation.

Marelli et al., in 2007, reported on data from the literature that the mean incidence of complications following TACE was liver failure in 13.6%, ascites in 14.7%, encephalopathy in 3.6%, renal failure in 1.8%, digestive bleed and abscesses [7]. Retrograde embolisation of the arteries of neighbouring organs may also lead to pancreatitis, cholecystitis or ischaemic damage to the digestive tract [8]. In the French cooperative trial, hepatic decompensation manifest as either ascites or encephalopathy was observed in 12% of cases [4]. Yamashita et al. also suggested that repeat courses of TACE could induce progressive liver atrophy [9].

The need to select patients for TACE, and the recognition of its contraindications, are universally admitted, although important discrepancies exist between authors. The major contraindications identified to avoid massive necrosis of the non-tumoural liver comprise inadequate portal flow as a result of portal obstruction, an arterio-portal fistula or hepato-fugal flow, and liver failure. The Child-Pugh class, serum bilirubin, prothrombin time and serum AST activity seem to be the most predictive parameters for decompensation [10,11] and it is well admitted, although not universally, that patients without cirrhosis or Child-Pugh A cirrhosis are the most likely to tolerate chemoembolisation.

What is still subject to uncertainty?

The technique itself

The selectiveness of embolisation is a factor in terms of tumour necrosis, and in diminishing ischaemic damage to the non-tumorous liver. Hyperselective embolisation is best used on single tumours or at most on less than four tumours

[12]. This remark also applies to doxorubicin-eluting bead, which are delivered by hyperselective catheterisation. However, the choice of cytotoxic drug if any remains debatable. Amphiphilic drugs, such as doxorubicin or cisplatin, have been selected because they can be mixed with Lipiodol, but the mixture is notoriously unstable, and cytotoxic drugs can induce severe secondary effects, such as fatigue, alopecia and cytopenia with doxorubicin, and renal failure with cisplatin [7]. Doxorubicin, due to its lesser toxicity, has been increasingly used, despite the absence of any demonstration of its benefits. It has been accepted since the paper by Llovet et al. [13] that chemoembolisation is superior to embolisation because survival in patients treated by chemoembolisation has been reported superior to controls. In that study, patients treated by embolisation alone did not receive Lipiodol, which being an oily emulsion, contributes to tumoural ischaemia. Furthermore, the survival of patients treated by embolisation alone even if not superior to controls was not inferior to those treated by chemoembolisation, despite a slight imbalance in the severity of liver function in favour of the chemoembolisation group. Two randomised studies have compared chemoembolisation, with or without cytotoxic drug, and failed to demonstrate any difference [14,15]. A recent still unpublished study from the United Kingdom seems to confirm these results. The use of cytotoxic drugs is, therefore, more controversial than ever.

Periodicity of procedure

The periodicity for procedures is also a subject of debate. On the one hand, the treatment must be repeated in cases of recurrence or an incomplete result; on the other hand, the repetition of procedures can lead to liver failure in cirrhotic patients. Moreover, the hope of preventing the growth of small satellite nodules seems unrealistic, as the smallest nodules are less prone to necrosis [6,13]. It is generally admitted that one or two procedures have to be performed according to the number and location of tumours and that subsequent procedures are indicated only in cases of recurrent tumoural growth when a significant antitumoural effect has been documented.

Criteria of selection for obtaining a tumoural response

Two conditions (hypervascularised and tumour size > 1 cm) are needed to expect a significant antitumoural effect. Very small nodules are poorly responsive [5]. Hypovascular HCCs are usually extremely malignant and have a rapidly unfavourable outcome, which seems uninfluenced by chemoembolisation. Very large tumours respond suboptimaly, probably because they are vascularised by many arterial pedicles, which preclude performing selective or hyperselective embolisation. Infiltrative forms are considered poorly sensitive. The best candidates for chemoembolisation would be medium-sized well-circumscribed hypervascularised tumours in limited number. But these tumours would better be treated by radiofrequency ablation (RFA) or other percutaneous treatments using a curative approach. In a recent practice-guideline update, Bruix and Sherman endorsed Barcelona Clinic Liver Cancer (BCLC) staging and recommended chemoembolisation in patients with Child-Pugh A or B cirrhosis and multinodular HCC, without portal invasion [16]. It is noteworthy that the two major randomised trials that provided the percentage of patients eligible for randomisation amongst HCC patients according to similar criteria gave the same value, i.e. both at 12% [4,13]. This percentage would be greater if patients initially eligible for curative options have secondary HCC recurrence and would then become candidates for chemoembolisation and lower if one considers the present indications for RFA.

Prognostic factors

The overall prognosis for patients with HCC is also dependent on the outcome of cirrhosis, which can be negatively influenced by repeated bouts of ischaemia. Due to limited precise data, it is difficult to identify all the factors predictive of liver decompensation. Not surprisingly, Chang et al. [10] identified several factors linked to liver function are serum bilirubin, prothrombin time and Child-Pugh class. The aetiology of the underlying liver disease could also be important. The benefit of chemoembolisation seems most striking in Chinese patients with HBV liver disease or without cirrhosis [17]. In contrast, several French randomised trials have provided negative results in terms of survival, despite significant tumour necrosis. This result is apparently due to the high rate of post-hepatic decompensation in patients with cirrhosis mainly caused by alcohol [4,18–20]. Although different techniques of embolisation were used in these trials, no benefits, in terms of survival, were demonstrated. Conversely, another trial from Barcelona demonstrated a significant benefit [13]. In the

Spanish study, the criteria for inclusion and the methods used were very similar to those of the French multicentre trial. Differences concerned the drug injected (cisplatin vs. Adriamycin), exclusion of patients with segmental portal-vein thrombosis (zero vs. very few) and, more strikingly, the cause of the underlying liver disease, which was mainly HCV in Spain. In the absence of meta-analysis taking in account individual data, the influence of underlying cirrhosis remains speculative. It is tempting to assume that HBV, HCV and alcoholic-liver disease, even when comparable in term of Child-Pugh class, are not similar. Alcoholic liver disease is usually accompanied by more extensive fibrosis, severe portal hypertension and may be more prone to ischaemic damage.

The influence of the chemoembolisation on survival

The overall influence of chemoembolisation on survival remains controversial (Table 18.1) and the most appropriate question is who could benefit? The answer to this question must take into account multiple individual parameters concerning the tumour itself, the severity of cirrhosis, portal hypertension and the cause of the underlying liver disease. A meta-analysis that takes into account these individual parameters would be needed but has not been performed and is virtually unfeasible as most randomised studies do not provide reliable and precise information. Despite the limitations, the meta-analysis performed by Llovet et al. [22], which concluded benefit survival has been widely considered as proof, these conclusions are fragile and could be different if they took the recent trial by Doffoël et al. [20] into account. Whatever the conclusions of future meta-analyses, the real question is given by the title of this chapter, who benefits? A question for which there has been no scientific answer as yet.

The absence of a definitive answer, despite the extensive number of chemoembolisation procedures performed throughout the world for the past 20 years represents a dramatic failure of the liver community.

Could new intra-arterial treatments improve the results?

The procedure of chemoembolisation has been refined, and is now more selective and less damaging to the non-tumorous liver. Recently, two promising related methods have emerged: drug-eluting beads (DEBs) and internal radiotherapy with yttrium-90.

TABLE 18.1 Randomised controlled trials comparing the overall survival between TACE and TAE vs. medical treatment for the treatment of HCC

Authors	Arms	Patients (number)	2-year survival rate	Survival benefit
Pelletier et al. [18]	TACE vs. control	21 21	24% 31%	NS
GRETCH [4]	TACE vs. control	50 46	38% 26%	NS
Pelletier et al. [19]	TACE+TMX vs. TMX	37 36	24% 26%	NS
Bruix et al. [21]	TAE vs. control	40 40	49% 50%	NS
Llovet et al. [13]	TAE vs. TACE vs. control	37 40 35	50% 63% 27%	$p = 0.02$
Lo et al. [17]	TACE vs. control	40 39	31% 11%	$p = 0.002$
Doffoël et al. [20]	TACE vs. control	62 61	25% 22%	NS

TACE, transarterial chemoembolisation; TAE, transarterial embolisation.

Chemoembolisation with drug-eluting beads

DEBs have been developed to enhance intratumoural delivery of doxorubicin and to reduce systemic side effects. In fact, the peak systemic levels of doxorubicin after DEB embolisation are approximately 5% of those after doxorubicin–Lipiodol embolisation, and levels remain stable over 7–10 days [23]. A pilot randomised controlled trial (RCT) reported a median time to disease progression of 42.2 and 36.2 weeks in patients treated with DEB–TACE and conventional TACE, respectively [24]. The large RCT study, which compared conventional TACE with DEBs, reported fewer systemic side effects from doxorubicin in patients treated with DEBs–TACE, though there was no statistically significant difference between tumour response and overall survival [25]. A beneficial effect of DEBs was observed in the subgroup of patients with more advanced cirrhosis, which may reflect the lesser toxicity of Adriamycin or less ischaemic damage to the liver because of more selective embolisation. Thus, embolisation with DEBs if used should be reserved for patients with a limited number of nodules allowing hyperselective embolisation and particularly for Child-Pugh B patients.

Internal endoarterial radiotherapy

This procedure delivers radiation to the tumour by infusion of radioactive substances embedded in glass or resin microspheres into the tumour's 'feeding' vessels. The most commonly used radioelement is yttrium-90 in microspheres. A good safety profile has been reported in observational studies. However, internal endoarterial radiotherapy (IER) is a costly and a complex procedure and is contraindicated in cases where there is significant hepatopulmonary shunting or aberrant digestive artery to prevent deposition of the radionuclide agents into the gastrointestinal tract. No RCTs have yet compared IER with TAE–TACE.

Two retrospective case-control studies have compared IER with TAE–TACE and did not observe a difference in overall survival between the two groups, despite a longer time to disease progression following IER. In the study of Salem et al. abdominal pain and increased transaminases levels were less frequently encountered in the radioembolisation group [26,27]. Except for cases of intermediate HCC (BCLC B), which have compromised portal flow or thrombosis, and perhaps patients with bilobar multifocal HCC, which can be treated in one session, the advantages of 90-Y IER over TACE are still to be defined.

Does chemoembolisation as neo-adjuvant therapy improve the results of curative treatments?

Prior to OLT

For HCC that is within the Milan criteria, the rationale for using chemoembolisation as a neo-adjuvant therapy prior to orthotopic liver transplantation (OLT) is to control tumour growth while the patient is on waiting list and for HCC outside the Milan criteria to downstage the tumour and make the patient eligible for OLT. Additionally, the response to chemoembolisation could provide information concerning the degree of malignancy of the tumour and the risk of recurrence. Although TAE–TACE can cause marked tumour necrosis and improve local control, the benefits of TAE–TACE performed systematically before OLT has not been demonstrated. No randomised controlled trials have compared the outcomes of patients with or without such neo-adjuvant therapy before OLT. Two case-control studies have shown that the high rate of tumour necrosis observed in pre-transplant TACE groups did not affect the 5-year survival and recurrence rates [28,29].

The advantage of chemoembolisation as a bridging tool to prevent dropout of patients listed for OLT remains unclear. The two prospective studies that used chemoembolisation before OLT reported a 15–46%, dropout rate with the higher rate being observed in more advanced HCCs, and when the mean waiting time was 12 months [30,31]. For HCCs within Milan criteria, pre-OLT chemoembolisation does not show any benefit if OLT is performed within 6 months. Furthermore, in this context, RFA allows better local control with a lower rate of complications.

Downstaging after chemoembolisation is observed in a small percentage of OLT candidates. Two prospective studies have reported high figures of 46% and 20%, and disease-recurrence rates after OLT of 40% and 30% in those groups. Overall disease-free and recurrence-free survival rates were not different between patients who did or did not respond to TACE [32,33]. However, for several authors one potential advantage of this sequential treatment is its ability to select patients with a good HCC profile in terms of postoperative recurrence who are those with an apparently complete response.

Prior resection

The result of three RCTs has not supported the routine use of pre-operative TAE–TACE for resectable HCCs

TABLE 18.2 Randomised controlled trials comparing the overall survival between combination therapy with TACE vs. resection alone

Authors	Arms	Patients (number)	3-year survival rate	
Wu et al. [34]	TACE+resection	24	38%	$p < 0.05$
	Resection	28	60%	
Yamasaki et al. [37]	TACE+resection	50	39%	NS
	Resection	47	31%	
Zhou et al. [36]	TACE+resection	52	40%	NS
	Resection	56	32%	

TACE, transarterial chemoembolisation.

(Table 18.2). Currently, there is no evidence that pre-TAE–TACE decreases the post-operative recurrence risk [34,36,37]. Furthermore, chemoembolisation can delay the time of resection, leading to drop out from surgery or may induce liver damage, such as perihepatic adhesions. Chemoembolisation is often performed before portal vein embolisation (PVE) as tumour progression, while non-embolised liver segments become hypertrophied, is an important issue. Because cessation of the portal flow induces a compensatory increase in arterial blood flow into embolised segments, arterio-portal shunts may attenuate the effects of PVE. Chemoembolisation before PVE has been shown to independently contribute to the atrophy and/or hypertrophy caused by PVE. Two observational studies have reported significantly increased disease-free survival of patients who received sequential selective TACE followed by PVE (performed 1–2 months after TACE), in comparison to those who received PVE alone [35,38]. However, results from such a sequential strategy have been not analysed on an intention-to-treat basis. The main advantage of this sequential management is to select the best candidates for hepatectomy.

Prior or following percutaneous treatments

To increase volume ablation, the combination of TAE–TACE with percutaneous ablation has been developed by some teams. This approach can increase the ablated zone by up to 6–7 cm. A meta-analysis of controlled trials that compared percutaneous treatment alone or combined with chemoembolisation showed a benefit of the combined treatment only, when TACE was associated with percutaneous ethanol ablation but not with RFA (Table 18.3)[44]. Improved local tumoural control and tumour-free survival rates have been reported by combining TAE–TACE with percutaneous ablation in large HCC tumours (>5 cm), but no impact on long-term survival was observed. Thus, currently, there is insufficient evidence for the systematic use of combined TACE + RFA in HCC patients, especially when the tumour is <5 cm [45]. Randomised controlled trials are ongoing 'but the development of new percutaneous techniques such as multipolar RFA that allows ablation areas more than 7 cm in diameter might be a better way of improvement'.

Finally who can benefit from chemoembolisation?

The answer to this question varies from one part of the world to another, and is subjective. There are reasons to think that patients without cirrhosis, or with well-compensated HBV cirrhosis, who are prevalent in Asia, could suffer less damage to the non-tumorous liver and benefit more from reduced tumoural growth. Conversely, the situation in Western countries is more ambiguous. According to the current criteria for patient selection, excluding those with poor general status, portal-vein thrombosis, or decompensated liver disease, results in the number of patients being reduced to 20% of all HCC cases at any time. However, this percentage does not take into account the tremendous progress made by percutaneous treatments and the fact that RFA and particularly multipolar RFA could be proposed to ablate up to three tumours of limited size and tumours larger than 5 cm in diameter with a curative purpose, as well as limited morbidity and mortality [46]. The selection of patients, based on contraindications for surgery, needs to be revisited and exclusion criteria must include all patients eligible for curative treatment, including RFA. The cause of the underlying liver disease must also be taken in account. There is no reason to rule out the results of the French trials that found an absence of benefit

TABLE 18.3 Randomised controlled trials comparing overall survival rates for combination therapy with TACE vs. percutaneous treatments

Authors	Arms	Patients (number)	Tumour size (mm)	Initial complete response	1-year survival rate	3-year survival rate	
Percutaneous ethanol injection							
Koda et al. [39]	TACE+PEI	26	≤30	ND	100%	80.8%	NS
	PEI	26		ND	91.3%	65.9%	
Francesco et al. [40]	TACE+PEI	19	54 ± 16	90%	89.5%	46%	$p < 0.05$
	TACE	21	55 ± 26	81.8%	47.6%	4.8%	
	PEI	20	52 ± 19	71.4%	50%	17.5%	
Percutaneous radiofrequency ablation							
Aikata et al. [41]	TACE+RFA	21	≤30	ND	95.2%	84%	NS
	RFA	23		ND	100%	73.9%	
Yang et al. [42]	TACE+RFA	24	66 ± 6	60.3%	68.3%	ND	
	TACE	11	64 ± 10	37.5%	53.2%	ND	
	RFA	12	52 ± 4	47.8%	57.6%	ND	
Shibata et al. [43]	TACE+RFA	46	<30	ND	100%	84.8%	NS
	RFA	43		ND	100%	84.5%	

TACE, transarterial chemoembolisation; PEI, percutaneous ethanol injection; RFA, radiofrequency ablation.

in terms of survival in those patients with cirrhosis mainly related to alcohol. However, a benefit might be expected for patients with HCV liver disease who are less prone to complications related to procedures.

Finally, the points of view expressed in this chapter cannot be considered as definitive as they represent a subjective interpretation of scarce randomised studies.

References

1. Yamashita Y, Takahashi M, Fukushima S, et al. Experimental study of hepatic artery embolization: evaluation of various embolic materials. *Radiat Med* 1987; 5:75–82.
2. Li X, Feng GS, Zheng CS, et al. Expression of plasma vascular endothelial growth factor in patients with hepatocellular carcinoma and effect of transcatheter arterial chemoembolization therapy on plasma vascular endothelial growth factor level. *World J Gastroenterol* 2004; 10:2878–2882.
3. Louha M, Poussin K, Ganne N, et al. Spontaneous and iatrogenic spreading of liver-derived cells into peripheral blood of patients with primary liver cancer. *Hepatology* 1997; 26:998–1005.
4. Groupe d'Etude et de Traitement du Carcinome Hépatocellulaire. A comparison of Lipiodol chemoembolization and conservative treatment for unresectable hepatocellular carcinoma. *N Engl J Med* 1995; 332:1256–1261.
5. Riaz A, Lewandowski RJ, Kulik L, et al. Radiologic-pathologic correlation of hepatocellular carcinoma treated with chemoembolization *Cardiovasc Intervent Radiol* 2010; 33:1143–1152.
6. Yamashita Y, Yoshimatsu S, Sumi M, et al. Dynamic MR imaging of hepatoma treated by transcatheter arterial embolization therapy. Assessment of treatment effect *Acta Radiol* 1993; 34:303–308.
7. Marelli L, Stigliano R, Triantos C, et al. Transarterial therapy for hepatocellular carcinoma: which technique is more effective? A systematic review of cohort and randomized studies. *Cardiovasc Intervent Radiol* 2007; 30:6–25.
8. Tarazov PG, Polysalov VN, Prozorovskij KV, et al. Ischemic complications of transcatheter arterial chemoembolization in liver malignancies. *Acta Radiol* 2000; 41:156–160.
9. Yamashita Y, Torashima M, Oguni T, et al. Liver parenchymal changes after transcatheter arterial embolization therapy for hepatoma: CT evaluation. *Abdom Imaging* 1993; 18:352–356.
10. Chan AO, Yuen MF, Hui CK, et al. A prospective study regarding the complications of transcatheter intraarterial lipiodol chemoembolization in patients with hepatocellular carcinoma. *Cancer* 2002; 94:1747–1752.
11. Chung JW, Park JH, Han JK, et al. Hepatic tumors: predisposing factors for complications of transcatheter oily chemoembolization. *Radiology* 1996; 198:33–40.
12. Golfieri R, Cappelli A, Cucchetti A, et al. Efficacy of selective transarterial chemoembolization in inducing tumor

necrosis in small (<5 cm) hepatocellular carcinomas. *Hepatology* 2011; 53(5):1580–1589.
13. Llovet JM, Real MI, Montana X, et al. Arterial embolisation or chemoembolisation versus symptomatic treatment in patients with unresectable hepatocellular carcinoma: a randomized controlled trial. *Lancet* 2002; 359:1734–1739.
14. Chang JM, Tzeng WS, Pan HB, et al. Transcatheter arterial embolization with or without cisplatin treatment of hepatocellular carcinoma. A randomized controlled study. *Cancer* 1994; 74:2449–2453.
15. Kawai S, Okamura J, Ogawa M, et al. Prospective and randomized clinical trial for the treatment of hepatocellular carcinoma – a comparison of lipiodol-transcatheter arterial embolization with and without adriamycin (first cooperative study). The Cooperative Study Group for Liver Cancer Treatment of Japan. *Cancer Chemother Pharmacol* 1992; 31: S1–S6.
16. Bruix J, Sherman M; Practice Guidelines Committee, American Association for the Study of Liver Diseases. Management of hepatocellular carcinoma. *Hepatology* 2005; 42:1208–1236.
17. Lo CM, Ngan H, Tso WK, et al. Randomized controlled trial of transarterial lipiodol chemoembolization for unresectable hepatocellular carcinoma. *Hepatology* 2002; 35:1164–1171.
18. Pelletier G, Roche A, Ink O, et al. A randomized trial of hepatic arterial chemoembolization in patients with unresectable hepatocellular carcinoma. *J Hepatol* 1990; 11:181–184.
19. Pelletier G, Ducreux M, Gay F, et al. Treatment of unresectable hepatocellular carcinoma with lipiodol chemoembolization: a multicenter randomized trial. *J Hepatol* 1998; 29:129–134.
20. Doffoël M, Bonnetain F, Bouché O, et al. Multicentre randomised phase III trial comparing tamoxifen alone or with transarterial lipiodol chemoembolisation for unresectable hepatocellular carcinoma in cirrhotic. *Eur J Cancer* 2008; 44:528–538.
21. Bruix J, Llovet JM, Castells A, et al. Transarterial embolization versus symptomatic treatment in patients with advanced hepatocellular carcinoma: results of a randomized, controlled trial in a single institution. *Hepatology* 1998; 27:1578–1583.
22. Llovet JM, Bruix J. Systematic review of randomized trials for unresectable hepatocellular carcinoma: Chemoembolization improves survival. *Hepatology* 2003; 37:429–442.
23. Varela M, Real MI, Burrel M, et al. Chemoembolization of hepatocellular carcinoma with drug eluting beads: efficacy and doxorubicin pharmacokinetics. *J Hepatol* 2007; 46:474–481.
24. Malagari K, Pomoni M, Spyridopoulos TN, et al. Safety Profile of Sequential Transcatheter Chemoembolization with DC Bead(TM): Results of 237 Hepatocellular Carcinoma (HCC) Patients. *Cardiovasc Intervent Radiol* 2011; 34:774–785.
25. Lammer J, Malagari K, Vogl T, et al. Prospective randomized study of doxorubicin-eluting-bead embolization in the treatment of hepatocellular carcinoma: results of the PRECISION V study. *Cardiovasc Intervent Radiol* 2010; 33:41–52.
26. Kooby DA, Egnatashvili V, Srinivasan S, et al. Comparison of yttrium-90 radioembolization and transcatheter arterial chemoembolization for the treatment of unresectable hepatocellular carcinoma. *J Vasc Interv Radiol* 2010; 21: 224–230.
27. Salem R, Lewandowski RJ, Mulcahy MF, et al. Radioembolization for hepatocellular carcinoma using Yttrium-90 microspheres: a comprehensive report of long-term outcomes. *Gastroenterology* 2010; 138:52–64.
28. Oldhafer KJ, Chavan A, Fruhauf NR, et al. Arterial chemoembolization before liver transplantation in patients with hepatocellular carcinoma: marked tumor necrosis, but no survival benefit? *J Hepatol* 1998; 29:953–959.
29. Decaens T, Roudot-Thoraval F, Bresson-Hadni S, et al. Impact of pretransplantation transarterial chemoembolization on survival and recurrence after liver transplantation for hepatocellular carcinoma. *Liver Transpl* 2005; 11:767–775.
30. Hayashi PH, Ludkowski M, Forman LM, et al. Hepatic artery chemoembolization for hepatocellular carcinoma in patients listed for liver transplantation. *Am J Transpl* 2004; 4:782–787.
31. Maddala YK, Stadheim L, Andrews JC, et al. Drop-out rates of patients with hepatocellular cancer listed for liver transplantation: outcome with chemoembolization. *Liver Transpl* 2004; 10:449–455.
32. Roayaie S, Frischer JS, Emre SH, et al. Long-term results with multimodal adjuvant therapy and liver transplantation for the treatment of hepatocellular carcinomas larger than 5 centimeters. *Ann Surg* 2002; 235:533–539.
33. Graziadei IW, Sandmueller H, Waldenberger P, et al. Chemoembolization followed by liver transplantation for hepatocellular carcinoma impedes tumor progression while on the waiting list and leads to excellent outcome. *Liver Transpl* 2003; 9:557–563.
34. Wu CC, Ho YZ, Ho WL, et al. Preoperative transcatheter arterial chemoembolization for resectable large hepatocellular carcinoma: a reappraisal. *Br J Surg* 1995; 82:122–126.
35. Yoo H, Kim JH, Ko GY, et al. Sequential transcatheter arterial chemoembolization and portal vein embolization versus portal vein embolization only before major hepatectomy for patients with hepatocellular carcinoma. *Ann Surg Oncol* 2011; 18(5):1251–1257.
36. Zhou WP, Lai EC, Li AJ, et al. A prospective, randomized, controlled trial of preoperative transarterial chemoembolization for resectable large hepatocellular carcinoma. *Ann Surg* 2009; 249:195–202.
37. Yamasaki S, Hasegawa H, Kinoshita HT, et al. A prospective randomized trial of the preventive effect of pre-operative

transcatheter arterial embolization against recurrence of hepatocellular carcinoma. *Jpn J Cancer Res* 1996; 87:206–211.

38. Ogata S, Belghiti J, Farges O et al. Sequential arterial and portal vein embolizations before right hepatectomy in patients with cirrhosis and hepatocellular carcinoma. *Br J Surg* 2006; 93:1091–1098.
39. Koda M, Murawaki Y, Mitsuda A, et al. Combination therapy with transcatheter arterial chemoembolization and percutaneous ethanol injection compared with percutaneous ethanol injection alone for patients with small hepatocellular carcinoma. *Cancer* 2001; 92:1516–1524.
40. Francesco S, Stella A, Gambacorta D, et al. Treatment of large hepatocellular carcinoma: comparison between techniques and long term results. *RadioMed* 2004; 108:356–371.
41. Aikata H, Shirakawa H, Takaki S, et al. Radiofrequency ablation combined with transcatheter arterial chemoembolization for small hepatocellular carcinoma. *Hepatology* 2006; 4:A487.
42. Yang P, Liang MH, Zhang YX, et al. Clinical application of a combination therapy of Lentinan, multi-electrode RFA and TACE in HCC. *Adv Ther* 2008; 25:787–794.
43. Shibata T, Isoda H, Hirokawa Y, et al. Small hepatocellular carcinoma: is radiofrequency ablation combined with transcatheter arterial chemoembolization more effective than radiofrequency ablation alone for treatment? *Radiology* 2009; 252:905–913.
44. Xu GH, Wen HC, Li ZW, et al. Evaluation of hepatic chemoembolization and percutaneous ethanol injection in the treatment of HCC. *Chin J Radiology* 2002; 1:66–68.
45. Wang W, Shi J, Xie WF. Transarterial chemoembolization in combination with percutaneous ablation therapy in unresectable hepatocellular carcinoma: a meta-analysis. *Liver Int* 2010; 30:741–749.
46. Seror O, N'Kontchou G, Ibraheem, et al. Large (>or= 5.0-cm) HCCs: multipolar RF ablation with three internally cooled bipolar electrodes–initial experience in 26 patients. *Radiology* 2008; 248:288–296.

19 Are drug-eluting beads worth using?

Christopher N. Hacking, Pradesh Kumar
Southampton University Hospitals NHS Trust, Southampton, UK

LEARNING POINTS

- To outline the basic principles of conventional and drug-eluting bead (DEB) transarterial chemoembolisation
- To describe the unique properties and pharmacokinetic profiles of available DEBs
- To review the current evidence comparing conventional and DEB transarterial chemoembolisation

Introduction

Hepatocellular carcinoma (HCC) is the sixth most common cancer worldwide, with more than 600,000 new cases diagnosed in 2002 [1]. It is the leading cause of death in cirrhotic patients. Historically, treatment options for HCC have been limited. While surgery can offer potential cure, it carries significant perioperative morbidity and mortality and is limited by tumour size, location and number of lesions [2,3]. Systemic chemotherapy has traditionally been the only alternative available to non-surgical candidates despite its lack of efficacy and significant toxicity profile in many patients. It is well established that HCC progression is strongly linked to neo-angiogenic activity. More importantly, it is well known that tumours, unlike healthy liver tissue, are supplied almost exclusively by hepatic arterial flow. This observation has led to active research into potential intra-arterial treatment. Over the last 20 years, transarterial chemoembolisation (TACE) has become increasingly used in patients with unresectable HCC.

Conventional TACE

Conventional TACE involves the selective intra-arterial delivery of a chemotherapeutic drug, emulsified with an oily agent such as Lipiodol (an iodised ester of poppy seed oil) with or without some other embolic agent (usually gelatin sponge or polyvinyl alcohol), into a target vessel supplying the tumour. The objective of the procedure is to deliver high concentration of drugs into the tumour and reduce the potential serious side effects seen with systemic chemotherapy. Embolic agents function to induce vascular occlusion in order to achieve tumour devascularisation, ischaemia and necrosis. Selective and/or superselective embolisation techniques using microcatheters are employed to ensure precise and safe delivery of embolic particles and preserve normal liver parenchyma. Despite the widespread use of this technique over the last two decades, their benefits in intermediate stage HCC were only recently proven with Level 1 evidence. Two randomised controlled trials showed that TACE has a significant and positive impact on survival in well-selected patients with preserved liver function when compared with supportive therapy [4,5]. In the Barcelona trial published in 2002, Llovet et al. set out to compare survival in patients treated with embolisation (with gelatin sponge) or TACE (with doxorubicin and gelatin sponge) with that of patients receiving supportive care. The study was terminated when a sequential analysis showed improvement in patients in the TACE group [5]. A systematic meta-analysis by the Barcelona group also confirmed a statistically significant survival benefit of TACE over supportive care or systemic chemotherapy [6]. Camma et al. compared overall 2-year mortality odds ratios (OR) to investigate the efficacy

Clinical Dilemmas in Primary Liver Cancer, First Edition. Edited by Roger Williams and Simon D. Taylor-Robinson.

of locoregional therapies. They pooled 13 studies involving 1777 patients who either received TACE or non-active treatment. The results demonstrated similar reduction in 2-year mortality in treated patients [7].

Drug-eluting bead-TACE

A more recent advance in locoregional therapy has been the development of DEBs. It has been shown previously that tumour extraction of chemotherapeutic drugs such as doxorubicin and 5-fluorouracil has been reported to be higher after hepatic artery infusion compared with systemic vein infusion [8]. This concept has been exploited further with the development of novel DEBs. DEBs are embolic agents that can be loaded with a chemotherapeutic drug. The two agents in common use currently are DC Beads® (Merit Medical – EMEA, Maastricht-Airport, the Netherlands) and HepaSphere™ Microspheres™ (Merit Medical – EMEA, Maastricht-Airport, the Netherlands) (Figure 19.1).

DC Beads

DC Beads or LC Beads® (USA) (Biocompatibles, UK) are polyvinyl alcohol microspheres that have the ability to sequester doxorubicin hydrochloride from solution through an ion-exchange mechanism and allow its slow and sustained release into the tumour bed whilst simultaneously inducing a calibrated arterial obstruction. DC Beads are the more widely used of these two agents. The embolisation particles are made from a unique drug-eluting technology based on a hydrogel that has been modified by a sulphonate group [9,10]. Doxorubicin binds in a stable manner to this sulphonate group. In a landmark pre-clinical study in 2006, Hong et al. elegantly designed a study to assess the pharmacokinetic profile and efficacy (tumour kill) of DEB as a new drug delivery system. In the study, DEB was found to provide a greater concentration of intratumoural doxorubicin over time, thereby maximising cytotoxic potency whilst limiting systemic toxicity when compared with conventional TACE (Figure 19.2).

DEB also resulted in a greater degree of tumour necrosis through slow, sustained elution in a locoregional fashion. There was an almost linear relationship between tumour necrosis and the 'dwell time' of DEB. More importantly, the peak plasma concentration of doxorubicin was significantly lower when administered with DEB and intra-arterially without DEB. As would be expected following conventional TACE, the DEB group demonstrated only minimal transient elevation of liver enzymes.

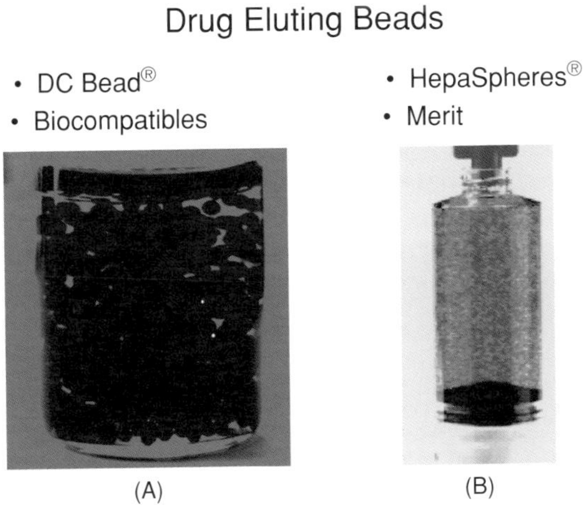

Drug Eluting Beads

- DC Bead®
- Biocompatibles

- HepaSpheres®
- Merit

(A) (B)

FIG 19.1 (A) A bottle of DC Beads or LC Beads [USA] (Biocompatibles, UK) of 100–300 μm size after mixing with doxorubicin solution. (B) A syringe of HepaSphere Microspheres [USA] (Merit Medical Systems, Inc.) of 200–400 μm microspheres after reconstitution with doxorubicin solution.

HepaSphere

HepaSphere Microspheres are expandable biocompatible microspheres made of sodium acrylate/vinyl alcohol copolymer. They differ from DC Beads in that they are sold in dehydrated form and must be reconstituted with non-ionic contrast media or physiologic saline solution before use. When exposed to aqueous media, they immediately absorb fluid and rapidly swell, the final size ranging from 200 to 800 μm. During the embolisation procedure, they conform to the occlusion site anatomy forming a moulded occlusion. The polymer contained within HepaSphere is anionic and carries a negative electrical charge. This property captures molecules with an opposite electrical charge such as doxorubicin, enabling them to act as a drug reservoir. Preliminary results from a multicentre Italian study suggest that DEB–TACE with HepaSphere is feasible, well tolerated, results in a promising tumour response and has a low complication rate [11].

Position statement for DEB–TACE

The Society of Interventional Radiology (SIR) currently recommends DEB–TACE as the first-line treatment for

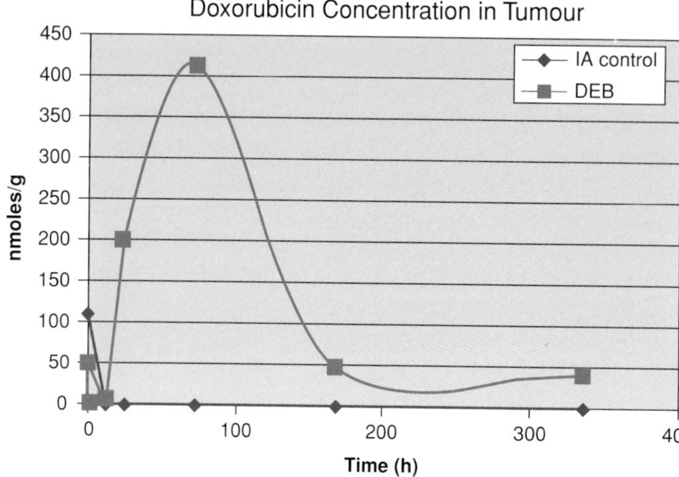

FIG 19.2 Doxorubicin levels in explanted liver tumour. In the DEB–TACE group (DEB), the greatest concentration of doxorubicin in the tumour was obtained at 3 days post-treatment and remained high at 7 days. In contrast, doxorubicin level within the tumour was nearly undetectable at all time points when administered intra-arterially (IA control). (Hong K, Khwaja A, Liapi E, et al. New intra-arterial drug delivery system for the treatment of liver cancer: preclinical assessment in a rabbit model of liver cancer. *Clin Cancer Res* 2006; 12(8): 2563–2567.)

intermediate stage inoperable HCC in patients with preserved liver function [12].

Staging of HCC

There are various staging systems for HCC, each having its own merits and weaknesses. The Barcelona Clinic Liver Cancer (BCLC) staging system is widely used in Western countries and in many clinical trials. The BCLC system (Figure 19.3) stages patients into very early stage, early stage, intermediate stage, advanced stage and end stage according to tumour size and number, vascular invasion and presence of metastases. Patients with very early and early stage are considered for curative treatment. Patients with intermediate stage, multinodular disease may be eligible for TACE. Patients with advanced stage disease with portal vein invasion or distant metastases can be considered for Sorafenib, an oral multikinase inhibitor.

Current evidence for DEB–TACE in HCC

DEB–TACE with doxorubicin-loaded DC Beads showed promising efficacy with low toxicity in a phase I/II trial in 2007 [13]. The study cohort included 35 Child-Pugh class A cirrhotics with unresectable HCC. Patients underwent two sessions of DEB–TACE over a 2-month period. In the phase I study involving 15 patients, no dose-limiting toxicity was observed up to 150 mg of doxorubicin. The peak plasma doxorubicin concentration was low and no systemic toxicity was observed. No treatment-related deaths were reported. According to the modified RECIST criteria, which also consider the volume of tumour necrosis, 19 (63.3%) patients achieved partial response while 2 (6.7%) achieved complete response.

Varela et al. reported their mid-term results concerning the safety and efficacy of DEB–TACE treatments in 27 Child-Pugh class A cirrhotic patients presenting with large or multifocal HCC [14]. Response rate was assessed with computed tomography at 6 months. DEB–TACE demonstrated an acceptable safety profile and was well tolerated. After a median follow-up of 27.6 months, the 1- and 2-year survival rates were 92.5% and 88.9%, respectively.

In a larger study in 2008, Malagari et al. studied 62 cirrhotic patients with solitary unresectable HCC. The purpose of the study was to assess the safety and efficacy of DEB–TACE. The investigators performed repeat chemoembolisations with a maximum dose of 150 mg doxorubicin loaded on to 100–300 μm microspheres at each session (maximum of 3 sessions). Follow-up was assessed using the European Association for the Study of the Liver (EASL) criteria. At 9 months, objective response (OR) was seen in 80.7%, complete response (CR) in 12.2%, progressive disease in 6.8% and stable disease in 12.2% [15].

Grosso et al. presented early results using HepaSphere Microsphere TACE in patients with unresectable HCC [11]. Fifty patients were treated with selective TACE loaded with either doxorubicin or epirubicin. Technical success was achieved in all procedures and no major complications were observed. Tumour response was evaluated according to the EASL criteria. The amended EASL criteria are an

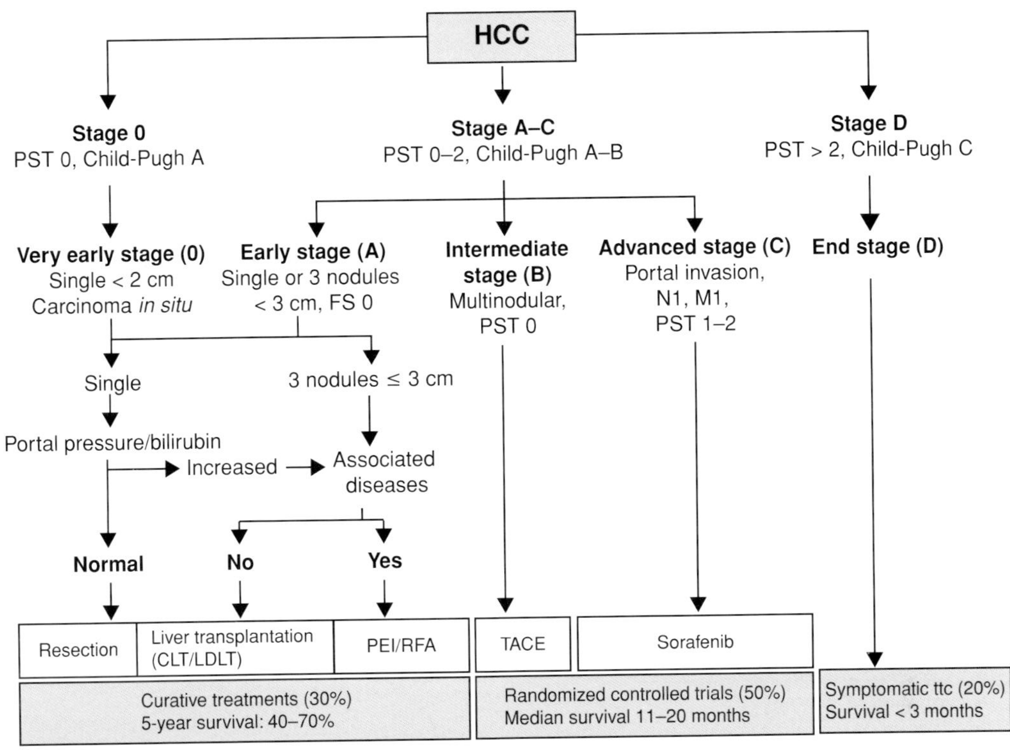

FIG 19.3 BCLC staging. BCLC, Barcelona Clinic Liver Cancer; PST, performance status; CLT, cadaveric liver transplantation; LDLT, living donor liver transplantation; PEI, percutaneous ethanol injection; RFA, radiofrequency ablation; TACE, transcatheter arterial chemoembolisation.

accepted method for assessing tumour necrosis following locoregional treatment [16]. At 6-month follow-up of 31 patients, complete tumour response was achieved in 16 of 31 (51.6%), partial response in 8 of 31 (25.8%) and progressive disease in 7 of 31 (22.6%) of patients. This initial Italian multicentre trial demonstrated that TACE with HepaSphere is feasible, well tolerated, has a low complication rate and is associate with a promising tumour response rate.

The PRECISION V trial is the first prospective, randomised controlled trial comparing the safety profile and efficacy of DEB–TACE with conventional TACE (cTACE) [17]. Two hundred and twelve patients with Child-Pugh A/B cirrhosis and large and/or multinodular unresectable HCC were randomised to receive either conventional TACE or doxorubicin-loaded DEB–TACE. The primary endpoint was 6-month tumour response rate according to the dimensions of residual viable tumour following independent blinded review of magnetic resonance imaging studies. The DEB–TACE group showed greater rates of complete response, objective response and disease control compared with the cTACE group (27% vs. 22%, 52% vs. 44% and 63% vs. 52%, respectively). Patients with Childs-Pugh B, bilobar disease and recurrent disease showed a significant response in objective response ($p = 0.038$) when compared with cTACE. Despite administration of a higher mean total dose, DEB–TACE resulted in a significant reduction in serious liver toxicity ($p < 0.001$) and doxorubicin side effects ($p = 0.0001$) compared with cTACE.

Current areas of research

The TACE-2 trial is an international, multicentre, randomised, placebo-controlled, double-blind, phase III trial of sorafenib in combination with doxorubicin-loaded DC Bead TACE. The trial aims to recruit a total of 412 patients. The primary outcome measure will be progression free survival.

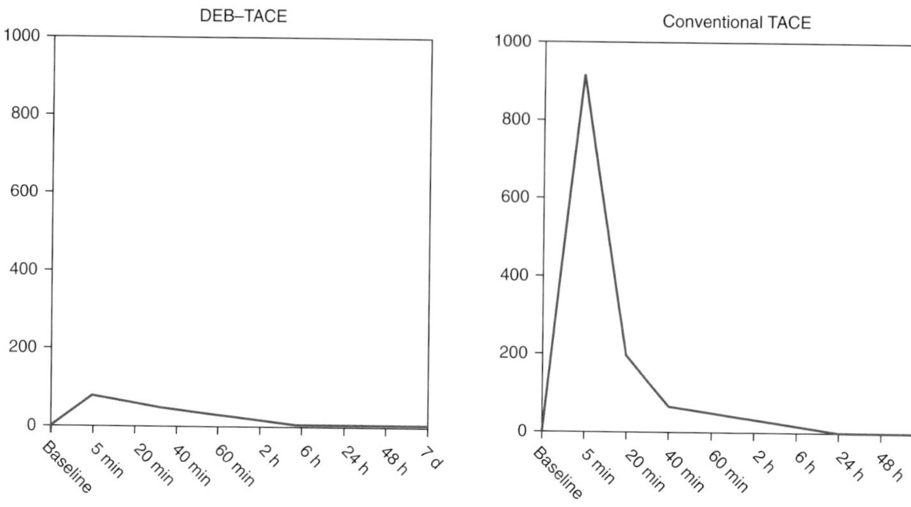

FIG 19.4 Pharmacokinetics of doxorubicin concentration in plasma. (Varela M, Real MI, Brunet M, et al. Chemoembolization of hepatocellular carcinoma with drug eluting beads: efficacy and doxorubicin pharmacokinetics. *J Hepatol* 2007; 46(3): 474–481.)

The sorafenib or placebo in combination with TACE for intermediate HCC (SPACE) trial is a phase II, randomized, double-blind, placebo-controlled study. The trial aims to assess the efficacy and tolerability of sorafenib as combination treatment in intermediate HCC. Their primary study endpoint will be time to progression (18).

The HiQuality Study (HepaSphere/QuadraSphere in Liver Cancer Treatment) is the first multinational phase III trial in the United States comparing HepaSphere Microspheres loaded with doxorubicin (hqTACE) and cTACE. This study will enrol 500 patients from 20 clinical sites in the United States, Europe and South America.

The results from these studies are eagerly anticipated as they have the potential to impact the future management of HCC.

Conclusion

Whilst staging in HCC is much debated, most western centres use the Barcelona Clinic Liver Cancer (BCLC) staging system (Figure 19.4). TACE or preferably DEB–TACE is now widely used for early stage disease as part of multimodality treatment, whilst on a transplant waiting list or to improve the results of surgical resection/thermal ablation. In intermediate stage disease, DEB–TACE is now the preferred option in Childs-Pugh class A and B cirrhotic patients with inoperable tumours. Multiple and bilateral disease can be treated, as can patients with unilateral portal vein invasion. DEB–TACE probably has no useful role in advanced disease, patients with bilobar disease or main portal vein invasion.

References

1. Parkin DM, Bray F, Ferlay J, et al. Global cancer statistics, 2002. *CA Cancer J Clin* 2005; 55(2):74–108.
2. Llovet JM, Burroughs A, Bruix J. Hepatocellular carcinoma. *Lancet* 2003; 362(9399):1907–1917.
3. Benzoni E, Molaro R, Cedolini C, et al. Liver resection for HCC: analysis of causes and risk factors linked to postoperative complications. *Hepatogastroenterology* 2007; 54(73): 186–189.
4. Lo CM, Ngan H, Tso WK, et al. Randomized controlled trial of transarterial lipiodol chemoembolization for unresectable hepatocellular carcinoma. *Hepatology* 2002; 35(5): 1164–1171.
5. Llovet JM, Real MI, Montana X, et al. Arterial embolisation or chemoembolisation versus symptomatic treatment in patients with unresectable hepatocellular carcinoma: a randomised controlled trial. *Lancet* 2002; 359(9319):1734–1739.
6. Llovet JM, Bruix J. Systematic review of randomized trials for unresectable hepatocellular carcinoma: chemoembolization improves survival. *Hepatology* 2003; 37(2):429–442.

7. Camma C, Schepis F, Orlando A, et al. Transarterial chemoembolization for unresectable hepatocellular carcinoma: meta-analysis of randomized controlled trials. *Radiology* 2002, 224:47–54.
8. Raoul JL, Heresbach MD, Bretagne JF et al. Chemoembolization of hepatocellular carcinomas, a study of biodistribution and pharmacokinetics of doxorubicin. *Cancer* 1992; 70:585–590.
9. Hong K, Khwaja A, Liapi E, et al. New intra-arterial drug delivery system for the treatment of liver cancer: preclinical assessment in a rabbit model of liver cancer. *Clin Cancer Res* 2006; 12(8):2563–2567.
10. Lewis AL, Gonzalez MV, Lloyd AW, et al. DC Bead: in vitro characterization of a drug-delivery device for transarterial chemoembolization. *J Vasc Interv Radiol* 2006; 17(2 Pt 1):335–342.
11. Grosso M, Vignali C, Quarretti P, et al. Transarterial chemoembolisation for hepatocellular carcinoma with drug-eluting microspheres: preliminary results from an Italian multicentre study. *Cardiovasc Intervent Radiol* 2008; 31(6):1141–1149
12. Brown DB, Geschwind JF, Soulen MC, et al. Society of Interventional Radiology position statement on chemoembolisation of hepatic malignancies. *J Vasc Interv Radiol* 2006; 17(2 Pt 1):217–223.
13. Poon RT, Tso WK, Pang RW, et al. A phase I/II trial of chemoembolization for hepatocellular carcinoma using a novel intra-arterial drug-eluting bead. *Clin Gastroenterol Hepatol* 2007; 5(9):1100–1108.
14. Varela M, Real MI, Brunet M, et al. Chemoembolization of hepatocellular carcinoma with drug eluting beads: efficacy and doxorubicin pharmacokinetics. *J Hepatol* 2007; 46(3):474–481.
15. Malagari K, Chatzimichael K, Alexopoulou E, et al. Transarterial chemoembolization of unresectable hepatocellular carcinoma with drug eluting beads: results of an open-label study of 62 patients. *Cardiovasc Intervent Radiol* 2008; 31(2):269–280.
16. Bruix J, Sherman M, Llovet JM, et al. Clinical management of hepatocellular carcinoma. Conclusions of the Barcelona-2000 EASL conference. European Association for the Study of the Liver. *J Hepatol* 2001; 35(3):421–430
17. Lammer J, Malagari K, Vogl T, et al. Prospective randomized study of doxorubicin-eluting bead embolization in the treatment of hepatocellular carcinoma: results of the PRECISION V study. *Cardiovasc Intervent Radiol* 2010; 33(1):41–52.
18. Lencioni R, Zhou J, Leberre M, et al. Sorafenib (SOR) or placebo (PL) in combination with transarterial chemoembolization (TACE) for intermediate-stage hepatocellular carcinoma (SPACE). *J Clin Oncol* 2010; 28(15):15.

20 What is the future of image-guided radiofrequency ablation for hepatocellular carcinoma?

Riccardo Lencioni

Division of Diagnostic Imaging and Intervention, University of Pisa School of Medicine, Pisa, Italy

LEARNING POINTS

- Radiofrequency ablation (RFA) is currently established as the standard of care for patients with early-stage hepatocellular carcinoma (HCC) when surgical options are precluded, and is considered a potentially radical treatment in properly selected candidates
- Uncontrolled investigations have suggested that RFA can achieve similar survival rates as surgical resection, particularly in patients bearing small, solitary tumours at the very early stage. However, there is no unequivocal data to back up RFA as a replacement for resection as first-line treatment for patients with early-stage HCC
- Newer thermal and non-thermal ablative techniques seem to have potential to overcome the limitations of RFA and warrant further clinical investigation
- The recent addition of molecular targeted drugs with anti-angiogenic and antiproliferative properties to the therapeutic armamentarium for HCC has prompted the design of clinical trials aimed at investigating the synergies between local ablation and adjuvant systemic treatments. The outcomes of these trials are eagerly awaited

Introduction

The term 'image-guided tumour ablation' is defined as the direct application of chemical or thermal therapies to a specific focal tumour (or tumours) in an attempt to achieve eradication or substantial tumour destruction [1]. Although tumour ablation procedures can be performed at laparoscopy or surgery, most procedures aimed at treating HCC are performed with a percutaneous approach. Hence, several authors refer to these procedures as 'percutaneous therapies'. The concept of image guidance is stressed in the title to highlight that image guidance is critical to the success of these therapies. Over the past 25 years, several methods for chemical or thermal tumour destruction have been developed and clinically tested [2]. Among these methods, RFA is currently established as the standard of care for patients with early-stage HCC when surgical options are precluded, and is considered a potentially radical treatment in properly selected candidates [3,4]. Nevertheless, newer thermal and non-thermal ablative techniques have been developed and promise to overcome some of the limitations of RFA in HCC treatment.

Percutaneous ethanol injection: the seminal technique

The seminal technique used for chemical ablation of HCC has been percutaneous ethanol injection (PEI). Although there have not been any randomised controlled trials (RCTs) comparing PEI and best supportive care or PEI and surgical resection, several retrospective studies have provided indirect evidence that PEI substantially improves the natural history of HCC in patients with Child-Pugh A cirrhosis and early-stage tumours; treatment with PEI has been shown to result in 5-year survival rates of 47–53% [5,6]. The major limitation of PEI is the high local recurrence rate that may reach 33% in lesions smaller than 3 cm and 43% in lesions exceeding 3 cm [7,8]. The injected ethanol does not always accomplish complete tumour ablation because of its inhomogeneous distribution within the

Clinical Dilemmas in Primary Liver Cancer, First Edition. Edited by Roger Williams and Simon D. Taylor-Robinson.

TABLE 20.1 Randomised controlled trials comparing RFA vs. PEI for the treatment of early-stage HCC

Author and year	Initial CR	Treatment failure[a]	Overall survival (%) 1 year	3 years	*P*
Lencioni et al. [13]					
RFA (n = 52)	91%	8%	88	81	NS
PEI (n = 50)	82%	34%	96	73	
Lin et al. [14]					
RFA (n = 52)	96%	17%	82	74	0.014
PEI (n =52)	88%	45%	61	50	
Shiina et al. [15]					
RFA (n = 118)	100%	2%	90	80	0.02
PEI (n = 114)	100%	11%	82	63	
Lin et al. [16]					
RFA (n = 62)	97%	16%	88	74	0.031
PEI (n = 62)	89%	42%	96	51	
Brunello et al. [17]					
RFA (n = 70)	96%	34%	88	59	NS
PEI (n = 69)	66%	64%	96	57	

RFA, radiofrequency ablation; PEI, percutaneous ethanol injection; HCC, hepatocellular carcinoma; CR, complete response; NS, not significant.
[a]Includes initial treatment failure (incomplete response) and late treatment failure (local recurrence).

lesion – especially in presence of intratumoural septa – and the limited effect on extracapsular cancerous spread. The recent introduction of a specific device for single-session PEI, a multipronged needle with three retractable prongs, each with four terminal side holes, has been shown to overcome some of these limitations by ensuring a more homogeneous ethanol perfusion throughout the whole tumour mass [9]. In a study including 141 patients with early-stage HCC, PEI performed with multipronged needles resulted in a rate of sustained complete response of 90% in tumours smaller than 3 cm and response of 75% in tumours ranging 3–5 cm in diameter [10]. Hence, PEI seems still to be able to offer a valuable treatment for early-stage HCC, especially for lesions in unfavourable locations for thermal ablation.

Radiofrequency ablation: the current standard of care

RFA has been the most widely assessed alternative to PEI for local ablation of HCC [11]. An important factor that affects the success of RFA is the ability to ablate all viable tumour tissue and possibly an adequate tumour-free margin. Ideally, a 360°, 0.5–1-cm-thick ablative margin should be produced around the tumour. This cuff would ensure that the peripheral portion of the tumour as well as any microscopic invasions located in its close proximity has been eradicated [12]. Five RCTs have compared RFA versus PEI for the treatment of early-stage HCC. These investigations consistently showed that RFA has higher anticancer effect than PEI, leading to a better local control of the disease [13–17] (Table 20.1). The assessment of the impact of RFA on survival has been more controversial. While a survival benefit was identified in the three RCTs performed in Asia, the two European RCTs failed to show statistically significant differences in overall survival between patients who received RFA and those treated with PEI, despite the trend favouring RFA (Table 20.1). In patients with early-stage HCC treated with percutaneous ablation, long-term survival is influenced by multiple different interventions, given that about 80% of the patients will develop recurrent intrahepatic HCC nodules within 5 years of the initial treatment and will receive additional therapies [18]. Nevertheless, three independent meta-analyses including all RCTs have confirmed that treatment with RFA offers a survival benefit as compared with PEI, particularly for tumours larger than 2 cm, thus establishing RFA as the standard percutaneous technique [19–21]. For studies that reported major complications, however, the incidence in RFA-treated patients

TABLE 20.2 Studies reporting 5-year survival of patients with early-stage HCC who received RFA as the sole first-line non-surgical treatment

Author and year	Number of patients	Overall survival (%)		
		1 year	3 years	5 years
Lencioni et al. [18]				
Child-Pugh A	144	100	76	51
Child-Pugh B	43	89	46	31
Tateishi et al. [23]				
Child-Pugh A	221	96	83	63
Child-Pugh B–C[a]	98	90	65	31
Choi et al. [24]				
Child-Pugh A	359	NA	78	64
Child-Pugh B	160	NA	49	38
N'Kontchou et al. [25]				
BCLC resectable[b]	67	NA	82	76
BCLC unresectable 168	NA	49	27	

HCC, hepatocellular carcinoma; RFA, radiofrequency ablation; NA, not available; BCLC, Barcelona Clinic for Liver Cancer.
[a]Only 4 of 98 patients had Child-Pugh C cirrhosis.
[b]BCLC criteria for resection include single tumour, normal bilirubin level (<1.5 mg/dL) and absence of significant portal hypertension.

was 4.1% (95% CI, 1.8–6.4%) compared with 2.7% (95% CI, 0.4–5.1%) observed in PEI-treated patients [22]. This difference was not statistically significant; nevertheless, this safety profile should be taken into consideration as part of the overall risk–benefit profile in each individual case.

Recent reports on long-term outcomes of RFA-treated patients have shown that in patients with Child-Pugh class A and early-stage HCC, 5-year survival rates are as high as 51–64%, and may reach 76% in patients who meet the Barcelona Clinic for Liver Cancer (BCLC) criteria for surgical resection [18,23–25] (Table 20.2). Therefore, an open question is whether RFA can compete with surgical resection as first-line treatment for patients with small, solitary HCC. Uncontrolled investigations have suggested that RFA can achieve similar survival rates as surgical resection, particularly in patients bearing small, solitary tumours at the very early stage of the BCLC classification [26]. On the other hand, a recent RCT comparing resection and RFA in patients who met the Milan criteria has reported superior overall survival and disease-free survival for the surgical arm (5-year survival, 75% for resection vs. 54% for RFA; $p = 0.001$) [27]. Of importance, patients in this study were divided into three subgroups: (a) solitary HCC smaller than or equal to 3 cm, (b) solitary HCC smaller than 5 cm, and (c) multifocal HCC. Survival analysis identified a benefit for resection in all subgroups ($p = 0.030$; $p = 0.046$; $p = 0.042$) [27]. Thus, at this point there is no unequivocal data to back up RFA as a replacement for resection as first-line treatment for patients with early-stage HCC.

The ability of RFA to achieve a complete tumour eradication appears to be dependent on tumour size and location. Histological studies performed in liver specimens of patients who underwent RFA as bridge treatment to transplantation showed that tumour size above 3 cm or the presence of large (3 mm or more) abutting vessels result in a drop of the rate of complete tumour necrosis to 50% or less [28]. Other clinical experiences have suggested that treatment of HCC tumours in sub-capsular location or adjacent to the gallbladder is associated with an increased risk of incomplete ablation and local tumour progression [29,30]. Treatment of tumours in such unfavourable locations has also been shown to result in a significant increase of major complications [31,32].

Novel methods for local ablation: the future?

Microwave ablation

Microwave ablation (MWA) is the term used for all electromagnetic methods of inducing tumour destruction by using devices with frequencies greater than or equal to 900 kHz [1]. MWA is emerging as a valuable alternative to RFA for thermal ablation of HCC. However, only one RCT has compared the effectiveness of MWA with that of RFA so far [33]. Although no statistically significant differences were observed with respect to the efficacy of the two procedures, a tendency favouring RFA was recognised in that study with respect to local recurrences and complications rates. However, it has to be pointed out that MWA technology has evolved significantly since the publication of this trial. Newer devices seem to overcome the limitation of the small volume of coagulation that was obtained with a single probe insertion in early experiences [34]. An important advantage of MWA over RFA is that treatment outcome is less affected by vessels located in the proximity of the tumour.

Laser ablation

The term laser ablation should be used for ablation with light energy applied via fibres directly inserted into the tissue. A great variety in laser sources and wavelength are available. In addition, different types of laser fibres, modified tips, and applicators can be used [35]. To date, few data are available concerning the clinical efficacy of laser ablation, as the treatment has been adopted by few centres worldwide. In particular, no RCTs to compare laser ablation with any other treatment have been published thus far. In a recent multicentre retrospective analysis including 432 non-surgical patients with early-stage HCC, 5-year overall survival was 34% (41% in Child-Pugh class A patients) [36].

Cryoablation

Cryoablation is a technique in which a liquid nitrogen cooled cryoprobe is placed into the tumour and an ice ball is created in the target tissue. The technique had limited application in HCC [37,38]. The complication rate is not negligible, particularly because of the risk for 'cryoshock', a life-threatening condition resulting in multi-organ failure, severe coagulopathy and disseminated intravascular coagulation following cryoablation. There are currently no RCTs that support the use of hepatic cryoablation for HCC treatment.

Irreversible electroporation

Irreversible electroporation (IRE) is a new, non-thermal ablation technique. Electroporation is a technique that increases cell membrane permeability by changing the transmembrane potential and subsequently disrupting the lipid bilayer integrity to allow transportation of molecules across the cell membrane via nano-size pores. This process – when used in a reversible fashion – has been used in research for drug or macromolecule delivery into cells. IRE is a method to induce irreversible disruption of cell membrane integrity resulting in cell death without the need for additional pharmacological injury [1]. IRE is administered under general anaesthesia with administration of a neuromuscular blocking agent to prevent undesirable muscle contraction [1]. IRE creates a sharp boundary between the treated and untreated area in vivo. This would suggest that IRE has the ability to sharply delineate the treatment area from the non-treated and that treatment planning can be precisely performed according to mathematical predictions. Moreover, because IRE is a non-thermal technique, there appears to be complete ablation to the margin of blood vessels without compromising the functionality of the blood vessels. Therefore, issues associated with perfusion-mediated tissue cooling or heating (a significant challenge with thermal methods) are not relevant. Preclinical investigation focused on HCC has shown promising results [39] and has prompted its clinical evaluation.

Combination therapies

Image-guided tumour ablation therapies have long been used in the setting of combined treatment strategies. An accepted indication is the use of these interventions in patients awaiting transplantation to prevent tumour progression when the waiting time exceeds 6 months [40]. The combined use of transcatheter treatments and tumour ablation techniques is very popular in the treatment of HCC tumours of intermediate (3–7 cm) size. A combination of chemoembolisation followed by RFA has been used to minimise heat loss due to perfusion-mediated tissue cooling and increase the therapeutic effect of RFA [41–44]. On the other hand, chemoembolisation with drug-eluting beads has been performed after an RFA procedure to increase tumour necrosis by exposing to high drug concentration the peripheral part of the tumour, where only sub-lethal temperatures may be achieved in a standard RFA treatment [45]. Unfortunately, despite several investigation reporting promising results, no definitive proof of clinical efficacy was reached, as no robust RCT comparing the efficacy of the combined use of transcatheter treatments and tumour ablation techniques over the one obtained with either therapy alone has been completed so far.

An important limitation of any local treatment is the high rate of tumour recurrence. After ablation of early-stage HCC, tumour recurrence rate exceeds 80% at 5 years, similar to post-resection figures [18]. Molecular studies have shown that early recurrences – occurring within the first 2 years after curative treatment – are mainly due to the spread of the original tumour, while late recurrences are more frequently due to the development of metachronous tumours independent of the previous cancer.

Increased understanding of the molecular signalling pathways involved in HCC has led to the development of molecular targeted therapies aimed at inhibiting tumour cell proliferation and angiogenesis. Sorafenib, a multikinase inhibitor with anti-angiogenic and antiproliferative properties, has been shown to prolong median overall survival and median time to radiological progression compared to placebo in RCTs and has become the current standard of care for patients with advanced-stage tumours not suitable for surgical or locoregional therapies [46,47]. To date, studies of sorafenib have demonstrated its efficacy in advanced HCC; however, there may also be a role for this agent – or other molecular targeted drugs – in earlier stage disease, such as in the setting of an adjuvant treatment after curative therapy. The first large studies in which an interventional locoregional treatment is evaluated in combination with a systemically active molecular targeted drug are already ongoing. Undertaking these studies has required an extraordinary effort due to the need to go beyond the boundaries of each discipline and to develop a common framework for the design of clinical trials to facilitate comparability of the results [4,48]. The outcomes of these trials are eagerly awaited, as they have the potential to revolutionise the treatment of HCC.

References

1. Lencioni R. Loco-regional treatment of hepatocellular carcinoma. *Hepatology* 2010; 52:762–773.
2. Lencioni R, Crocetti L. Image-guided thermal ablation of hepatocellular carcinoma. *Crit Rev Oncol Hematol* 2008; 66:200–207.
3. Bruix J, Sherman M. Management of hepatocellular carcinoma. *Hepatology* 2005; 42:1208–1236.
4. Llovet JM, Di Bisceglie AM, Bruix J, et al. Panel of Experts in HCC-Design Clinical Trials. Design and endpoints of clinical trials in hepatocellular carcinoma. *J Natl Cancer Inst* 2008; 100:698–711.
5. Lencioni R, Bartolozzi C, Caramella D, et al. Treatment of small hepatocellular carcinoma with percutaneous ethanol injection. Analysis of prognostic factors in 105 Western patients. *Cancer* 1995; 76:1737–1746.
6. Livraghi T, Giorgio A, Marin G, et al. Hepatocellular carcinoma and cirrhosis in 746 patients: long-term results of percutaneous ethanol injection. *Radiology* 1995; 197:101–108.
7. Khan KN, Yatsuhashi H, Yamasaki K, Yamasaki M, Inoue O, Koga M, Yano M. Prospective analysis of risk factors for early intrahepatic recurrence of hepatocellular carcinoma following ethanol injection. *J Hepatol* 2000; 32:269–278.
8. Koda M, Murawaki Y, Mitsuda A, et al. Predictive factors for intrahepatic recurrence after percutaneous ethanol injection therapy for small hepatocellular carcinoma. *Cancer* 2000; 88:529–537.
9. Lencioni R, Crocetti L, Cioni D, et al. Single-session percutaneous ethanol ablation of early-stage hepatocellular carcinoma with a multipronged injection needle: results of a pilot clinical study. *J Vasc Interv Radiol* 2010; 21:1533–1538.
10. Kuang M, Lu MD, Xie XY, et al. Percutaneous ethanol ablation of early-stage hepatocellular carcinoma by using a multi-pronged needle with single treatment session and high-dose ethanol injection. *Radiology* 2009; 253:552–561.
11. Lencioni R, Crocetti L. Radiofrequency ablation of liver cancer. *Tech Vasc Interv Radiol* 2007; 10:38–46.
12. Crocetti L, De Baere T, Lencioni R. Quality improvement guidelines for radiofrequency ablation of liver tumours. *Cardiovasc Intervent Radiol* 2010; 33:11–17.
13. Lencioni R, Allgaier HP, Cioni D, et al. Small hepatocellular carcinoma in cirrhosis: randomized comparison of radiofrequency thermal ablation versus percutaneous ethanol injection. *Radiology* 2003; 228:235–240.
14. Lin SM, Lin CJ, Lin CC, Hsu CW, Chen YC. Radiofrequency ablation improves prognosis compared with ethanol injection for hepatocellular carcinoma < or = 4 cm. *Gastroenterology* 2004; 127:1714–1723.
15. Shiina S, Teratani T, Obi S, et al. A randomized controlled trial of radiofrequency ablation versus ethanol injection for small hepatocellular carcinoma. *Gastroenterology* 2005; 129:122–130.
16. Lin SM, Lin CJ, Lin CC, Hsu CW, Chen YC. Randomised controlled trial comparing percutaneous radiofrequency thermal ablation, percutaneous ethanol injection, and percutaneous acetic acid injection to treat hepatocellular carcinoma of 3 cm or less. *Gut* 2005; 54:1151–1156.
17. Brunello F, Veltri A, Carucci P, et al. Radiofrequency ablation versus ethanol injection for early hepatocellular carcinoma: a randomized controlled trial. *Scand J Gastroenterol* 2008; 43:727–735.
18. Lencioni R, Cioni D, Crocetti L, et al. Early-stage hepatocellular carcinoma in cirrhosis: long-term results of

percutaneous image-guided radiofrequency ablation. *Radiology* 2005; 234:961–967.

19. Orlando A, Leandro G, Olivo M, Andriulli A, Cottone M. Radiofrequency thermal ablation vs. percutaneous ethanol injection for small hepatocellular carcinoma in cirrhosis: meta-analysis of randomized controlled trials. *Am J Gastroenterol* 2009; 104:514–524.
20. Cho YK, Kim JK, Kim MY, Rhim H, Han JK. Systematic review of randomized trials for hepatocellular carcinoma treated with percutaneous ablation therapies. *Hepatology* 2009; 49:453–459.
21. Germani G, Pleguezuelo M, Gurusamy K, Meyer T, Isgrò G, Burroughs AK. Clinical outcomes of radiofrequency ablation, percutaneous alcohol and acetic acid injection for hepatocelullar carcinoma: A meta-analysis. *J Hepatol* 2010; 52:380–388.
22. Bouza C, López-Cuadrado T, Alcázar R, Saz-Parkinson Z, Amate JM. Meta-analysis of percutaneous radiofrequency ablation versus ethanol injection in hepatocellular carcinoma. *BMC Gastroenterol* 2009; 9:31.
23. Tateishi R, Shiina S, Teratani T, et al. Percutaneous radiofrequency ablation for hepatocellular carcinoma. *Cancer* 2005; 103:1201–1209.
24. Choi D, Lim HK, Rhim H, et al. Percutaneous radiofrequency ablation for early-stage hepatocellular carcinoma as a first-line treatment: long-term results and prognostic factors in a large single-institution series. *Eur Radiol* 2007; 17:684–692.
25. N'Kontchou G, Mahamoudi A, Aout M, et al. Radiofrequency ablation of hepatocellular carcinoma: long-term results and prognostic factors in 235 Western patients with cirrhosis. *Hepatology* 2009; 50:1475–1483.
26. Livraghi T, Meloni F, Di Stasi M, et al. Sustained complete response and complications rates after radiofrequency ablation of very early hepatocellular carcinoma in cirrhosis: Is resection still the treatment of choice? *Hepatology* 2008; 47:82–89.
27. Huang J, Yan L, Cheng Z, et al. A randomized trial comparing radiofrequency ablation and surgical resection for HCC conforming to the Milan criteria. *Ann Surg* 2010; 252:903–912.
28. Lu DS, Yu NC, Raman SS, et al. Radiofrequency ablation of hepatocellular carcinoma: treatment success as defined by histologic examination of the explanted liver. *Radiology* 2005; 234:954–960.
29. Komorizono Y, Oketani M, Sako K, et al. Risk factors for local recurrence of small hepatocellular carcinoma tumors after a single session, single application of percutaneous radiofrequency ablation. *Cancer* 2003; 97:1253–1262.
30. Kim SW, Rhim H, Park M, et al. Percutaneous radiofrequency ablation of hepatocellular carcinomas adjacent to the gallbladder with internally cooled electrodes: assessment of safety and therapeutic efficacy. *Korean J Radiol* 2009; 10:366–376.
31. Llovet JM, Vilana R, Brú C, et al. Increased risk of tumor seeding after percutaneous radiofrequency ablation for single hepatocellular carcinoma. *Hepatology* 2001; 33:1124–1129.
32. Teratani T, Yoshida H, Shiina S, et al. Radiofrequency ablation for hepatocellular carcinoma in so-called high-risk locations. *Hepatology* 2006; 43:1101–1108.
33. Shibata T, Iimuro Y, Yamamoto Y, et al. Small hepatocellular carcinoma: comparison of radio-frequency ablation and percutaneous microwave coagulation therapy. *Radiology* 2002; 223:331–337.
34. Yu NC, Lu DS, Raman SS, et al. Hepatocellular carcinoma: microwave ablation with multiple straight and loop antenna clusters – pilot comparison with pathologic findings. *Radiology* 2006; 239:269–275.
35. Vogl TJ, Straub R, Eichler K Woitaschek D, Mack MG. Malignant liver tumors treated with MR imaging-guided laser-induced thermotherapy: experience with complications in 899 patients (2,520 lesions). *Radiology* 2002; 225: 367–377.
36. Pacella CM, Francica G, Di Lascio FM, et al. Long-term outcome of cirrhotic patients with early hepatocellular carcinoma treated with ultrasound-guided percutaneous laser ablation: a retrospective analysis. *J Clin Oncol* 2009; 27:2615–2621.
37. Orlacchio A, Bazzocchi G, Pastorelli D, et al. Percutaneous cryoablation of small hepatocellular carcinoma with US guidance and CT monitoring: initial experience. *Cardiovasc Intervent Radiol* 2008; 31:587–594.
38. Shimizu T, Sakuhara Y, Abo D, et al. Outcome of MR-guided percutaneous cryoablation for hepatocellular carcinoma *J Hepatobiliary Pancreat Surg* 2009; 16:816–823.
39. Guo Y, Zhang Y, Klein R, et al. Irreversible electroporation therapy in the liver: longitudinal efficacy studies in a rat model of hepatocellular carcinoma. *Cancer Res* 2010; 70:1555–1563.
40. Belghiti J, Carr BI, Greig PD, Lencioni R, Poon RT. Treatment before liver transplantation for HCC. *Ann Surg Oncol* 2008; *Ann Surg Oncol* 2008; 15:993–1000.
41. Rossi S, Garbagnati F, Lencioni R, et al. Percutaneous radiofrequency thermal ablation of nonresectable hepatocellular carcinoma after occlusion of tumor blood supply. *Radiology* 2000; 217:119–126.
42. Yamasaki T, Kurokawa F, Shirahashi H, Kusano N, Hironaka K, Okita K. Percutaneous radiofrequency ablation therapy for patients with hepatocellular carcinoma during occlusion of hepatic blood flow. Comparison with standard percutaneous radiofrequency ablation therapy. *Cancer* 2002; 95:2353–2360.

43. Veltri A, Moretto P, Doriguzzi A, et al. Radiofrequency thermal ablation (RFA) after transarterial chemoembolization (TACE) as a combined therapy for unresectable non-early hepatocellular carcinoma (HCC). *Eur Radiol* 2006; 16:661–669.
44. Helmberger T, Dogan S, Straub G, et al. Liver resection or combined chemoembolization and radiofrequency ablation improve survival in patients with Hepatocellular carcinoma. *Digestion* 2007; 75:104–112.
45. Lencioni R, Crocetti L, Petruzzi P, et al. Doxorubicin-eluting bead-enhanced radiofrequency ablation of hepatocellular carcinoma: a pilot clinical study. *J Hepatol* 2008; 49: 217–222.
46. Llovet JM, Ricci S, Mazzaferro V, et al. Sorafenib in advanced hepatocellular carcinoma. *N Engl J Med* 2008; 359:378–390.
47. Cheng AL, Kang YK, Chen Z, et al. Efficacy and safety of sorafenib in patients in the Asia-Pacific region with advanced hepatocellular carcinoma: a phase III randomised, double-blind, placebo-controlled trial. *Lancet Oncol* 2009; 10:25–34.
48. Lencioni R, Llovet JM. Modified RECIST (mRECIST) assessment for hepatocellular carcinoma. *Semin Liver Dis* 2010; 30:52–60.

21 Alternative ablation techniques for hepatocellular carcinoma

John Karani
King's College Hospital, London, UK

LEARNING POINTS

- Alternative techniques are based on proven physical principles of thermal or non-thermal ablation
- Radiofrequency ablation (RFA) remains the technique with the best evidence base
- The applicability of the alternative techniques separately or in combination with chemoembolisation is yet to be established in controlled trials
- Non-invasive ablation techniques are now being developed that have the potential to reduce the morbidity and mortality of intervention but with an equivalent biological effect

The last decade has seen the emergence of local ablative therapies for the treatment of hepatocellular carcinoma (HCC) and a developing evidence base for their efficacy. These techniques have been used as the primary therapy or in combination with other locoregional therapies principally chemoembolisation or as adjunct to liver resection or transplantation. Two broad categories exist based on either thermal or non-thermal principles of ablation. Most of the techniques in current practice are based on heat ablation, which when targeted at tumours leads to coagulative necrosis of cells. These include, microwave, focussed ultrasound (FUS), laser, cryoablation and radiofrequency (RF). These ablation methods can be delivered percutaneously at open surgery or laparoscopy. The non-thermal techniques are those of chemical ablation with direct injection of ethanol or acetic acid. An emerging non-thermal therapy deploys the physical principle of irreversible electroporation (IRE) where tumour necrosis is induced by application of an electric current.

The guiding therapeutic principle of all these techniques is to deliver an energy force to a target HCC that reliably results in macro and microscopic destruction of the tumour whilst preserving the adjacent tissue. Successful ablation with reduced marginal tumour recurrence requires that the technique and image guidance delivers an ablative margin of normal tissue surrounding the tumour of 5–10 mm. The techniques should carry a low morbidity and be deliverable through systems that allow for accurate image guidance. Ultrasound, computed tomography and magnetic resonance imaging (MRI) singularly or in combination provide accurate guidance with the development of faster scan acquisitions and software development for fusion imaging, allowing more accurate targeting and parameters for measuring treatment response. Comparing the outcome of all these techniques is limited as many studies lack randomisation and have a selection bias. This criticism is particularly applicable to the newer techniques. Unquestionably, RFA is the most popular and provides the strongest evidence base in favour of its use in small tumours.

To date, there is a limit to the size of a tumour that can be successfully treated but multiple overlapping ablations or positioning of multiple applicators coupled with development in the applicators is expanding the size of tumour to which this technique can be applied. In addition, the anatomical location of tumours to the intrahepatic vasculature and biliary tree may limit the degree of coagulative necrosis because of 'heat sink' and, therefore, the potential for incomplete treatment and disease recurrence. Therefore, competitive newer technologies are emerging although

Clinical Dilemmas in Primary Liver Cancer, First Edition. Edited by Roger Williams and Simon D. Taylor-Robinson.

their efficacy is yet to be tested in studies that would provide evidence for a change in practice.

This chapter reviews the basic physical principles, delivery systems and evidence to date of the applicability of these techniques.

Chemical ablation

Direct intratumoural injection of chemical substances, such as ethanol or acetic acid, is the ablative method with has the longest history in clinical practice. It provided the evidence for the principle for all subsequent ablative techniques in the treatment paradigm of HCC [1–3]. The biological principle is that ethanol diffuses into the tumour cells and results in dehydration of the cytoplasm, protein denaturation and coagulative necrosis. Common to most of the ablative techniques, there is vascular endothelial damage that leads to platelet aggregation and thrombosis. The diffusion of the alcohol and its biological effect may be limited if the tumour has a fibrous capsule or pseudo capsule. Acetic acid induces necrosis through the same biological mechanism [4]. However, animal studies have shown that it is able to diffuse through fibrous tissue more effectively than ethanol [5] and, therefore, may have the potential to induce more effective ablation. This is yet to be proven by an evidence base that justifies a change in practice. Combination thermal and non-thermal techniques may be used in combination. Whereas the anatomical location of a tumour or proximity to a vessel may reduce the efficacy of RFA, adjunctive injection of ethanol may ensure a more effective tumour-free ablation margin. A randomised comparison of RF thermal ablation versus percutaneous ethanol injection (PEI) has demonstrated that RFA is superior to PEI with respect to local recurrence survival rates [6]. In a series of 102 patients with cirrhosis and either single HCC 5 cm in diameter or smaller or up to three HCCs each 3 cm or smaller, 1 and 2-year survival rates were 100% and 98% in the RFA group and 96% and 88% in the PEI group. One and 2-year local recurrence-free survival rates were 98% and 96% in the RFA group and 83% and 62% in the PEI group, respectively.

Cryoablation

The principle of cryotherapy is of rapid cooling, slow thawing and repetition of the cool/thaw cycle. There are two main effects of cryo-destruction. Firstly, there is direct cellular injury, and secondly post-thaw ischaemia that results in endothelial vascular injury. Tissues undergoing cryoablation develop crystallisation of intra- and extracellular water including the vascular space. At cellular level at temperatures of −40°C or less, there is destruction of the cell membrane and tissue necrosis. In the vascular space at extracellular level, there is stasis, platelet aggregation and thrombus formation. This accentuates the cell necrosis by induction of microvascular ischaemia. Whilst early cryoablation systems were only applicable to open-operative use, the more modern systems allow treatment by a percutaneous or laparoscopic approach. However, the ablation zone correlates to the probe diameter so that the zone of ablation is limited by the size of the probe that can be safely placed in the liver. Most of the systems with a historical base and literature use the Joule–Thomson effect. This physical principle describes the change in temperature of a gas that results from expansion or compression of the gas. Argon can generate temperatures as low as −140°C. Newer systems use nitrogen near its critical point to induce cooling, and this method is now the focus of development and experimentation.

Experience of cryoablation in the treatment of HCC is limited to relatively small series. A series of 65 patients treated by a combination of cryoablation and ethanol injection with a mean follow-up of 14 months reported a 50.8% survival without recurrence, 33% alive with recurrence but in only 3 patients was there evidence of recurrence at the site of the ablation [7].

Microwave ablation

The term microwave defines electromagnetic energy in the 300 MHz to 300 GHz with devices for tissue ablation typically operating at either 915 MHz or 2.45 GHz. Heat is produced as a result of dielectric hysteresis (rotating dipoles) When electromagnetic energy is applied to tissue there is rotation of molecules as they continuously align with the applied field and this induced kinetic energy results in generation of local heat within the tissue. Microwaves readily penetrate all tissues even those with low electrical conductivity including dehydrated or burned tissue and can produce extremely high temperatures (>150°C). Microwave can heat tissue more effectively than RF by increasing the thermal conduction in surrounding tissue and the volume of ablation.

Most reports of the applicability and results of microwave in the treatment of HCC come from China and Japan. In a large series of 288 patients with 477 tumours treated by microwave ablation, survival rates of 93%, 72% and 51% were achieved at 1, 3 and 5 years, respectively [8]. The average tumour size was 4 cm or less. In the analysis of the study, there was a local recurrence of 8%, recurrence in same segment of 9% and in other liver segments of 12%. Extrahepatic metastatic disease developed in 6% of patients culminating in a total recurrence or metastatic incidence of 35%. Most comparative studies of RF and microwave have concluded that both these techniques have an equivalent performance in inducing necrosis and preventing local tumour recurrence. In a comparative study of 72 patients with 94 HCCs with a follow-up of 6–27 months, recurrence of tumour occurred in 4 patients treated by microwave and 8 with RF [9]. A further study of 98 nodules of HCC in 49 patients of which 72 were treated with microwave found a recurrence rate of 11.8% with microwave and 21% with RF [10].

Laser ablation

The physical principle of laser therapy using light energy to induce tissue hyperthermia has wide clinical application, but in the treatment of HCC, it has few advantages over more established techniques. Laser sources including pumped neodymium-doped yttrium aluminium garnet (Nd-YAG lasers) emit approximately 600–1000-nm wavelength light energy provide an efficient method for tissue heating. However, because light is scattered and absorbed rapidly by tissues, lasers have limited energy penetration and create smaller ablation zones. Light does not penetrate dessicated tissues. Adaptation of the technology with deployment of diffuser tips and multiple applicators can partially overcome the disadvantage of the physical principle but not to the extent where the outcome and ease of use outweigh the other techniques. However, one advantage is that laser energy may be coupled through optical fibres and delivery systems, which are MR compatible with less imaging artefact. Therefore, MR temperature mapping to gauge the zone of thermal ablation in 'real time' can be readily conducted. Laser ablation has been used in conjunction with other techniques including chemoembolisation and operative vascular occlusion to increase the zone of ablation, but analysis of the data is such that a clear recommendation for the use of laser-based techniques has not emerged.

High-intensity focused ultrasound

The first of the emerging technologies to be considered is ultrasonic ablation.

Ultrasound energy can be used to elevate tissue temperatures by using interstitial ultrasound applicators [11–13]. In this technique, high-intensity ultrasound with time-averaged intensities of 100–10,000 W/cm^2 are directed to a focus. This energy level compares with time-averaged intensities of 0.1–100 mW/cm^2 in diagnostic ultrasound. The focus rapidly heats due to molecular vibration leading to a rapid rise in temperature, which results in coagulative tissue necrosis. Other phenomena that occur at high intensities are cavitation, microstreaming and radiation forces. The advantage of this local therapy is that it is non-invasive. The evidence base for this technique as an alternative therapy is yet to be established, but any technique that can be delivered externally without the inherent risks and complications of percutaneous targeting demands development and critical analysis.

Irreversible electroporation

The second of the emerging technologies is percutaneous IRE, which is a non-thermal technique. Cells are destroyed by being subjected to programmed consecutive micro- to millisecond long pulses of electrical energy. The pulses generate electric fields of up to 3 kV/cm, which result in irreversible damage to the cell membrane and induction of apoptosis and cell death. As a non-thermal technique, it is not limited by heat sink, and therefore, there is a theoretical advantage that tumours close to vessels may be more effectively treated [14,15]. The electrodes are of insulated needles with an exposed active portion with most tumours potentially requiring multiple needles to provide sufficient field strength for effective cell death. The potential complications of this technique include the generation of electrical energy that could induce cardiac arrhythmias or muscle contraction. At present, this is an experimental technique. As with all the new developments in ablation, it is only the results from comparative controlled trials that will determine whether it becomes accepted into routine clinical practice.

The future of these techniques

There will inevitably be modification of all these techniques to create larger and more uniform zones of ablation with a lower morbidity and with equipment and applicators that are more flexible and easily deployed. However, there is an increasing emphasis to research methods that modulate tissue response to these techniques. A second line of development is to examine the efficacy of combination locoregional therapies in the treatment of HCC.

The primary factors that limit the effect of thermal ablation are tissue perfusion and thermal conductivity. If there are intrahepatic vessels greater than 3 mm adjacent to the HCC then these can act as a heat sink and limit the zone of coagulative necrosis. It is often this physical limitation that prevents the complete eradication of tumour cells, which then form the focus of tumour recurrence. Pharmacological or intravascular mechanical techniques that modulate and reduce the perfusion of the liver will reduce the adverse effect of heat sink. Balloon occlusion techniques and neoadjuvant chemoembolisation that reduce local tissue perfusion are now part of clinical practice. Further strategies that alter the climate for ablation are pre-conditioning of the tumour and peri-tumoural perfusion by combining thermal ablation with chemotherapeutic agents and radiation. There is increasing evidence of a therapeutic synergy in combining thermal ablation techniques with chemotherapy (free or contained within liposomes). Drugs that are directed towards reducing angiogenesis may enhance the apoptosis that results from ablation [16]. Combining irradiation and thermal ablation is in an experimental phase, but there are theoretical biological mechanisms. Radiation induces inhibition of tissue repair and secondly the increased sensitisation of the tumour to radiation owing to the increased oxygenation in the tumour zone from hyperthermic injury [17].

Conclusion

Ablation techniques are now an accepted part of the treatment paradigm for HCC, improving the survival in selected patients. However, the dilemmas are currently those of which of the competing techniques should be used and should they be deployed singularly or in combination with other locoregional and systemic therapies. Most observers would agree that RFA is the technique by which others should be judged, given its worldwide adoption and extensive literature providing the evidence base for its use. The pace of change in the other techniques is driven by the technological manipulation of principles of physics and computer science. The extrapolation of this science into translational research to benefit patients demands the governance of controlled trials with exacting comparative studies that are not yet available.

References

1. Blendis L. Percutaneous ethanol ablation of small hepatocellular carcinomas: twenty years on. *Gastroenterology* 2006; 130(1):280–282 (discussion 282).
2. Taniguchi M, Kim SR, Imoto S, et al. Long-term outcome of percutaneous ethanol injection therapy for minimum sized hepatocellular carcinoma. *World J Gastroenterol* 2008; 14(13):1997–2002.
3. Andruilli A, de Sio I, Solmi L, et al. Survival of cirrhotic patients with early hepatocellular carcinoma or liver transplantation. *Liver Transpl* 2004; 109110:1355–1363.
4. Ohnishi K, Ohyama N, Ito S, Fujiwara K. Small hepatocellular carcinoma: treatment with US-guided intratumoral injection of acetic acid. *Radiology* 1994; 193(3):747–752.
5. Ohnishi K. Comparison of percutaneous acetic acid injection and percutaneous ethanol injection for small hepatocellular carcinoma. *Hepatogastroenterology* 1998; 45(suppl 3): 1254–1258.
6. Lencioni R, Allgaier H-P, Cioni D, et al. Small hepatocellular carcinoma in cirrhosis: randomized comparison of radiofrequency thermal ablation versus percutaneous ethanol injection. *Radiology* 2003; 288:235–240.
7. Xu KC, Niu LZ, He WB, et al. Percutaneous cryoablation in combination with ethanol for unresectable HCC. *World J Gastroenterol* 2003; 9:2686–2689.
8. Liang P, Dong B, Yu X. Prognostic factors for survival in patients with hepatocellular carcinoma after percutaneous microwave ablation. *Radiology* 2005; 235:299–307.
9. Shibata T, Iiumoro Y, Yamamoto Y, et al. Small hepatocellular carcinoma; comparison of radiofrequency ablation and microwave therapy. *Radiology* 2002; 223:331–337.
10. Lu Md, Xu HX, Xie XY, et al. Percutaneous microwave therapy and radiofrequency ablation: a retrospective comparative study. *J Gastroenterol* 2005; 40:1054–1060.
11. Dubinsky T, Cuevas C, Dighe M. High intensity focused ultrasound: current potential and oncological applications. *Am J Roentgenol* 2008; 190:191–199.
12. Fischer K, Gedroyc W, Jolesz F. Focused Ultrasound as a Local Therapy for Liver Cancer. *Cancer J* 2010; 16(2):118–124.
13. Li Y, Sha W, Zhou Y. Short and long term efficacy of high intensity focused ultrasound therapy for advanced hepatocellular carcinoma. *J Gastroenterol Hepatol* 2007; 22:2148–2154.

14. Lee EW, Loh CT, Kee ST. Imaging guided percutaneous irreversible electroporation; ultrasound and immunohistological correlation. *Technol Cancer Res Treat* 2007; 6(4):287–294.
15. Rubinsky B, Onik G, Mikus P. Irreversible electroporation; a new ablation modality-clinical implications. *Technol Cancer Res Treat* 2007; 6(1):37–48.
16. Ahmed M, Goldberg SN. combination radiofrequency ablation and adjuvant IV liposomal doxorubicin increases tissue coagulation and intratumoural drug accumulation. *Int J Hyperthermia* 2004; 20(7):781–802.
17. Solazzo S, Mertyna P, Peddi H, Ahmed M, et al. RF ablation with adjuvant therapy: comparison of external beam irradiation and liposomal doxorubicin on ablation efficacy in an animal model. *Int J Hyperthermia* 2008; 24(7):560–567.

22 Justification for sorafenib and chemotherapy

Philip J. Johnson
Cancer Research UK Clinical Trials Unit, University of Birmingham, Birmingham, UK

LEARNING POINTS

- The use of sorafenib in patients with advanced hepatocellular carcinoma (HCC) illustrates how the perception of cost-effectiveness varies in different societies and health care systems
- Similarly, there is wide variation in tolerability of the drug reflecting the price patients are prepared to pay, in terms of attributable toxicity and the survival improvement

The last 25 years have seen major advances in the treatment of HCC. These have included the actual treatments themselves, predominantly locoregional, and the rigor with which new treatments are tested to establish an evidence base. Several therapeutic approaches can now achieve complete local control. Whether these equate to 'cure' is a matter of definition. Whilst liver transplantation may effectively remove the tumour and the underlying associated liver disease, other local therapies still leave most patients with some degree of underlying liver disease and the possibility of death therefrom, and the possibility of developing a new 'second' tumour. Treatments that might reverse the underlying liver disease are current areas of intensive research.

Any justification for systemic treatment must be based on the clinical need, the balance of benefit and toxicity and the balance of cost against perceived utility. Each of these aspects is now considered.

The need for systemic chemotherapy

The limitations of the newer radical local treatments are apparent. Whether we consider surgical resection, radiofrequency ablation (RFA) or percutaneous ethanol injection, there are limitations as to the size/volume of tumour that can be dealt with. Such limitations partly reflect technical aspects secondary to the associated chronic liver disease (CLD) or, in the case of RFA, the difficulty in generating sufficient temperature to be tumouricidal. More importantly, the size limitations occur because size is probably a surrogate for microvascular tumour invasion and the consequent likelihood of metastatic disease. This being the case we can envisage two solutions; early diagnosis (i.e. diagnosis at a time when tumours are small enough to be amenable to 'curative' therapies) that might be achieved by surveillance programmes and systemic agents to deal with metastatic disease at the sub-clinical stage or when grossly apparent. If we assume that currently available local therapies *are* potentially curative for patients with small tumours, then it is pertinent to ask 'how would an effective systemic therapy be of benefit'?

1. In some patients, HCC is the first presentation of CLD, and even for those entering a surveillance programme, a proportion will still only be detected when the disease is advanced, and many treated with locoregional therapies will have at time of recurrence advanced disease.
2. Adjuvant systemic treatment after a local therapy might reduce the risk of development of subsequent

Clinical Dilemmas in Primary Liver Cancer, First Edition. Edited by Roger Williams and Simon D. Taylor-Robinson.

recurrence. The latter is the major cause of failure of locoregional therapies. It might also permit the treatment to be administered to patients with tumours outside current size limitations.

3. It might be used in a neo-adjuvant setting, such that tumours currently excluded from locoregional treatment on size grounds might be 'downsized'.
4. It might become part of a combination therapy.

For all these reasons, it seems justified to seek an effective systemic treatment.

Conventional cytotoxic chemotherapy

Response rates for single-agent cytotoxic chemotherapy are low, and significant durable remission is uncommon. The most widely used agent has been doxorubicin. An early prospective randomised trial comparing doxorubicin with best supportive care reported significantly increased survival [1]. Mitoxantrone gave similar results, with perhaps less toxicity and was subsequently licensed for use in HCC [2] although it has never been widely accepted as 'standard of care'. In two recent large-scale trials of drugs that had shown promising activity in early phase trials, Ti67, a novel tubulin-binding drug [3], and nolatrexed, a thymidylate synthase inhibitor [4], were tested with doxorubicin as the control arm. In the former, there was no survival improvement; in the latter, the patients in the doxorubicin arm survived significantly longer (32.3 weeks compared with 22.3 weeks) [3,4]. The European Medical Agency (EMEA) considered this trial in their Public Assessment Report on sorafenib and observed that, on the basis of the 10-week improvement in survival, 'it [Doxorubicin] was likely to be an effective agent'.

Combination chemotherapy appears to give a higher response rate, although again the duration of remission is usually short. In general, even for well-selected patients, the expected objective response is only around 20–30%. A phase II study of a four-drug systemic combination regimen (cisplatin, recombinant interferon α-2b, doxorubicin and 5-fluorouracil (PIAF)) was encouraging, showing that although the response rate was not high (25%), 9 of the 13 partial responders had their disease rendered resectable [5]. However, a prospective randomised study comparing the PIAF regimen to conventional systemic doxorubicin showed that although the expected response rates for doxorubicin and PIAF were achieved (10% and 20%, respectively) and survival was in line with the phase II trial experience (8.5 months), this did not translate into a significant improvement in survival when compared with doxorubicin alone. It was suggested that any benefit in terms of the increased response rate was counteracted by increased toxicity [6]. A recent phase II trial of a similar combination, cisplatin, doxorubicin and capecitibine, showed similar results in terms of activity with a response rate of 24% [7]. Thus conventional cytotoxic therapy has undoubted activity in the advanced disease setting, and the feasibility of the neo-adjuvant approach has been suggested; whether or not this translates into a survival advantage remains unproven.

Much has been made of the toxicity of drugs such as doxorubicin in patients with cirrhosis but in the largest reported trial, involving 222 patients receiving doxorubicin, it was reported to be 'well tolerated'. There were no treatment related deaths and only 7% were withdrawn because of adverse events.

Is there now any justification for using cytotoxic chemotherapy? Certainly first-line treatment is now widely accepted as being sorafenib, but there are some situations where cytotoxics may be considered. In some countries, sorafenib is not considered cost-effective (see Section 'Cost-effectiveness') and thus not available through public health systems. In such circumstances, provided it is made clear to the patient that survival benefit has not been rigorously proven, it may be justified in those patients who are keen for some form of therapy. Also there are situations where the tumour is on the borderline of being resectable and here cytotoxic chemotherapy has been shown, in some cases, to shrink the tumour sufficiently to permit resection [5].

Sorafenib as a single agent in the advanced setting

The evidence base comprises three key papers [8–10], the most important of which reports the SHARP trial [8]. The most critical and independent review of data is that provided by NICE [11,12]. The SHARP trial, which was stopped early on the grounds of clear efficacy, showed that in patients with advanced, non-resectable disease sorafenib 400 mg b.i.d. resulted in an improvement in survival of 2.8 months (10.7 vs. 7.9), when compared with a placebo-treated control group. As such this was the first study to show a statistically significant improvement in survival in a rigorously designed, placebo-controlled clinical trial.

Having said this, there were a number of limitations:

1. Firstly, with a view to identifying the true antitumour effect of the drug, the study was confined to patients with good liver function (95% were classified as Child's grade A) so that the competing effect of death from the underlying liver disease would be minimised. The results of the study are strictly speaking, therefore, only applicable to patients with good liver function. There is some evidence that the agent is less effective in those with worse liver function; this matter is considered in Section 'Toxicity and tolerability'.
2. Secondly, one of the primary outcome measures, time to symptomatic progression, was not achieved. The authors suggest, quite reasonably, that this may be attributable to the lack of sensitivity of the instrument used (FHSI-8) to measure time to symptomatic disease progression. This instrument may fail to differentiate between drug toxicity, the underlying liver disease and the symptoms of HCC. The EORTC QLQ-C30 instrument is currently being validated and is likely to be a more useful instrument in the clinical trial setting [13,14]. However, the position remains that, at present, it is not clear whether or not patients experience any improvement in their quality of life. Some workers, particularly those with a hepatological background, consider that survival figures should be the focus of the evidence base [15]. Many oncologists would argue otherwise; namely that whilst a focus on survival is a comfortable position for investigators, for patients with a terminal disease, quality of life is more important.
3. The patients in the SHARP study were predominantly of European extraction with underlying disease aetiology of excessive alcohol consumption and/or chronic hepatitis C virus infection. Whether these results would be applicable to that majority of patients worldwide where chronic hepatitis B virus infection was the major aetiological factor was unanswered. This limitation was extended by the 'Asia Pacific' (AP) study [10]. This was a less rigorously designed trial but the results were remarkably similar. There was a significant improvement in survival, with a very similar reduction in hazard ratio, although the overall survival in both arms was less than in the SHARP study.
4. The median survival improvement of 2.8 months (in the West [9]) and 1.7 months (in the East [10]) is, to many outside the field of oncology, regarded as minimal progress, and to patients, classifying such a treatment as 'clinically effective' causes some dismay. Against this, it should be recognised that because the SHARP trial was stopped early, the figures given for survival improvement potentially underestimate the benefit and are, as such, the minimum figure. Equally, although the absolute figure is small, when expressed in terms of percentage increase in life expectancy, the quoted figure of 44% is much more impressive. Finally, experience shows that in the development of chemotherapy such small improvements have often been key to the subsequent development of effective regimes, the classical example being secondary liver cancer.

On the basis of these data, the clinician has to determine, without the consideration of cost, whether the use of sorafenib is justified. The conclusion of the NICE review [12], and that of most of those in field, was that it *is* a clinically effective treatment for advanced HCC in patients for whom surgical or locoregional therapy had failed or was not suitable. There is, as yet, insufficient evidence to justify treatment in those with poor liver function (see Section 'Toxicity and tolerability'). Patients should be told that they may suffer side effects of diarrhoea, Hand Foot Skin (HFS) syndrome and general lethargy and that there is no guarantee that they will feel any better in themselves. Furthermore, and in practice this is difficult for patients to accept, it is unlikely that their physician will be able to tell if 'the drug is working' since major change in tumour size is uncommon. At most the physician can usually only say that 'there is disease stabilisation'.

Toxicity and tolerability

The two large placebo-controlled trials involving a broad spectrum of disease aetiologies and ethnic backgrounds have given a clear picture of the toxicity and agreed with the figures reported in the phase II trial [16]. Thus, the main toxicities in the SHARP and AP trials were HFS reaction (sorafenib vs. placebo: 8% vs. <1% and 8% vs. 2%, respectively) and diarrhoea (sorafenib vs. placebo: 8% vs. 2% and 6% vs. 0%, respectively). The comparable figures for the phase II study were 9.5% and 5%. On this basis, a starting dose of 400 mg b.i.d. was established and the drug was considered as being well tolerated. The percentage of patients requiring dose reduction or permanent discontinuation was 22% and 34%, respectively, in the AP study.

Subsequently the question of tolerability seems less clear. In the Japanese/Korean study [17], over 40% of patients had their drug permanently discontinued and in the combination study of sorafenib versus sorafenib plus AMG 479, only 2 of 13 patients could tolerate the full dose [18]. The remainder required a dose reduction from 400 mg b.i.d. to 400 mg daily due to sorafenib-related adverse events, mainly HFS syndrome and fatigue. In an investigation of the importance of the cirrhosis stage, the preliminary studies suggest little difference between tolerability between Child's Grade A and B [19,20], but a recent review of the toxicity of sorafenib in HCC concluded that '... although not life-threatening, toxicity of sorafenib can severely impact on the physical, psychological and social well-being of patients' [21].

Of course, the term 'tolerable' is not absolute. A physician may encourage a patient to persevere with a medication in the face of side effects if the outcome is likely to be highly beneficial and the patient is likely to comply. For example, cisplatin-based regimens may impact severely on quality of life but these are usually 'tolerated' if, as in the case of metastatic germ cell tumours, the outcome is likely to be cure. On the other hand, oncologists are reluctant to recommend perseverance with a toxic treatment if the improvement is only perceived to be marginal. It may be that this is the case when, as in HCC, the improvement is only a small number of months and the overall survival is often less than 1 year. Thus, patients will probably vary widely as to the degree of toxicity they are prepared to accept vis-à-vis the perceived benefit in terms of improved life expectancy.

The matter is complicated by suggestions that toxicity might itself be a marker of efficacy, i.e. those developing toxicity may be precisely the same group that achieve maximum benefit as assessed by survival improvement [22,23]. The functional impairment consequent on grade 3 HFS syndrome is significant, and patients may not be able to walk or use their hands effectively. Physicians are reacting in two ways. Firstly, there is an increasing understanding of how to manage the toxicity, and secondly, some physicians are starting patients off on 400 mg daily and then increasing to 800 mg if the drug is well tolerated.

The landscape with respect to targeted agents such as sorafenib is, thus, starting to appear very similar to that seen with old-fashioned cytotoxic treatments. The overall toxicity is no less, just different in nature. The art of administration is similarly to administer the maximum dose consistent with acceptable side effects, and those side effects may, in reality, be markers for drug efficacy.

Cost-effectiveness

Cost-effectiveness analysis (sometimes called cost-utility analysis) compares the costs and health effects of an intervention to assess the extent to which it can be regarded as providing value for money, and thereby offers health care providers the quantitative information with which to allocate limited health care resources. The most commonly used outcome measure is quality-adjusted life years (QALY).

On the basis of figures relating to the purchase of sorafenib in the United Kingdom, the base-case incremental cost-effectiveness ratio (ICER) is around £64,800 ($100,000) per QALY gained. However, the precise figures depend on several assumptions – particularly how overall survival is extrapolated beyond the SHARP study timeframe, the pricing structure offered by the manufacturer and the duration of treatment. On the basis of different probability distributions, particularly toward the tail, and other assumptions, the figures ranged from £50,000 to £76,000. In any event, the conclusion was: '[A]s a treatment for advanced HCC or where locoregional therapies had failed or were not suitable, [Sorafenib] would not be a cost-effective use of NHS resources.' The committee to evaluate drugs for Ontario, Canada, also came to the same conclusion based on a quoted price of C$175 per day (24).

However, studies for the United States [25] and Canada [26] that have undertaken economic analyses examining cost-effectiveness compared with best supportive care arrived at different conclusions. In the American study, life years gained with sorafenib was 1.58 ± 0.17 compared with 1.05 ± 0.10 for best supportive care and the incremental cost-effectiveness ratio was $US62,473 per life-year gained. The cost-effectiveness ratio was considered to fall within the threshold that US society is willing to pay (i.e. $US50,000–$US100,000). The Canadian study came to broadly similar conclusions.

In the standard model of oncological drug development, new agents are developed and tested in the advanced disease setting, and once some degree of activity has been demonstrated, they progress to application in the adjuvant, then neo-adjuvant setting and in combination with other agents. Such argument justifies the use and development of sorafenib further and the approach is outlined briefly in the following.

Adjuvant therapy

Sorafenib might be administered after apparently complete eradication of tumour by resection or RFA with a view to decreasing the recurrence rate, and thereby improving overall survival. This is the design of the STORM trial. Recruitment has been completed and final results are awaited. It might also be administered after transarterial chemoembolisation (TACE), which is given with palliative intent. Several such trials are under way with design varying in respect of when the sorafenib is administered in relation to TACE. One such study has recently been reported in abstract form. In a phase III study of sorafenib in 458 patients from Japan and Korea with advanced (Child-Pugh A disease) HCC treated after TACE who had ≥25% tumour necrosis/shrinkage at 1–3 months following one or two TACE procedures, patients were randomised to sorafenib 400 mg b.i.d. or placebo (P). There was no improvement in overall survival or time to progression.

Combination therapy

There are numerous trials of sorafenib either 'head to head' with other targeted agents or in combination but none of these have, to date, been reported. A single randomised phase II trial of sorafenib in combination with doxorubicin compared with doxorubicin alone has recently been reported [11] with overall survival in the doxorubicin arm of 6.9 months (similar to that reported in other large studies in which doxorubicin was the control arm) compared with 13.5 months in the combination arm.

Clearly, there is no evidence to support sorafenib in the adjuvant setting to date. Furthermore, in the setting of potentially curative treatment any long-term toxicity needs to be considered carefully as a significant fraction of patients will have been cured and will not achieve any benefit from adjuvant treatment. The sorafenib/doxorubicin setting is more controversial. The trial was a randomised phase II design, not a definitive randomised study, and as such only undertaken to determine if there is a case for progression to a phase III trial. Furthermore from the single agent data now available it is clear that the phase III trials should be sorafenib versus sorafenib plus doxorubicin. This trial is currently under way (Trial Number: CALGB 80802). How hepatologists and oncologists proceed prior to the reporting of this trial, and on the basis of the evidence in the literature, remains to be seen.

Conclusions

The answer to the question posed in the title rests on two difficult balancing acts and in neither is there a clear objective answer. In the first, there is the balance between the survival benefit and the high cost. This is ultimately a question for the individual, society and politicians as to the value they are prepared to place on a particular degree of improvement in survival. The second is the balance between prolongation of survival and toxicity. This balance, being reported in terms of 'tolerability', will also vary from patient to patient and amongst different cultural groups.

References

1. Lai CL, Wu PC, Chan GC, et al. Doxorubicin versus no antitumor therapy in inoperable hepatocellular carcinoma. A prospective randomized trial. *Cancer* 1988; 62(3):479–483.
2. Dunk AA, Scott SC, Johnson PJ, et al. Mitozantrone as single agent therapy in hepatocellular carcinoma: a phase II study. *J Hepatology* 1985; 1:395–404.
3. Posey J, Johnson P, Mok T, et al. Results of a phase 2/3 open-label, randomized trial of T138067 versus doxorubicin (DOX) in chemotherapy-naïve, unresectable hepatocellular carcinoma (HCC). *Proc Am Soc Clin Oncol* 2005; 23: 4035a.
4. Gish RG, Porta C, Lazar L, et al. A Phase II randomized controlled trial comparing the survival of patients with unresectable hepatocellular carcinoma treated with nolatrexed or doxorubicin. *J Clin Oncol* 2007; 25(21):3069–3075.
5. Leung TWT, Patt YZ, Lau WY, et al. Complete pathological remission is possible with systemic combination chemotherapy for inoperable hepatocellular carcinoma. *Clin Cancer Research* 1999; 5:1676–1681.
6. Yeo W, Mok TS, Zee B, et al. A randomized phase III study of doxorubicin versus cisplatin/interferon alpha-2b/doxorubicin/fluorouracil (PIAF) combination chemotherapy for unresectable hepatocellular carcinoma. *J Natl Cancer Inst* 2005; 97:1532–1538.
7. Park SH, Lee Y, Han SH, et al. Systemic chemotherapy with doxorubicin, cisplatin and capecitabine for metastatic hepatocellular carcinoma. *BMC Cancer* 2006; 6:3.
8. Llovet JM, Ricci S, Mazzaferro V, et al. SHARP Investigators Study Group. Sorafenib in advanced hepatocellular carcinoma. *N Engl J Med* 2008; 359(4):378–390.
9. Cheng AL, Kang YK, Chen Z, et al. Efficacy and safety of sorafenib in patients in the Asia-Pacific region with advanced hepatocellular carcinoma: a phase III randomised, double-blind, placebo-controlled trial. *Lancet Oncol* 2009; 10(1): 25–34.

10. Abou-Alfa GK, Johnson P, Knox JJ, et al. Doxorubicin plus sorafenib vs. doxorubicin alone in patients with advanced hepatocellular carcinoma: a randomized trial. *JAMA* 2010; 304(19):2154–2160.
11. Hepatocellular carcinoma (advanced and metastatic) – Sorafenib (first line): appraisal consultation 2. NATIONAL INSTITUTE FOR HEALTH AND CLINICAL EXCELLENCE. Appraisal consultation document.
12. Connock M, Round J, Bayliss S, et al. Sorafenib for the treatment of advanced hepatocellular carcinoma. *Health Technol Assess* 2010; 14(suppl 1): 17–21.
13. Aaronson NK, Ahmedzai Bergman B, et al. The European Organization of Research and Treatment of Cancer QLQ-C30: a quality of life instrument for use in international clinical trials in oncology. *J Natl Cancer Inst* 1993; 85:365–376.
14. Yeo W, Mo FKF, Koh J, et al. Quality of life is predictive of survival in patients with unresectable hepatocellular carcinoma. *Ann Oncology* 2006; 17:1083–1089.
15. Bruix J, Sherman M. Management of hepatocellular carcinoma. Practice Guidelines Committee, American Association for the Study of Liver Diseases. *Hepatology* 2005; 42(5):1208–1236.
16. Abou-Alfa GK, Schwartz L, Ricci S, et al. Phase II study of Sorafenib in patients with advanced hepatocellular carcinoma. *J Clin Oncol* 2006; 24(26):4293–4300.
17. Okita K, Imanaka K, Chida N, et al. Phase III study of sorafenib in patients in Japan and Korea with advanced hepatocellular carcinoma (HCC) treated after transarterial chemoembolization (TACE). 2010 Gastrointestinal Cancers Symposium 2010 LBA 128.
18. Puzanov ISJ, Gilbert J, Mahalingam D et al. Safety and pharmacokinetics of AMG479 in erlotinib or sorafenib in patients with advanced solid tumors. *J Clin Oncology* 2010; 28:15s (abstract 3018).
19. Schütte K, Zimmermann L, Bornschein J, et al. Sorafenib therapy in patients with advanced hepatocellular carcinoma in advanced liver cirrhosis. *Digestion* 2011 83(4):275–282.
20. Ozenne V, Paradis V, Pernot S, et al. Tolerance and outcome of patients with unresectable hepatocellular carcinoma treated with sorafenib. *Eur J Gastroenterol Hepatol* 2010; 22(9):1106–1110.
21. Blanchet B, Billemont B, Barete S, et al. Toxicity of sorafenib: clinical and molecular aspects. *Expert Opin Drug Saf* 2010; 9(2):275–287.
22. Jain L, Sissung TM, Danesi R, et al. Hypertension and hand-foot skin reactions related to VEGFR2 genotype and improved clinical outcome following bevacizumab and sorafenib. *J Exp Clin Cancer Res* 2010; 29:95.
23. Vincenzi B, Santini D, Russo A, et al. Early skin toxicity as a predictive factor for tumor control in hepatocellular carcinoma patients treated with sorafenib. *Oncologist* 2010; 15(1):85–92.
24. Sorafenib (for hepatocellular carcinoma) Committee to Evaluate Drugs, Ministry of Health and Long Term Care, Ontario (CED) January 2009
25. Carr BI, Carroll S, Muszbek N, et al. Economic evaluation of sorafenib in unresectable hepatocellular carcinoma. *J Gastroenterol Hepatol* 2010; 25(11):1739–1746.
26. Muszbek N, Shah S, Carroll S, et al. Economic evaluation of sorafenib in the treatment of hepatocellular carcinoma in Canada. *Curr Med Res Opin* 2008; 24(12):3559–3569.

23 When to consider surgery?

Emmanuel Melloul, Mickaël Lesurtel, Pierre-Alain Clavien

Department of Visceral and Transplantation Surgery, University Hospital Zurich, Zurich, Switzerland

LEARNING POINTS

- Since liver transplantation can only be proposed for approximately 30% of patients with hepatocellular carcinoma (HCC), liver resection appears as one of the best alternatives in therapy
- The decision-making process for liver resection in patients with HCC should integrate tumour stage, quality and function of the underlying liver parenchyma, volume of the future liver remnant and general condition of the patient
- In patients with the best features (solitary tumour, compensated cirrhosis, no portal hypertension), the reported 5-year survival rates range from 50% to 70%
- Recurrence rate after liver resection for HCC is still high (>50% at 5 year). It is related to the underlying liver disease and the biological characteristics of HCC tumours, which recur most often away from the primary site of resection
- In patients with a normal liver parenchyma, the liver function is not altered, and even extensive liver resections are well tolerated. Recurrence is then only associated with tumour biology

Introduction

Among curative treatment options for HCC, liver resection and transplantation are considered the mainstay of curative therapy. However, liver transplantation (LT) can only be proposed in approximately 30% of patients with HCC because of donor scarcity and the limitations of transplant criteria in this particular context [1].

The selection of the primary treatment for HCC depends on the tumour stage, functional status of the liver and general condition of the patient. When the liver parenchyma is normal, which is the less frequent situation, the treatment of choice consists of a major hepatectomy. However, most patients with HCC have an underlying chronic liver disease at the time of diagnosis. In this situation, LT is considered as the treatment of choice because it takes care of both the tumour and the underlying disease. While progress performed in the screening of patients with chronic liver diseases has increased the detection rate of HCC, the low availability of liver grafts and the allocation system in Europe and the United States preclude proposing LT in many patients with HCC and underlying chronic liver disease.

Formerly, liver resections in patients with cirrhosis were few in number due to high morbidity and mortality rates, and a high recurrence rate related to the associated liver disease. However, development of new techniques and a better knowledge of risk factors associated with partial hepatectomy have considerably improved the short-term and long-term results of liver resection in these patients [2,3]. This better scenario, together with the scarcity of donors, led to a renewed interest in liver resection for HCC patients. Indeed, liver resection appears as one of the best therapeutic options in cases with an otherwise normal liver and in patients with underlying chronic liver disease who do not meet the accepted transplant criteria.

This chapter focuses on the indications for liver resection in patients with HCC associated with a normal parenchyma or with an underlying chronic liver disease.

Clinical Dilemmas in Primary Liver Cancer, First Edition. Edited by Roger Williams and Simon D. Taylor-Robinson.

Selection criteria for liver resection in patients with HCC

To consider a liver resection in patients with HCC, three factors need to be integrated in the decision-making: (1) tumour stage, (2) quality and function of the underlying liver parenchyma and (3) volume of the future liver remnant (FLR).

Tumour stage

Assessment of tumour extent is the primary step in determining resectability and the type of surgical resection in HCC patients. Triphasic contrast-enhanced computed tomography (CT) is essential to define number and size of the tumour. It detects the presence of satellite nodules, tumour macrovascular invasion and extra hepatic metastases. Magnetic resonance imaging is a valuable alternative, particularly when contrast agents are contraindicated or for better lesion characterisation with more specific enhancement.

Tumour-associated predictors of poor outcome after liver resections include satellite nodules, size of lesion >5 cm, serum alpha-fetoprotein level >2000 ng/mL, positive resection margins, vascular invasion and Union for International Cancer Control (UICC) stages III or IV (tumours with direct invasion of adjacent organs, regional lymph node metastases or distant metastases) [4].

According to the Japanese Registry, which has one of the largest series of HCC resections worldwide, the presence of multiple intrahepatic tumours is associated with a worse outcome [5]. In this series, the 5-year survival rate was 57% when the tumour was simple and decreased to 26% when multiple. In addition, Vauthey et al. have previously reported that patients with a solitary tumour of 5 cm or less have a 5-year survival rate of 43%, whereas it fell to 32% when the tumour is over 5 cm [6]. These results possibly related with the strong correlation between the size of the tumour and the risk of microvascular invasion. Microvascular invasion is an important prognostic factor, which can only be assessed on the resected specimen. It occurs in 20% of cases for tumours of 2 cm in diameter, and in 60–90% of cases when the tumour reaches more than 5 cm [7]. A multicentre study of 300 patients with HCC >10 cm reported a 5-year overall survival rate of 27% [8]. Major liver resections for large or multinodular HCC should be restricted to selected patients with preserved liver function.

Three situations deserve special attention in the tumour staging – HCC with biliary or vascular extension and ruptured HCC:

- A tumour thrombus (macrovascular invasion) into one of the main portal branches (sectorial or lobar), or into a hepatic vein, is observed in a small proportion of advanced HCC. These vascular invasions are associated with a worse prognosis due to intrahepatic and systemic tumour dissemination originating from the portal and hepatic veins thrombi, respectively. In a multicentre study including 102 patients, Pawlik et al. demonstrated that HCCs with invasion of a major portal branch have 1-, 3- and 5-year survival rates of 47%, 17% and 10%, respectively [9]. In the study from Vauthey et al., 5-year survival in patients with and without macrovascular invasion was 15% versus 41%, respectively [6].
- HCC can cause a fistula into the biliary tree. This is associated with jaundice, and the treatment consists of a liver resection with biliary desobstruction to remove the tumour extension.
- Ruptured HCC usually presents with a haemoperitoneum. The first treatment consists of arterial embolisation to control the bleeding. When the patient is stabilised and in good condition, a secondary liver resection can be considered.

Liver parenchyma: quality and function

Almost 90% of HCC develop on a chronic liver disease. The most common liver diseases encountered are viral hepatitis B and C, alcoholic liver disease, haemochromatosis and non-alcoholic steatohepatitis (NASH). The risk of a resection when there is an underlying chronic liver disease is related to a decrease in the capacity of the remnant liver to regenerate [10]. The major risk for the patient is post-operative liver failure, which can lead to death or decompensate cirrhosis. According to the recent results from the main Asian and occidental series (Table 23.1), the mortality after liver resection for HCC in cirrhotic patients has significantly decreased since the past 20 years. In the series from Poon et al., which included 50% of cirrhosis, the in-hospital mortality decreased from 13% to 2.5% between the early and late 90s [2]. In the series from Wu et al. (100% of cirrhosis), mortality rate decreased from 3.7% to less than 1% over the same period of time [11].

Before considering resection, liver function tests should be carried out to fully assess the putative underlying liver

TABLE 23.1 Main Asian and occidental published series of patients resected for HCC from 2000 to 2010

Authors	Year of publication	Study period	*N*	Cirrhosis (%)	Diameter HCC <5 cm (%)	Perioperative mortality (%)	1-year survival (%)	3-year survival (%)	5-year survival (%)	3-year recurrence rate (%)	5-year recurrence rate (%)
Asian series											
Zhou et al. [25]	2001	1967–1998	1000	88	100	1.5	91	76	64	–	–
Poon et al. [2]	2001	1989–1993	136	50	29	13	68	47	36	–	–
		1994–1999	241	43	45	2.5	82	62	49	–	–
Yamamoto et al. [26]	2001	1990–1994	58	70	100	–	96	84	61	–	–
Shimozawa and Hanazaki [27]	2004	1987–2001	135	71	100	2	95	73	55	50	70
Wu et al. [11]	2005	1991–1996	161	100	–	3.7	–	–	46	–	72
		1997–2002	265	100	–	0.4	–	–	61	–	66
Taura et al. [28]	2007	1990–2003	293	54	100	3.8	89	78	61	58	71
Wang et al. [29]	2010	1991–2004	438	100	38	7.5	72	53	43	47	56
Lee et al. [30]	2010	1997–2007	130	100	–	0.8	80	65	52	46	50
Occidental series											
Grazi et al. [31]	2001	1983–1998	264	100	64	4.9	–	63	41	36	56
Wayne et al. [32]	2002	1980–1998	249	73	100	6.1	–	–	41	–	–
Belghiti et al. [33]	2002	1990–1999	300	82	47	6	81	57	37	–	–
Grazi et al. [34]	2003	1981–2002	308	100	–	2.9	86	64	42	33	50
			135	0	–	1.1	84	68	51	32	39
Ercolani et al. [35]	2003	1983–1999	224	100	81	3	83	63	42	38	54
Lang et al. [14]	2005	1998–2003	33	0	–	6	87	50	–	–	–
Lubrano et al. [13]	2008	1986–2005	20	0	–	5	85	70	64	34	42
Cherqui et al. [36]	2009	1990–2007	67	73	100	4.5	–	–	72	48	56

disease. One of the commonest used scoring systems is the Child-Pugh classification. However, this score provides only a rough estimation of the metabolic activity of the liver, stratifying patients into three groups only: those with compensated (class A) cirrhosis, and those with moderate (class B) or severe (class C) decompensated cirrhosis. In Eastern countries, more sophisticated quantitative liver function tests have been developed to refine patient selection for liver resection, including the indocyanine green (ICG) clearance test. ICG is a dark bluish-green tricarbocyanine dye that rapidly binds to plasma beta-lipoprotein and is completely and exclusively cleared by hepatocytes. ICG is excreted into bile in unmodified form and does not enter the enterohepatic circulation [10]. Usually, the percentage of ICG retention is measured at 15 minutes after its injection allows the extent of liver resection to be defined; for example, a major hepatectomy up to 15% ICG retention and limited resection if retention is beyond 20% [3].

Portal vein hypertension is another important risk factor for post-operative liver failure and is usually considered as a contraindication to major liver resection. The best way to determinate the porto-systemic venous gradient is by the catheterism of hepatic veins. A gradient pressure between portal vein and hepatic vein >10 mmHg defines portal hypertension. This cut-off identifies cirrhotic patients who are likely to decompensate after liver resection [12]. However, this method is invasive and not routinely used. A less invasive method to diagnose portal hypertension is the detection of oesophageal varices at gastroscopy, splenomegaly and/or venous collateral channels on the pre-operative CT scan imaging. If in doubt, a biopsy of the non-tumoural liver may be performed to detect fibrosis/cirrhosis or active disease in the liver prior to surgery.

In patients with a normal liver parenchyma and liver function, even extensive liver resections are well tolerated, provided that the FLR volume is sufficient (see Section 'Future liver remnant volume'). According to the most recent series of liver resection for HCC in normal liver parenchyma, the reported peri-operative mortality ranged from 0% to 6.4% with a morbidity of 10–21% [13–15].

Future liver remnant volume

Whereas young patients (<40 years of age) with a good general condition tolerate the removal of up to 75% of the whole liver volume, the cirrhotic liver tolerates tissue loss poorly due to its impaired function and decreased ability to regenerate after resection [10]. Assessment of FLR volume is performed by CT volumetry. In patients with chronic liver disease, it has been shown that liver resection can be performed safely when the FLR accounts for more than 40% of the whole liver volume. If too small, an attempt through the regenerative capacity of the liver is made to increase the FLR volume before resection by pre-operative portal vein embolisation (PVE) of the hemi-liver to be resected. This may be sufficient to prevent post-operative life-threatening liver failure due to insufficient residual liver. Resection can then be considered 3–6 weeks after portal vein occlusion, when the maximal changes in volume have been reached. PVE is also becoming more commonly used to identify patients in whom liver regeneration is impaired.

On the basis of our current practice and available data, we proposed the decision tree shown in Figure 23.1, for major hepatectomy in patients with normal liver parenchyma (A) and those with cirrhosis (B); for cirrhotic liver with an ICG test less than 14% at 15 minutes, we apply the algorithm for normal liver parenchyma with a higher cut-off point for the volume of the FLR (35–40%).

Another strategy in cirrhotic patients consists in the sequential use of transarterial chemoembolisation (TACE) and PVE, prior to a major liver resection [4]. TACE (see Chapter 17) directly affects the tumour and embolises arterioportal shunts that are frequent in the context of cirrhosis. This approach allows a better tumour control during the period between PVE and the planned surgery, and has been associated with more efficient hypertrophy of the FLR.

Since the decision to perform a liver resection in patients with HCC implies the assessment of numerous pre-operative factors, several prognostic staging models accounting for both the extent of HCC and the functional reserve of the liver have been developed to predict survival and assess outcomes of liver resection. One of the most widely used models is the Barcelona Clinic Liver Cancer (BCLC) staging system [16] (see Chapter 10). Patients with very early stage (stage A) disease are optimal candidates for a radical treatment for a possible cure. According to this classification system, patients with a single tumour and with normal serum bilirubin levels and portal pressure are the best candidates for liver resection.

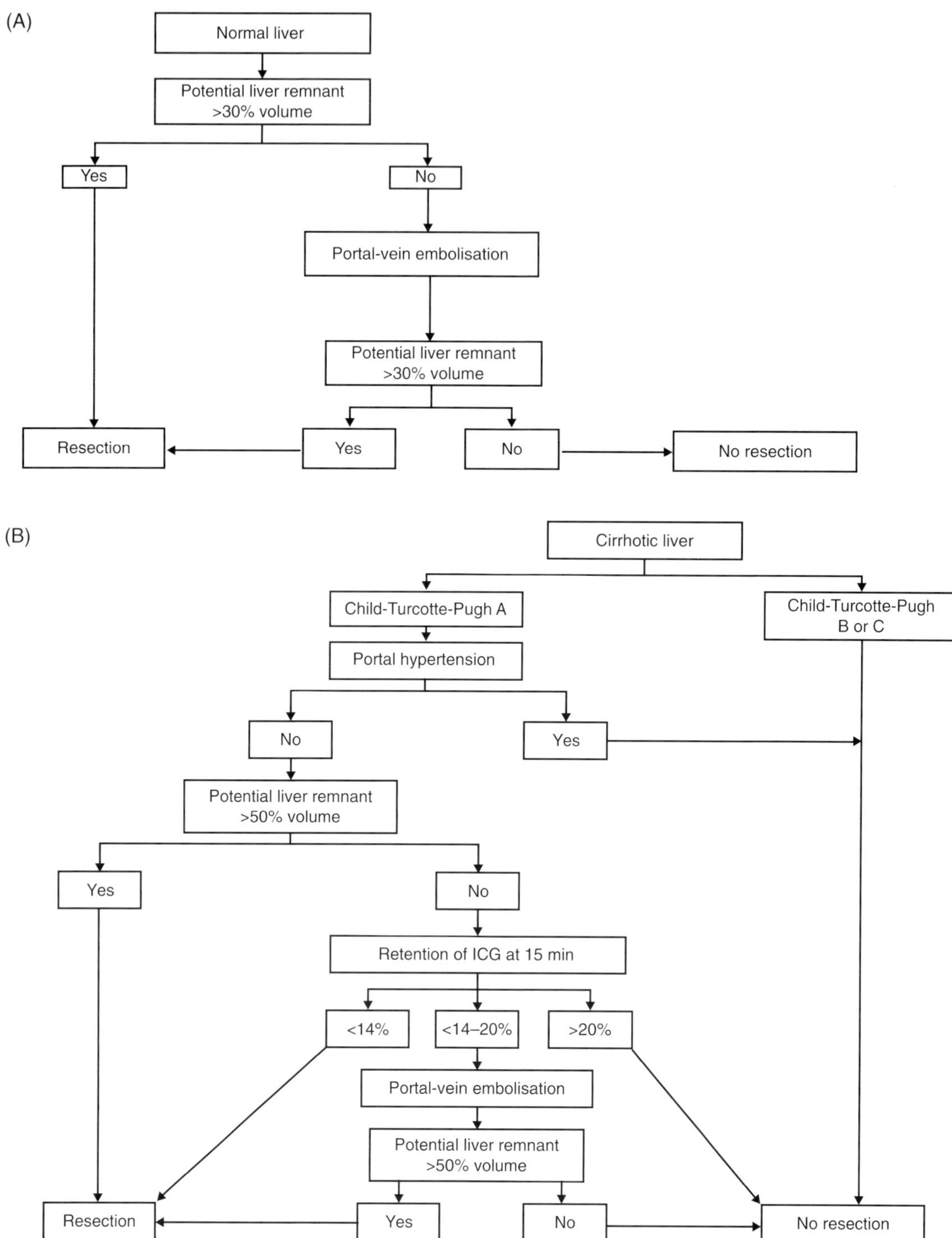

FIG 23.1 Proposed decision tree for major hepatectomy in patients with normal liver parenchyma (A) and those with cirrhosis (B).

Long-term outcome and recurrence after liver resection for HCC

Due to the heterogeneity of published series (Table 23.1), the results of long-term survival for patients with underlying chronic liver disease are variable. In patients with the best features (solitary tumour, Child A, no portal hypertension), the reported 5-year survival rates range from 50% to 70%. The 3- and 5-year recurrence rates range from 36% to 58% and from 39% to 70%, respectively. Recurrence is usually related to the underlying liver disease and the biology of HCC tumours, and occurs most often far away from the primary site of resection.

In series restricted to resection with normal liver parenchyma (Table 23.1), the 1- and 5-year survival rates ranged from 62% to 97% and from 25% to 81%, respectively [13–15]. The 1- and 5-year disease-free survival rates ranged from 49% to 84% and from 24% to 54%, respectively. The 5-year reported incidence of tumour recurrence, which most frequently – though less than in cirrhotic patients – occurs in the liver, ranged from 30% to 73%.

Liver resection as a bridge to liver transplantation

In patients with HCC and compensated cirrhosis and with a long anticipated time on the waiting list for a transplant, a strategy consisting of liver resection followed by listing for LT can be applied. This strategy allows control of the tumour and a better assessment of its pathological features. In case of negative prognosis factors (poor differentiation, microvascular invasion, absence of capsule), a short-term LT may still be proceeded with (bridging strategy), but if the tumour does not show any such risk factors for recurrence, LT may be postponed and offered only in presence of tumour recurrence (salvage procedure). Some authors have shown, in selected patients with early-stage HCC, that liver resection followed by salvage LT at the time of recurrence share similar outcomes as strategies using primary LT [17]. For others [18], liver resection used as a bridge to LT is associated with higher operative mortality, increased recurrence and worse outcome than primary LT. Therefore, liver resection as a bridge to LT and salvage LT are not yet adopted in many centres, which still offer primary LT as the initial choice of treatment in cirrhotic patients with HCC, even when the tumour is initially resectable [4].

Technical considerations

Anatomic versus non-anatomic resection

HCC cells can infiltrate the portal vein and spread via the portal blood flow, resulting thereafter in intrahepatic metastases. Anatomic liver resection aims at the complete removal of at least one Couinaud's segment containing the tumour, together with the portal vein related to the neoplasm and the corresponding hepatic territory.

Regimbeau et al. have shown in a small but homogenous study that overall and disease-free survival rates were significantly longer and recurrence rate lower after anatomic resection [19]. The results of a recent meta-analysis have shown that in patients with HCC, anatomic resection is superior to non-anatomic resection in terms of disease-free survival [20]. However, there was no significant difference in overall survival and local recurrence between the two techniques. These results should be taken cautiously as all the series included were retrospective in nature. Despite this low level of evidence, anatomic resection seems to be associated with a better outcome and should be preferred in HCC patients with preserved liver function.

Laparoscopic liver resection

The place of laparoscopy in liver surgery is increasing worldwide. Many types of liver resections, including major hepatectomies, are now performed by laparoscopy in specialised centres. According to the 2008 International Consensus Conference on laparoscopic liver surgery (the Louisville Statement), this technique is a safe and effective approach to the management of surgical liver disease in the hands of trained surgeons with experience in both hepato-biliary and laparoscopic surgery [21]. Recently, Dagher et al. have shown in a large prospective multicentre study that laparoscopic resection for HCC is feasible in selected patients, with good operative and oncologic results [22]. In this series, 74% of patients were cirrhotic, of which 90% had Child A. Liver resection was anatomic in 65% of patients and major in 10%. The conversion rate to open surgery was 9%, and less than 10% of patients received blood transfusion. The in-hospital mortality rate was 1.2% and overall morbidity 10%. Finally, the overall and recurrence-free survival rates at 1, 3 and 5 years were 92.6%, 68.7% and 64.9%, and 77.5%, 47.1% and 32.2%, respectively, comparable to open surgery [22].

Hanging manoeuvre and the anterior approach

Two specific surgical techniques have been shown to be useful for HCC resection: the anterior approach and liver hanging manoeuvre.

The anterior approach is based on performing parenchyma transection prior to liver mobilisation aiming to reduce tumour mobilisation and seeding of tumour cells. In a prospective controlled study, this strategy was associated with better short-term and long-term outcomes than standard approach in HCC patients who underwent right hepatectomy [23]. In this series, the median overall survival was 68 months after anterior approach versus 22 months after standard approach, and disease-free survivals were 15.5 months versus 13.9 months, respectively.

The liver hanging manoeuvre was described at the end of the 90s to facilitate the anterior approach by using a tape in the avascular retrohepatic precaval space to guide the direction of the parenchyma transection and minimise bleeding by elevation of the liver along its deeper parenchyma plane [24]. Albeit this technique is helpful for safer liver resection, data based on the long-term survival when the hanging manoeuvre is used with the anterior approach are still lacking.

Conclusion

Because of the current allocation system in Europe and the United States, only one-third of the patients with HCC occurring in an underlying chronic liver disease have access to LT. Liver resection has taken an important place in the curative treatment for HCC with acceptable post-operative mortality and 3- and 5-year survival rates. This surgery can be performed with low mortality, providing adequate liver function, FLR volume and absence of high portal pressure. The main principles of liver resection in this setting are anatomic resection with pre-operative PVE in the case of a too small calculated FLR volume. For large HCC occupying the right hemi-liver, anterior approach, with or without hanging manoeuvre, should be preferred. The laparoscopic approach has shown good preliminary results in selected patients and trained hands. However, the recurrence rate after liver resection for HCC is still high (>50% at 5 year), mostly related to the biological characteristics of the tumour and the underlying liver disease.

References

1. Llovet JM, Burroughs A, Bruix J. Hepatocellular carcinoma. *Lancet* 2003; 362(9399):1907–1917.
2. Poon RT, Fan ST, Lo CM, et al. Improving survival results after resection of hepatocellular carcinoma: a prospective study of 377 patients over 10 years. *Ann Surg* 2001; 234(1):63–70.
3. Imamura H, Seyama Y, Kokudo N, et al. One thousand fifty-six hepatectomies without mortality in 8 years. *Arch Surg* 2003; 138(11):1198–1206.
4. McCormack L, Petrowsky H, Clavien PA. Surgical therapy of hepatocellular carcinoma. *Eur J Gastroenterol Hepatol* 2005; 17(5):497–503.
5. Ikai I, Arii S, Kojiro M, et al. Reevaluation of prognostic factors for survival after liver resection in patients with hepatocellular carcinoma in a Japanese nationwide survey. *Cancer* 2004; 101(4):796–802.
6. Vauthey JN, Lauwers GY, Esnaola NF, et al. Simplified staging for hepatocellular carcinoma. *J Clin Oncol* 2002; 20(6):1527–1536.
7. Pawlik TM, Delman KA, Vauthey JN, et al. Tumor size predicts vascular invasion and histologic grade: implications for selection of surgical treatment for hepatocellular carcinoma. *Liver Transpl* 2005; 11(9):1086–1092.
8. Pawlik TM, Poon RT, Abdalla EK, et al. Critical appraisal of the clinical and pathologic predictors of survival after resection of large hepatocellular carcinoma. *Arch Surg* 2005; 140(5):450–457.
9. Pawlik TM, Poon RT, Abdalla EK, et al. Hepatectomy for hepatocellular carcinoma with major portal or hepatic vein invasion: results of a multicenter study. *Surgery* 2005; 137(4):403–410.
10. Clavien PA, Petrowsky H, DeOliveira ML, et al. Strategies for safer liver surgery and partial liver transplantation. *N Engl J Med* 2007; 356(15):1545–1559.
11. Wu CC, Cheng SB, Ho WM, et al. Liver resection for hepatocellular carcinoma in patients with cirrhosis. *Br J Surg* 2005; 92(3):348–355.
12. Burroughs AK, Thalheimer U. Hepatic venous pressure gradient in 2010: optimal measurement is key. *Hepatology* 2010; 51(6):1894–1896.
13. Lubrano J, Huet E, Tsilividis B, et al. Long-term outcome of liver resection for hepatocellular carcinoma in noncirrhotic nonfibrotic liver with no viral hepatitis or alcohol abuse. *World J Surg* 2008; 32(1):104–109.
14. Lang H, Sotiropoulos GC, Domland M, et al. Liver resection for hepatocellular carcinoma in non-cirrhotic liver without underlying viral hepatitis. *Br J Surg* 2005; 92(2):198–202.
15. Capussotti L, Muratore A, Amisano M, et al. Liver resection for large-size hepatocellular carcinomas in 47 non-cirrhotic

patients – no mortality and long-term survival. *Hepatogastroenterology* 2006; 53(71):768–772.

16. Bruix J, Llovet JM. Prognostic prediction and treatment strategy in hepatocellular carcinoma. *Hepatology* 2002; 35(3):519–524.
17. Belghiti J, Cortes A, Abdalla EK, et al. Resection prior to liver transplantation for hepatocellular carcinoma. *Ann Surg* 2003; 238(6):885–892.
18. Adam R, Azoulay D, Castaing D, et al. Liver resection as a bridge to transplantation for hepatocellular carcinoma on cirrhosis: a reasonable strategy? *Ann Surg* 2003; 238(4):508–518.
19. Regimbeau JM, Kianmanesh R, Farges O, et al. Extent of liver resection influences the outcome in patients with cirrhosis and small hepatocellular carcinoma. *Surgery* 2002; 131(3):311–317.
20. Chen J, Huang K, Wu J, et al. Survival after anatomic resection versus nonanatomic resection for hepatocellular carcinoma: a meta-analysis. *Dig Dis Sci* 2010; 56(6):1626–1633.
21. Buell JF, Cherqui D, Geller DA, et al. The international position on laparoscopic liver surgery: The Louisville Statement, 2008. *Ann Surg* 2009; 250(5):825–830.
22. Dagher I, Belli G, Fantini C, et al. Laparoscopic hepatectomy for hepatocellular carcinoma: a European experience. *J Am Coll Surg* 2010; 211(1):16–23.
23. Liu CL, Fan ST, Cheung ST, et al. Anterior approach versus conventional approach right hepatic resection for large hepatocellular carcinoma: a prospective randomized controlled study. *Ann Surg* 2006; 244(2):194–203.
24. Ogata S, Belghiti J, Varma D, et al. Two hundred liver hanging maneuvers for major hepatectomy: a single-center experience. *Ann Surg* 2007; 245(1):31–35.
25. Zhou XD, Tang ZY, Yang BH, et al. Experience of 1000 patients who underwent hepatectomy for small hepatocellular carcinoma. *Cancer* 2001; 91(8):1479–1486.
26. Yamamoto J, Okada S, Shimada K, et al. Treatment strategy for small hepatocellular carcinoma: comparison of long-term results after percutaneous ethanol injection therapy and surgical resection. *Hepatology* 2001; 34(4 Pt 1):707–713.
27. Shimozawa N, Hanazaki K. Longterm prognosis after hepatic resection for small hepatocellular carcinoma. *J Am Coll Surg* 2004; 198(3):356–365.
28. Taura K, Ikai I, Hatano E, et al. Influence of coexisting cirrhosis on outcomes after partial hepatic resection for hepatocellular carcinoma fulfilling the Milan criteria: an analysis of 293 patients. *Surgery* 2007; 142(5):685–694.
29. Wang J, Xu LB, Liu C, et al. Prognostic factors and outcome of 438 Chinese patients with hepatocellular carcinoma underwent partial hepatectomy in a single center. *World J Surg* 2010; 34(10):2434–2441.
30. Lee KK, Kim DG, Moon IS, et al. Liver transplantation versus liver resection for the treatment of hepatocellular carcinoma. *J Surg Oncol* 2010; 101(1):47–53.
31. Grazi GL, Ercolani G, Pierangeli F, et al. Improved results of liver resection for hepatocellular carcinoma on cirrhosis give the procedure added value. *Ann Surg* 2001; 234(1): 71–78.
32. Wayne JD, Lauwers GY, Ikai I, et al. Preoperative predictors of survival after resection of small hepatocellular carcinomas. *Ann Surg* 2002; 235(5):722–730.
33. Belghiti J, Regimbeau JM, Durand F, et al. Resection of hepatocellular carcinoma: a European experience on 328 cases. *Hepatogastroenterology* 2002; 49(43):41–46.
34. Grazi GL, Cescon M, Ravaioli M, et al. Liver resection for hepatocellular carcinoma in cirrhotics and noncirrhotics. Evaluation of clinicopathologic features and comparison of risk factors for long-term survival and tumour recurrence in a single centre. *Aliment Pharmacol Ther* 2003; 17 Suppl 2:119–129.
35. Ercolani G, Grazi GL, Ravaioli M, et al. Liver resection for hepatocellular carcinoma on cirrhosis: univariate and multivariate analysis of risk factors for intrahepatic recurrence. *Ann Surg* 2003; 237(4):536–543.
36. Cherqui D, Laurent A, Mocellin N, et al. Liver resection for transplantable hepatocellular carcinoma: long-term survival and role of secondary liver transplantation. *Ann Surg* 2009; 250(5):738–746.

24 Transplant considerations

Myron Schwartz
The Mount Sinai Medical Center, New York, NY, USA

LEARNING POINTS

- Liver transplantation is the treatment of choice for patients with unresectable hepatocellular carcinoma (HCC) within the Milan criteria
- While recurrence of HCC is more common after resection than after transplant, post-operative 5-year patient survival is similar between resection and transplantation for patients with solitary HCC, Child's A cirrhosis and no portal hypertension; depending on organ availability, transplant waiting list dropout may result in higher intention-to-treat survival with resection than with transplantation
- Based on tumour size and number, the risk of post-transplant HCC recurrence is a continuum; broadened criteria will result in higher recurrence rates
- Downstaging, that is, non-surgical treatment of HCC in patients awaiting transplantation to reduce viable tumour size/number to within Milan criteria followed by a period of observation during which progression is not observed, is increasingly being practiced and appears to yield post-transplant survival rates similar to those achieved with patients initially within Milan criteria
- Living donor transplantation (LDT) provides a source of donor organs for which there is no competition. While controversial, in the view of many centres, this reasonably allows transplantation of patients with higher risk of HCC recurrence that would otherwise be acceptable

Introduction

Liver transplantation has a high likelihood of curing patients with early HCC, and in patients with early HCC who have liver dysfunction that precludes resection and who are otherwise suitable candidates transplantation is universally accepted as the treatment of choice, subject to donor organ availability. However, there are many patients with HCC who do not fall neatly within this definition of the ideal HCC transplant candidate but who nevertheless are likely best-served with transplantation. This chapter examines this diverse group of patients to try and refine our understanding of when transplantation should be considered.

Definition of early HCC

From the standpoint of liver transplantation, what we really need to know is whether or not a patient has HCC outside of the liver; since the entire native liver will be removed, the extent of tumour within the liver is irrelevant except as a predictor of extrahepatic spread. Among the identifiable characteristics of HCC within the liver, the presence of vascular invasion (VI) correlates most closely with the likelihood of occult metastasis and, thus, post-transplant HCC recurrence [1]. However, it should be noted that VI is not an all-or-none issue; gross VI implies an overwhelming likelihood of metastasis, whereas microscopic VI, depending on the size of vessels invaded and their distance from the tumour presents a spectrum of risk ranging from as high as that associated with gross VI to as low as that seen when VI is absent [2]. While gross VI is commonly identifiable on pre-transplant imaging, microscopic VI by definition is not; since decisions about transplant candidacy of needs must be based on imaging, we must rely on surrogates for VI,

Clinical Dilemmas in Primary Liver Cancer, First Edition. Edited by Roger Williams and Simon D. Taylor-Robinson.

and the size and number of tumours seen on imaging has emerged as the most practical surrogate for this purpose.

While not based on a highly sophisticated statistical analysis, the criteria employed by Mazzaferro et al., in his 1996 publication [3] (one nodule ≤5 cm, or 2–3 nodules all <3 cm), when applied to findings on pre-transplant imaging, have been repeatedly demonstrated to yield a pool of candidates who can be transplanted with a likelihood of recurrence around 10%, and for practical purposes these Milan criteria may be considered to define early HCC.

Resection versus transplantation

Hepatic resection is a potentially curative treatment for HCC that can be performed with low morbidity and mortality in the range of 1% in patients with cirrhosis and HCC who have preserved liver function (Child's A) and no portal hypertension [4]. When such patients present with HCC within the Milan criteria, in particular with a solitary HCC ≤5 cm (since patients with multiple HCC's are more likely to develop subsequent new tumours), resection and transplantation become competing options [5]. While resection can certainly be performed in patients who do not meet these strict criteria [6], the increased morbidity/mortality and decreased long-term survival diminish its appeal when the transplant alternative is available.

There is no question that HCC recurrence is far less frequent after transplantation than after resection, where the majority of patients will experience recurrence within 5 years. This is the result of both intrahepatic metastasis and de novo tumour development, both of which are obviated by transplant. However, HCC recurrence after resection does not equate with death; repeat resection [7], percutaneous tumour ablation [8] and transplantation [9] remain as potentially curative options. With a transplant, while HCC recurrence is a relative rarity, there are non-tumour-related issues that affect the overall outcome and must be weighed against post-resection HCC recurrence in choosing the best option for a particular patient.

As opposed to the perioperative mortality rate of around 1% in properly selected resection candidates, the mortality associated with transplantation over the first year, related to technical, immunologic, and infectious complications and regardless of the reason for transplant, is around 10%. Furthermore, for patients with hepatitis C, who constitute the majority of patients with HCC undergoing transplant in the West, post-transplant hepatitis C recurrence leads to the accelerated development of cirrhosis (roughly 25% within 5 years) and 5-year patient survival rates around 10% lower than for patients with other causes of cirrhosis [10]. The fact is that patients with hepatitis C-related HCC have worse outcomes after resection than patients with other underlying diseases (particularly hepatitis B) as well; but our Mount Sinai data, as well as a number of other studies, demonstrate no significant difference in patient survival at 5 years after resection versus transplantation [11].

Unlike resection, transplantation requires donor organs, the limited availability of which dictates a variable waiting period depending on the local organ supply. Even with the priority typically accorded patients with HCC meeting the Milan criteria, waiting times can exceed 1 year in many locales. Despite efforts using a variety of non-surgical approaches and, occasionally, even resection, to limit HCC progression, dropout from the waiting list over a 1 year waiting period is in the range of 20–25% [12]. In choosing resection or transplantation for a patient who is eligible for both, outcomes must be viewed on an intention-to-treat basis incorporating waiting list dropout. In the Mount Sinai experience in New York, similar to other reports from centres where transplant waiting times are lengthy, resection yields significantly better intention-to-treat survival than transplantation and is thus the preferred treatment for patients with Child's A cirrhosis, no portal hypertension, and a solitary HCC ≤5 cm.

Very early HCC

Transplantation is an accepted treatment for early HCC; as HCC progresses beyond the Milan criteria within the liver the likelihood of unrecognised extrahepatic spread and subsequent post-transplant recurrence rises, limiting the benefit and thus constituting inefficient use of the scarce donor resource [13]. There is also room for concern at the other end of the spectrum: Are there some patients with HCC that is so early that transplantation fails to provide adequate benefit vis-à-vis alternative ablation treatments, that is, use is not justified? While liver pathologists have debated the definition of very early HCC, from the liver transplant perspective, attention has focused on those patients with solitary HCC <2 cm; a group that has come to be called T1 based on a classification initially devised by the American Liver Tumor Study Group. This was subsequently adopted in the United States and elsewhere as the basis for liver allocation to patients with HCC (within this classification the remaining patients within the Milan criteria are designated as T2) [14].

The first and foremost concern about the suitability of patients with T1 HCC as transplant candidates grew out of reports of the early US experience using the Model for End-stage Liver Disease (MELD) system beginning in 2002, which granted waiting list priority to patients with T1 HCC, demonstrating that in nearly a third of patients transplanted priority pathology failed to reveal the presence of a tumour [15]. The difficulty in making a definitive diagnosis of liver nodules under 2 cm is widely discussed in the literature [16]. There have been improvements in liver imaging technology, and criteria for imaging-based diagnosis have been refined, such that when both arterial enhancement and venous washout are demonstrated on a high-quality CT or MR study, HCC may be confidently diagnosed when sized between 1and 2 cm [17]. Biopsy remains a viable way to establish the diagnosis in lesions not meeting imaging criteria. The basis for concern over organ wastage due to transplanting patients for mistaken HCC diagnosis has thus to a large extent been dissipated over recent years.

The other issue raised concerning very early HCC is that the benefit resulting from transplant may not be great enough to justify its use relative to patients with later-stage HCC or with other accepted indications for transplant. The incidence of micro-VI related to HCC <2 cm is very low; this fact, along with the technical ease with which most small HCCs can be treated with radiofrequency ablation (RFA), explains why multiple reports have shown that long-term local control of HCC <2 cm by RFA can be achieved in 95% or more of patients [18,19]. This being the case, the need for transplant on the basis of such a lesion is dubious. Another argument relates to the philosophical basis underlying the prioritisation of HCC patients within the MELD allocation system. In developing this system, the waiting list dropout for HCC patients was equated with death on the waiting list for non-tumour patients, and the priority score assigned to HCC patients was chosen to equalise the respective endpoints between the two groups. The risk of waiting list dropout for patients with T1 HCC has been repeatedly shown to be very low, and thus prioritising them before their tumours reach T2 unfairly directs organs to the HCC patient cohort. On the basis of the foregoing reasons, patients with T1 HCC are no longer granted priority for transplantation in the United States and many other countries.

HCC beyond the Milan criteria

The Milan criteria provide a convenient, easily reproducible way of selecting a subset of patients with HCC who will do well with transplantation. However, it is clear to all involved in the field that there are many patients with HCC beyond the Milan criteria who could also be cured with a transplant. In 2002, Roayaie et al. demonstrated 5-year survival of 55% in a cohort of patients with HCC between 5 and –7 cm transplanted within the context of a multidisciplinary treatment protocol [20]. A number of authors have proposed modest expansion of the Milan criteria, based on either simple measurement of tumour diameter and number of nodules or on resultant volume calculations. The University of California, San Francisco (UCSF) criteria (one tumour ≤6.5 cm, or 2–3 nodules ≤4.5 cm with total tumour diameter ≤8 cm) developed by Yao et al. represent the most widely publicised and best-validated among these efforts [21]. Initially based on retrospective data from the pathology of explanted livers, the UCSF criteria have been validated prospectively based on pre-transplant imaging and in the single-centre UCSF experience [22].

However, not all subsequent analyses at other centres have provided confirmatory evidence of the utility of UCSF criteria [23]. It is an inescapable fact that the risk of post-transplant recurrence is directly related to tumour size and number. This has been most clearly and definitively demonstrated by Mazzaferro et al. in the 'Metroticket' paper wherein 1112 patients with HCC beyond the Milan criteria were studied [13]. A linear relation was observed between tumour diameter and recurrence throughout the observed range. The number of tumours also correlated significantly with recurrence, with the effect tending to plateau after three tumours. An elegant graphic (Figure 24.1) provided a simple means of estimating the likelihood of recurrence for a patient with any given size/number combination. On the basis of this analysis, Mazzaferro proposed the 'up-to-7' criteria, wherein the sum of the number of tumours and the diameter of the largest tumour in cm should not exceed 7.

The subject of expansion of criteria has engendered endless debate based not on whether patients with HCC beyond the Milan criteria could benefit, but rather on the impact that transplanting them has on the rest of the candidate pool. It is a fact of transplant life that there is significant geographical variability in the availability of donor organs and it is only natural, then, that there is

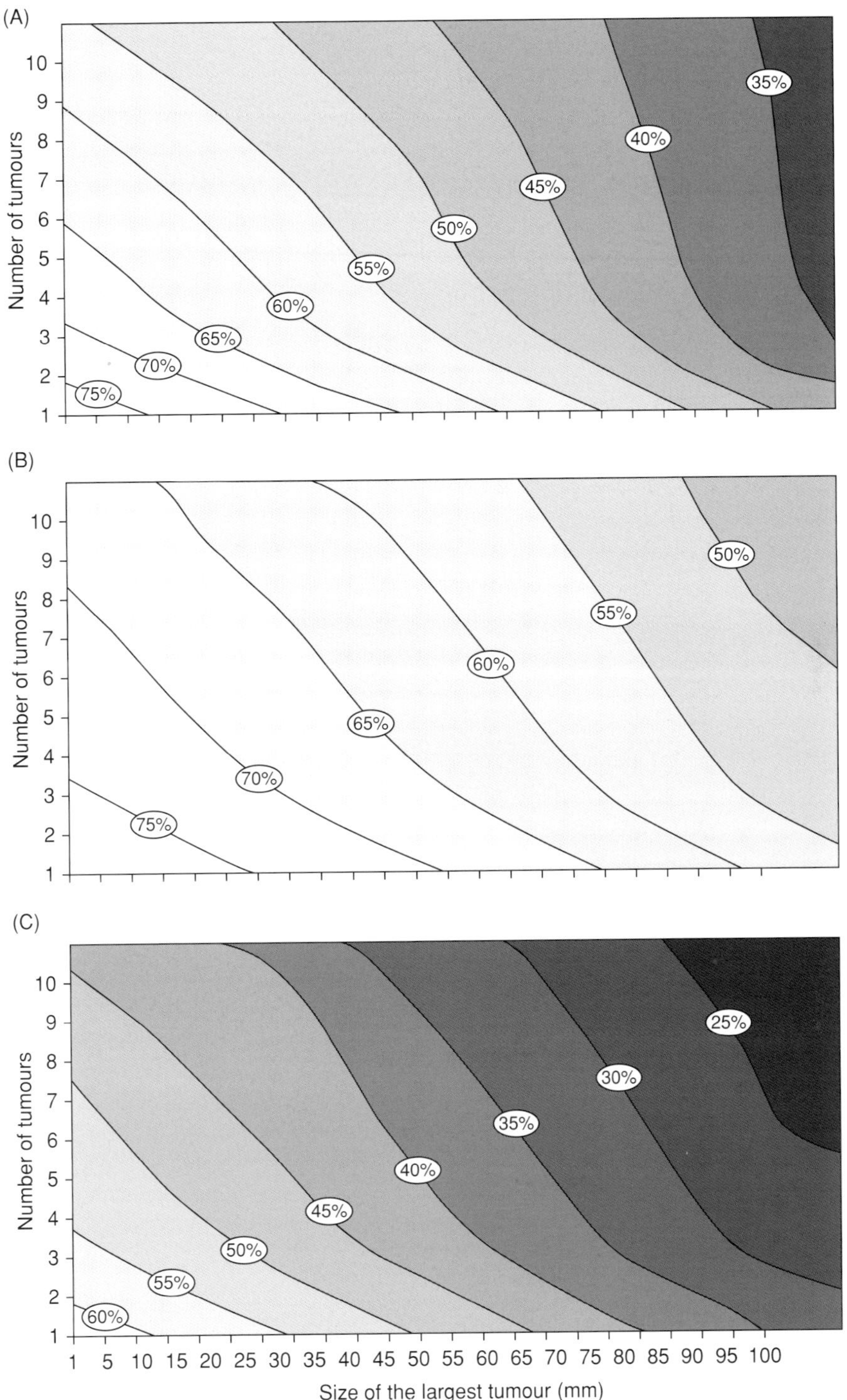

FIG 24.1 From Mazzaferro V, Llovet JM, Miceli R, et al. Predicting survival after liver transplantation in patients with hepatocellular carcinoma beyond the milan criteria: a retrospective, exploratory analysis. *Lancet Oncol* 2009; 10(1):35–43.

corresponding variability in the willingness of centres to expand criteria for transplanting patients with HCC [24].

Downstaging

Over the past few years, interest concerning the transplantation of patients with HCC beyond the Milan criteria has shifted from expanded criteria to downstaging. This we may define as treatment of HCC, generally by non-surgical means, to reduce the size and/or number of tumours from beyond to within acceptable criteria. Inherent in this discussion is an understanding that non-surgical HCC treatment does not typically reduce the diameter of treated lesions; indeed, RFA usually results in a larger lesion than was originally present. Along the lines of the modified response evaluation criteria in solid tumours (RECIST) criteria for measuring tumour response [25], HCC that originally demonstrated arterial enhancement and is rendered non-enhancing by treatment is considered to have been effectively treated. The portion of the tumour with persistent enhancement is taken to be the viable remnant. Typical downstaging protocols require reduction of the size/number of enhancing lesions to within the Milan criteria, though the aim is to render all detectable HCC non-enhancing.

The concept of downstaging at first look seems quite irrational in the transplant setting. The entire liver will be removed at transplant, rendering the extent of tumour within the liver irrelevant except insofar as it serves as a surrogate marker for extrahepatic spread. If patients with HCC beyond the Milan criteria are not granted priority because their likelihood of having occult extrahepatic spread is unacceptably high, how could treating the primary tumour alter occult spread that may have already taken place? The answer, most all with an interest in this area agree, lies in a waiting period that, either by design or by circumstance, is built into a downstaging protocol, giving a 3–6 month period after effectively controlling the primary site to observe both for the development of extrahepatic spread and for early progression of the primary tumour, which is believed by many to be an indicator of aggressive tumour biology. Another element of downstaging protocols often considered relevant is the establishment of entry criteria in terms of tumour size and number beyond which patients may not be enrolled.

A number of authors have reported excellent results with downstaging protocols [26], most notably the UCSF group who have abandoned the use of their own UCSF criteria in favour of a downstaging strategy [27]. With entry limited to patients with solitary HCC between 5–8 cm, 2–3 tumours between 3–5 cm, or 4–5 tumours $\leq$3 cm and with the sum of tumour diameters $\leq$8 cm, and with ablative tumour treatment to reduce enhancing tumour to within the Milan criteria, and a minimum 3-month observation period, they reported that downstaging was successful in 43/61 patients (29.5% dropout rate, mostly due to tumour progression). Four-year survival was 92.1% among the 35 patients who had been transplanted without a single instance of post-transplant HCC recurrence. Data such as these have engendered considerable debate among policy makers [24]. Whilst the concept of downstaging has gained considerable credibility and is widely practiced, it has to this point not been formally incorporated into the allocation system in most countries.

Living donor transplantation

The limited supply of deceased donor livers is the primary constraint on transplantation for HCC, leading to both long waiting times for initially suitable candidates with resultant dropout and decreased intent-to-treat survival and the exclusion of many patients with potentially curable HCC beyond the Milan criteria from candidacy in the first place. LDT, which provides an organ to a specific candidate without impacting organ availability for other patients, enables timely transplantation of suitable candidates, thereby eliminating the risk of dropout. LDT also changes the equation for candidates with HCC beyond the Milan criteria. Such patients are denied a transplant not because transplantation would not be the best possible treatment for them – it clearly would be for many such patients with tumour confined to the liver and without macro-VI – but, rather, because allocating organs to these patients who have a somewhat diminished likelihood of cure is an inefficient use of a scarce resource. This scarcity is not an issue with LDT; it is replaced by concern over donor risk, the justification of which depends on the likelihood that the recipient will benefit as a result.

With deceased donor transplantation the analysis is simple. If, for example, a scarce liver can provide a 75% chance of 5-year survival for a patient without HCC or with HCC within the Milan criteria versus a 50% chance for a patient with more advanced HCC, the organ should be assigned to the patient more likely to benefit. With LDT, on the other hand, we must weigh the likelihood of survival of the recipient against the risk of donor mortality, which in adult LDT is estimated in the range of 0.2–0.5% [28]. The considerations here are more philosophical than statistical, depending on the views of doctors, patients, and society on whether donors are to be protected from themselves, or granted autonomy to decide. The current consensus seems to be that LDT may be offered to candidates with HCC outside the Milan criteria as long as the estimated likelihood of long-term recipient survival is in the range of 50%.

Some early analyses of the results of LDT for HCC suggested that the procedure was associated with an increased risk of post-transplant HCC recurrence attributed to ill-defined growth factors present as the result of the regenerative milieu in recipients of small grafts [29]. This concern has been largely eliminated by a recent report from the A2ALL multicentre US LDT study group, not yet published, showing that in a multivariate analysis, graft type (deceased vs. living donor) was not an independent predictor of recurrence. Another concern about LDT has been 'fast-tracking', pushing patients to transplantation so rapidly that biologically unfavourable HCCs do not have time to manifest their adverse characteristics until they do so in the form of post-transplant recurrence [30]. For patients with HCC within Milan criteria, who have repeatedly been shown to have low likelihood of post-transplant recurrence, the greater concern seems to be with dropout from the waiting list, and the expeditious performance of LDT. For patients with HCC beyond the Milan criteria, however, most centres approach patients with the possibility for LDT similarly to other such patients, with non-surgical treatment to downstage the tumour and a period of observation without tumour progression or the appearance of extrahepatic spread before proceeding to LDT.

Assessing tumour biology: present and future

Current HCC transplant selection criteria rely on surrogate markers for what we really want to know, which is the essential biological nature of the tumour and whether, despite the absence of detectable spread, metastasis has in fact begun. The histologic appearance of cancer has long been identified as correlating with tumour behaviour. For HCC, the Edmondson-Steiner grading system is in widespread use. Poorly differentiated (G3) HCC as defined in this system has been repeatedly identified as a predictor of poor outcome in HCC, and some programmes have included tumour grade in their candidate selection criteria. Cillo et al. [31] reported excellent results transplanting patients with HCC without regard to tumour size or number but eliminating patients with G3 HCC from candidacy. Alpha-fetoprotein (AFP) is a simple serum marker that has long been identified as correlating with prognosis in HCC; although it has been available for many years, there is heightened recent interest in the role of AFP in discriminating among candidates otherwise considered suitable for transplantation. While there is, at this point, no general consensus as to the appropriate cut-off above which AFP elevation should be considered a contraindication to transplant, a number of recent papers have called for its inclusion in criteria for selecting HCC patients for transplant [32].

As with many common cancers, molecular studies of HCC are now starting to appear that offer promise beyond simple clinical and radiologic criteria to predict tumour behaviour. Minguez et al. have identified a molecular signature for VI in HCC that has independent predictive ability in a multivariate model along with clinical and imaging variables [33]. Marsh et al. have published a number of studies demonstrating that losses or gains of chromosomal DNA in HCCs removed at transplant correlate with tumour recurrence and survival [34]; expanding on the work, Schwartz et al. reported that an index of allelic imbalance (gain or loss of DNA in tumour compared with non-tumour tissue) at the loci of nine microsatellites situated in the genome adjacent to known cancer-related genes correlated very strongly with post-transplant recurrence [35]. In this study, among 35 patients with HCC beyond the Milan criteria, recurrence was observed in 1/11 patients who had an index <0.27 (the best cut-off, as determined by ROC curve analysis), as compared with 21/24 patients with an index ≥ 0.27. In a multivariate analysis, the index of allelic imbalance was by far the most significant predictor of recurrence (HR $= 17$, $p = .0002$).

The primary issue standing in the way of clinical application of molecular markers is concern whether results based, as were those described above, on sampling of entire tumours removed at surgery can be duplicated with pre-transplant percutaneous tumour biopsies. Pawlik et al. showed in a retrospective review of patients biopsied for diagnosis and then taken for resection that in only 35% of patients ultimately found at pathology to harbour G3 HCC was this identified on the pre-operative biopsy [36]. An additional concern with transplantation is the evolution of molecular alterations over time. If a patient is studied at time of listing, and then waits 9–12 months for a transplant, will the original molecular profile of the tumour reflect the tumour's current status? Ongoing research will need to address these concerns before the potential of molecular studies to enhance our decision-making can begin to be realised.

References

1. Jonas S, Bechstein WO, Steinmuller T, et al. Vascular invasion and histopathologic grading determine outcome after liver transplantation for hepatocellular carcinoma in cirrhosis. *Hepatology* 2001; 33(5):1080–1086.
2. Roayaie S, Blume IN, Thung SN, et al. A system of classifying microvascular invasion to predict outcome after resection in patients with hepatocellular carcinoma. *Gastroenterology* 2009; 137(3):850–855.
3. Mazzaferro V, Regalia E, Doci R, et al. Liver transplantation for the treatment of small hepatocellular carcinomas in patients with cirrhosis. *N Engl J Med* 1996; 334(11):693–699.
4. Imamura H, Seyama Y, Kokudo N, et al. One thousand fifty-six hepatectomies without mortality in 8 years. *Arch Surg* 2003; 138(11):1198–1206.
5. Poon RT, Fan ST, Lo CM, Liu CL, Wong J. Long-term survival and pattern of recurrence after resection of small hepatocellular carcinoma in patients with preserved liver function: implications for a strategy of salvage transplantation. *Ann Surg* 2002; 235(3):373–382.
6. Ishizawa T, Hasegawa K, Aoki T, et al. Neither multiple tumors nor portal hypertension are surgical contraindications for hepatocellular carcinoma. *Gastroenterology* 2008; 134(7):1908–1916.
7. Minagawa M, Makuuchi M, Takayama T, Kokudo N. Selection criteria for repeat hepatectomy in patients with recurrent hepatocellular carcinoma. *Ann Surg* 2003; 238(5):703–710.
8. Choi D, Lim HK, Kim MJ, et al. Recurrent hepatocellular carcinoma: percutaneous radiofrequency ablation after hepatectomy. *Radiology* 2004; 230(1):135–141.
9. Belghiti J, Cortes A, Abdalla EK, et al. Resection prior to liver transplantation for hepatocellular carcinoma. *Ann Surg* 2003; 238(6):885–893.
10. Berenguer M, Prieto M, Rayon JM, et al. Natural history of clinically compensated hepatitis C virus-related graft cirrhosis after liver transplantation. *Hepatology* 2000; 32: 852–858.
11. Schwartz M, Roayaie S, Konstadoulakis M. Strategies for the management of hepatocellular carcinoma. *Nat Clin Pract Oncol* 2007; 4(7):424–432.
12. Llovet JM, Sala M, Fuster J, et al. Predictors of dropout and survival of patients with hepatocellular carcinoma candidates for liver transplantation. *Hepatology* 2003; 38: 763A.
13. Mazzaferro V, Llovet JM, Miceli R, et al. Predicting survival after liver transplantation in patients with hepatocellular carcinoma beyond the milan criteria: a retrospective, exploratory analysis. *Lancet Oncol* 2009; 10(1):35–43.
14. UNOS policy 3.6.4.4: liver transplant candidates with hepatocellular carcinoma [Internet]; 2005 [updated 6/24/2005. Available from: http:www.optn.org/policiesAndBylaws/policies.asp.
15. Wiesner RH, Freeman RB, Mulligan DC. Liver transplantation for hepatocellular cancer: the impact of the MELD allocation policy. *Gastroenterology* 2004; 127(5 suppl 1):S261–267.
16. Burrel M, Llovet JM, Ayuso C, et al. MRI angiography is superior to helical CT for detection of HCC prior to liver transplantation: an explant correlation. *Hepatology* 2003; 38(4):1034–1042.
17. Bruix J, Sherman M. Practice Guidelines Committee, American Association for the Study of Liver Diseases. Management of hepatocellular carcinoma. *Hepatology* 2005; 42(5):1208–1236.
18. Shiina S, Teratani T, Obi S, et al. A randomized controlled trial of radiofrequency ablation with ethanol injection for small hepatocellular carcinoma. *Gastroenterology* 2005; 129(1):122–130.
19. Livraghi T, Meloni F, Di Stasi M, et al. Sustained complete response and complications rates after radiofrequency ablation of very early hepatocellular carcinoma in cirrhosis: is resection still the treatment of choice? *Hepatology* 2008; 47(1):82–89.
20. Roayaie S, Frischer JS, Emre SH, et al. Long-term results with multimodal adjuvant therapy and liver transplantation for the treatment of hepatocellular carcinomas larger than 5 centimeters. *Ann Surg* 2002; 235(4):533–539.
21. Yao FY, Ferrell L, Bass NM, et al. Liver transplantation for hepatocellular carcinoma: expansion of the tumor size limits does not adversely impact survival. *Hepatology* 2001; 33(6):1394–1403.
22. Yao FY, Xiao L, Bass NM, Kerlan R, Ascher NL, Roberts JP. Liver transplantation for hepatocellular carcinoma: validation of the UCSF-expanded criteria based on preoperative imaging. *Am J Transplant* 2007; 7(11): 2587–2596.
23. Decaens T, Roudot-Thoraval F, Hadni-Bresson S, et al. Impact of UCSF criteria according to pre- and post-OLT tumor features: analysis of 479 patients listed for HCC with a short waiting time. *Liver Transpl* 2006; 12(12): 1761–1769.

24. Pomfret EA, Washburn K, Wald C, et al. Report of a national conference on liver allocation in patients with hepatocellular carcinoma in the united states. *Liver Transpl* 2010; 16(3):262–278.
25. Lencioni R, Llovet JM. Modified RECIST (mRECIST) assessment for hepatocellular carcinoma. *Semin Liver Dis* 2010; 30(1):52–60.
26. Chapman WC, Majella Doyle MB, Stuart JE, et al. Outcomes of neoadjuvant transarterial chemoembolization to downstage hepatocellular carcinoma before liver transplantation. *Ann Surg* 2008; 248(4):617–625.
27. Yao FY, Kerlan RK Jr, Hirose R, et al. Excellent outcome following down-staging of hepatocellular carcinoma prior to liver transplantation: an intention-to-treat analysis. *Hepatology* 2008; 48(3):819–827.
28. Ringe B, Strong RW. The dilemma of living liver donor death: to report or not to report? *Transplantation* 2008; 85(6):790–793.
29. Lo CM, Fan ST, Liu CL, Chan SC, Ng IO, Wong J. Living donor versus deceased donor liver transplantation for early irresectable hepatocellular carcinoma. *Br J Surg* 2006; 94(1):78–86.
30. Roberts JP, Venook A, Kerlan R, Yao F. Hepatocellular carcinoma: ablate and wait versus rapid transplantation. *Liver Transpl* 2010; 16(8):925–929.
31. Cillo U, Vitale A, Bassanello M, et al. Liver transplantation for the treatment of moderately or well-differentiated hepatocellular carcinoma. *Ann Surg* 2004; 239(2):150–159.
32. Merani S, Majno P, Kneteman NM, et al. The impact of waiting list alpha-fetoprotein changes on the outcome of liver transplant for hepatocellular carcinoma. *J Hepatol* 2011.
33. Minguez B, Hoshida Y, Toffanin S, Lachenmayer A, Cabellos L, Bruix J, Mandeli J, Thung S, Savic R, Roayaie S, Mazzaferro V, Schwartz M, Golub T, Friedman S, Llovet J. Gene-expression signature of vascular invasion inHepatocellular carcinoma. *J Hepatol* 2011 (in press).
34. Marsh JW, Finkelstein SD, Demetris AJ, et al. Genotyping of hepatocellular carcinoma in liver transplant recipients adds predictive power for determining recurrence-free survival. *Liver Transpl* 2003; 9(7):664–671.
35. Schwartz M, Dvorchik I, Roayaie S, et al. Liver transplantation for hepatocellular carcinoma: extension of indications based on molecular markers. *J Hepatol* 2008; 49(4): 581–588.
36. Pawlik TM, Gleisner AL, Anders RA, Assumpcao L, Maley W, Choti MA. Preoperative assessment of hepatocellular carcinoma tumor grade using needle biopsy: implications for transplant eligibility. *Ann Surg* 2007; 245(3):435–442.

PART 6
What Does the Future Hold?

25 Dipstick markers for diagnosis: feasible or not?

Mohamed I.F. Shariff, Simon D. Taylor-Robinson

Department of Medicine, Imperial College London, London, UK

LEARNING POINTS

- Urine contains a wealth of diagnostic information, and dipstick markers are widely used in the clinical setting to diagnose a number of conditions.
- For a marker molecule to be present in urine it must be small enough and of correct ionic charge to avoid renal glomerular repulsion and tubular re-absorption.
- The ideal biomarker for hepatocellular carcinoma (HCC) would be highly sensitive and specific but also applicable in resource-poor settings in the developing world.
- Urinary markers of HCC have been identified since the 1970s and include nucleosides, nucleotides, small proteins, polyamines and most recently metabolites. None as yet shows perfect sensitivity and specificity.
- It is likely that a combination of urinary markers, rather than a single one, will hold the key.

Introduction

Sweet urine

Urine has long been known to possess diagnostic attributes, its sweet taste recorded in ancient Indian scriptures being probably the earliest documentation of this. Subsequently, Thomas Willis (1621–1675) differentiated diabetes from other causes of polyurea from the sweet tasting urine of diabetics. These attributes have been exploited in clinical practice including the diagnosis of microscopic haematuria, through peroxidise activity of lysis-released haemoglobin with dipstick reagents; proteinuria, through reaction of protein amine groups with acid base indicators on the dipstick strip; glycosuria, through conversion to hydrogen peroxide by glucose oxidase; urinary tract infection, based on the presence of leukocytes, or more specifically, leukocyte esterase, and nitrites, formed by bacterial conversion of nitrates, in the urine and pregnancy, through a strip-based immunoassay for beta human chorionic gonadotrophin (βHCG), to name only a few examples of the diagnostic potential of urine [1,2].

Urinary biomarkers

To be present in the urine, a biomarker must avoid being too large or of incorrect ionic charge to allow plasma filtration through the renal glomerulus and then avoid tubular re-absorption to eventually pass through the renal collecting system, into the urine and into the outside world. The filtration barrier in the renal glomerulus is highly permeable to water, small solutes and ions and poorly permeable to larger plasma proteins. Molecules of <20 kDa or 1.8 nm in size may pass through, though the barrier also repels those proteins, like albumin, which are negatively charged. If a biomarker is successful in running this gauntlet, it must finally be stably present in large enough quantities for disease detection at the patient's bedside.

What makes a good diagnostic test?

Independent of the disease, a diagnostic test should meet certain criteria. It should primarily be sensitive to detect the disease when present, and specific, to confirm its absence in a target population. Ideally, a test would display 100% sensitivity and specificity. However, this is very rarely possible, given limitations in technology, cost and disease variability.

Clinical Dilemmas in Primary Liver Cancer, First Edition. Edited by Roger Williams and Simon D. Taylor-Robinson.

The most accurate tests are dubbed the 'gold standard', often too expensive and time consuming to use for rapid diagnostics at the patient's bedside. The test should detect the disease at an early stage, allowing for the most successful treatment. This is particularly germane to HCC as lesions below 2 cm are curable with resection or transplant.

HCC is most prevalent in the developing world [3], particularly developing countries in sub-Saharan Africa. Expense, therefore, is of paramount importance as the test should be available to those most at risk, irrespective of monetary wealth. The test should be rapid to provide the clinician and patient with the information quickly, so that a management plan can be instituted. Again, this is of vital importance in the developing world where patients may live many days journey from the health clinic and have limited resources for travel. The test should also be as minimally invasive and lowest risk to the patient as possible. Finally, HCC occurs in diverse world populations, usually where hepatitis B virus or hepatitis C virus are high in incidence. The test should, therefore, be applicable across all patient groups and ethnicities.

A urine dipstick test for HCC would fill many of these criteria. It has the potential to be quick, would be non-invasive and can be interpreted by the medical practitioner attending the patient at the bedside. Research by our group and others is exploring the diagnostic capabilities of urine from patients with HCC, with a view to such a test, and there have been recent promising developments.

How could cancer be detected in the urine?

For any urine biomarker three central attributes are necessary for it to fulfil. First, the biomarker, if produced pre-renally, needs to be small enough and of the correct ionic charge to be filtered by the renal glomerulus and not re-absorbed by the tubules. Therefore, it has to be roughly less than 20 kDa in atomic weight. Second, the marker should be specific to the cancer in question and not secondary to the effects of cancer on general physiology. Finally, the marker should be secreted in adequate amounts for accurate, repeatable detection in early disease. Large, complex proteins are unlikely to enter the urinary stream, so are not candidates for urinary biomarkers. The key lies in the detection of metabolites, small molecules from 50 to 1000 Da, which include amino acids, peptides, bile acids and nucleotides. Individually, because these metabolites are ubiquitous in most cellular functions, they possess minimal diagnostic attributes; in combination with other altered metabolites, however, a metabolic profile can be built that may be highly specific. Such metabolic profiling has been termed 'metabonomics', describing the altered metabolic state in response to a drug or disease stimuli in the mammalian system [4].

Urinary biomarkers in HCC

Nucleosides

The quest to identify urinary markers of HCC began in the 1970s when early reports of levels of methylated purines (7-methylguanine, 1-methylguanine, N-dimethylguanine, 1-methylhypoxanthine and adenine) were found to be elevated in the urine of patients with HCC compared with both healthy controls and disease controls with cirrhosis [5] (see Table 25.1). This may have indicated rapid ribonucleic acid (RNA) turnover indicative of HCC and methylation of nucleic acid as a potential carcinogenic mechanism. In 1976, using immunoassay technology, urine levels of cyclic guanosine 3′:5′ monophosphate (cGMP) were observed to be higher in rats with transplanted liver and renal tumours [6]. In 1982, Dusheiko and colleagues repeated the study in human subjects and observed that urinary cGMP excretion was elevated in 80% of patients with HCC, 75% of patients with hepatic disease and 68% of patients with other neoplasms [7]. cGMP levels were also observed to be elevated in plasma and ascitic fluid. These results supported the hypothesis of a shift in cyclic nucleotide metabolism toward cGMP in malignant diseases. However, urinary cGMP did

TABLE 25.1 Urinary markers of hepatocellular carcinoma

Year	Urinary biomarker
Nucleosides and nucleotides	
1974	Methylated purines [5]
1976	Cyclic GMP [6,7]
1986	Pseudouridine [8]
Proteins and polyamines	
1990	TGFα and β [9–11]
1998	Neopterin [12–15]
2004	Urinary trypsin inhibitor [16,17]
1998	Spermine, putrescine, spermidine [18]
Metabolite profiles	
2009	Octanedioic acid, glycine and hypoxanthine [19]
2010	Creatinine, carnitine, creatine [20]

not detect progression of cirrhosis to HCC, nor was it specific to HCC.

The case for nucleoside derivatives as tumour markers was enforced in 1986 when Tamura and colleagues detected elevated levels of urinary pseudouridine using high performance liquid chromatography (HPLC) in patients with HCC. Pseudouridine is a C-glycoside isomer of the nucleoside uridine and it is the most prevalent of the over 100 different modified nucleosides found in RNA. When combined with serum alpha-fetoprotein (AFP), sensitivity for HCC diagnosis reached 83% [8]. However, urinary pseudouridine levels have also been shown to be elevated in other malignancies, such as non-Hodgkin's lymphoma, probably as an indicator of overall cellular proliferation of tumour growth.

Jeng and colleagues proposed the use of the urinary nucleosides adenosine, cytidine and inosine as markers of HCC, following an HPLC-based study in Taiwanese subjects [21]. It was observed that these markers were raised in the urine of HCC patients. When combined with serum AFP, sensitivity for tumour diagnosis improved to 80%; however, the study was only conducted with one healthy subject group as controls and no patients with cirrhosis, substantially reducing the validity of the findings.

Transforming growth factor α and β

In 1990, transforming growth factor α (TGFα) was detected in the urine of patients with HCC through a modified enzyme-linked immunosorbent assay (ELISA) assay [9]. The following year Chuang and colleagues identified low molecular weight epidermal growth factor-related TGFs with functional activity in HCC patient urine, although subject numbers were only seven in each group [10]. This was confirmed by the same group in a larger study in 1997, identifying urinary TGFβ1 as the main marker, which also correlated with prognosis and survival [11]. A functional link was attractive as TGFs are known to reversibly stimulate non-transformed cells to grow as colonies in vitro, suggesting their carcinogenic role. Whether these findings are unique to HCC, and not to malignancies in general, remains to be explored.

Neopterin

In 1998, a Japanese study observed neopterin, a protein now known to be released from macrophages following inflammatory stimulation, to be elevated in the urine of patients with advanced HCC, and although correlating with tumour size, it was not detected in those with early disease [12,13]. Interestingly, in these studies, urinary neopterin levels were not correlated with serum AFP. Neopterin has since been shown to be elevated in a number of malignancies and pro-inflammatory conditions such as human immunodeficiency virus (HIV) related disease [14]. As such, its use in the precise diagnosis of HCC is not valid. Indeed, the simultaneous HPLC measurement of urinary pseudouridine, neopterin and creatinine has been shown to be an indicator of RNA turnover, indicative of malignant growth, in adenocarcinoma, HCC and non-Hodgkin's lymphoma [15].

Polyamines

The polyamines putrescine, spermine, spermidine are required for cellular proliferation, though their exact role is unclear. Putrescine acts on *S*-adenosylmethionine (SAMe), a methylating molecule, to produce spermine that in turn acts on further SAMe molecules to produce spermidine [22]. Antionella and colleagues reported increased urinary levels of free and acetylated polyamines using reverse phase liquid chromatography (RPLC) in HCC patients compared with healthy controls and patients with cirrhosis (disease controls) [18]. Unfortunately, as with other markers, polyamines are not sensitive enough for accurate early tumour detection and may not be specific to HCC.

Urinary trypsin inhibitor

In 2004, an ELISA-based study investigated the correlation of urinary trypsin inhibitor (UTI), with HCC and liver cirrhosis [16]. UTI is a 25-kDa trypsin inhibitor believed to be produced by hepatocytes and, therefore, a marker of hepatocyte function. UTI was elevated in patients with HCC. However, there was no significant difference between patients with cirrhosis and those with HCC, negating its usefulness in early tumour detection. Further studies have found correlations with severity of liver disease and in 2009 Kikuchi and colleagues demonstrated a decrease in plasma UTI levels post-tumour resection and a significant correlation of tumour tissue UTI with risk of tumour recurrence post-resection ($p = 0.006$) [17]. UTI may certainly be a marker of liver disease and HCC but lacks sensitivity in detecting tumours at an early stage.

Metabolic profiling

Wu and colleagues recently reported a urinary gas chromatography mass spectrometry study of 20 HCC patients, which identified a marker panel of 18 metabolites

(A)

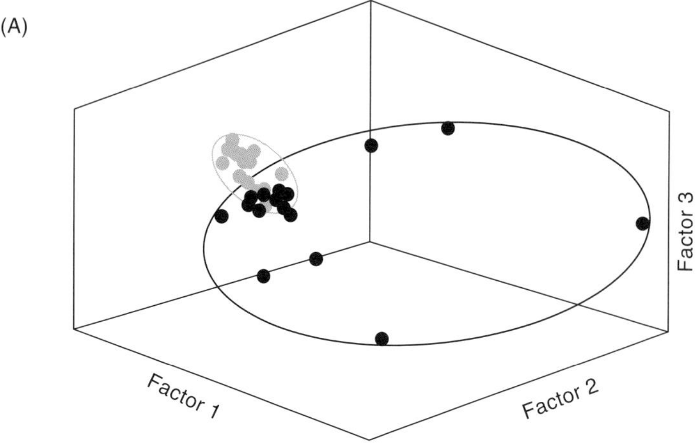

(B)

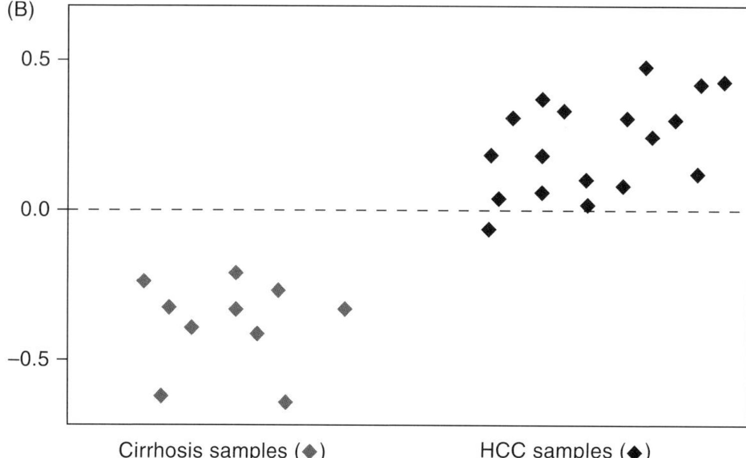

FIG 25.1 (A) Principal components analysis scatter plot of HCC subjects (•) vs. healthy controls (•) and (B) partial least squared discriminant analysis of HCC subjects vs. cirrhosis subjects.

discriminating HCC and healthy Chinese controls [19]. This panel of discriminatory metabolites included octanedioic acid, glycine and hypoxanthine. Unfortunately, no cirrhosis disease control group was included, reducing the applicability of any findings to the most at risk target population.

Most recently, Shariff and colleagues, using proton magnetic resonance spectroscopy combined with multivariate statistical analysis, identified a set of urinary metabolite markers which could distinguish patients with HCC from healthy controls with 100% sensitivity and 93% specificity and HCC from cirrhosis with 89.5% sensitivity and 88.9% specificity in a Nigerian cohort of subjects (Figure 25.1) [20]. This metabolite set consisted of creatinine, creatine, carnitine and acetone, implicating altered energy metabolism and cellular proliferation in patients with hepatomas and, in the form of creatine, a marker of cancer cachexia and increased global muscle breakdown. Larger studies, from diverse populations are required to confirm these findings are applicable to the diverse spectrum of patients that develop this tumour.

Conclusions

Urine contains a wealth of information that can be utilised for the diagnosis of underlying pathology. The use of urinary dipstick markers is established in clinical practice for the diagnosis of many different diseases from urinary tract infections to ketonuria, allowing the medical practitioner to institute rapid informed treatment decisions. A reliable urinary dipstick test for HCC would be of immense value both in the developed world, whereby surveillance could be carried out in the community by general practitioners, and in the developing world, allowing the diagnosis to be made in resource-poor settings that may not have access to imaging or serological tests. Diagnostic urinary markers have been identified since the 1970s and include nucleosides, small proteins, polyamines and most recently metabolites, and although advances have been made, accurate, repeatable and specific, biomarkers are still yet to be produced. Metabolic profiling may offer the answer in identifying groups of markers potentially increasing the accuracy of the test. Large, multinational studies are required to validate initial pilot study findings and ensure that any markers identified are applicable across aetiologies and populations. With the correct approach, dipstick diagnosis of HCC is, therefore, a tangible possibility in diagnosing this devastating tumour.

References

1. Simerville JA, Maxted WC, Pahira JJ. Urinalysis: a comprehensive review. *Am Fam Physician* 2005; 71(6):1153–1162.
2. Subramonian K, MacDonald H, Vijapurapu R, Yadav S. Urine dipstick tests. *Student BMJ* 2009; 17: b260.
3. Shariff MI, Cox IJ, Gomaa AI, Khan SA, Gedroyc W, Taylor-Robinson SD. Hepatocellular carcinoma: current trends in worldwide epidemiology, risk factors, diagnosis and therapeutics. *Expert Rev Gastroenterol Hepatol* 2009; 3(4):353–367.
4. Nicholson JK, Lindon JC. Systems biology: metabonomics. *Nature* 2008; 455(7216):1054–1056.
5. Ho Y, Lin HJ. Patterns of excretion of methylated purines in hepatocellular carcinoma. *Cancer Res* 1974; 34(5):986–990.
6. Criss WE, Murad F. Urinary excretion of cyclic guanosine 3′:5′-monophosphate and cyclic adenosine 3′:5′-monophosphate in rats bearing transplantable liver and kidney tumors. *Cancer Res* 1976; 36(5):1714–1716.
7. Dusheiko GM, Levin J, Kew MC. Cyclic nucleotides in biological fluids in hepatocellular carcinoma. *Cancer* 1981; 47(1):113–118.
8. Tamura S, Amuro Y, Nakano T, et al. Urinary excretion of pseudouridine in patients with hepatocellular carcinoma. *Cancer* 1986; 57(8):1571–1575.
9. Katoh M, Inagaki H, Kurosawa-Ohsawa K, Katsuura M, Tanaka S. Detection of transforming growth factor alpha in human urine and plasma. *Biochem Biophys Res Commun* 1990; 167(3):1065–1072.
10. Chuang LY, Tsai JH, Yeh YC, et al. Epidermal growth factor-related transforming growth factors in the urine of patients with hepatocellular carcinoma. *Hepatology* 1991; 13(6):1112–1116.
11. Tsai JF, Jeng JE, Chuang LY, et al. Clinical evaluation of urinary transforming growth factor-beta1 and serum alpha-fetoprotein as tumour markers of hepatocellular carcinoma. *Br J Cancer* 1997; 75(10):1460–1466.
12. Kawasaki H, Watanabe H, Yamada S, Watanabe K, Suyama A. Prognostic significance of urinary neopterin levels in patients with hepatocellular carcinoma. *Tohoku J Exp Med* 1988; 155(4):311–318.
13. Daito K, Suou T, Kawasaki H. Clinical significance of serum and urinary neopterin levels in patients with various liver diseases. *Am J Gastroenterol* 1992; 87(4):471–476.
14. Sucher R, Schroecksnadel K, Weiss G, Margreiter R, Fuchs D, Brandacher G. Neopterin, a prognostic marker in human malignancies. *Cancer Lett* 2010; 287(1):13–22.
15. Motyl T, Traczyk Z, Holska W, niewska-Michalska D, Ciesluk S, Kukulska W, et al. Comparison of urinary neopterin and pseudouridine in patients with malignant proliferative diseases. *Eur J Clin Chem Clin Biochem* 1993; 31(4):205–209.
16. Lin SD, Endo R, Kuroda H, et al. Plasma and urine levels of urinary trypsin inhibitor in patients with chronic liver diseases and hepatocellular carcinoma. *J Gastroenterol Hepatol* 2004; 19(3):327–332.
17. Kikuchi I, Uchinami H, Nanjo H, et al. Clinical and prognostic significance of urinary trypsin inhibitor in patients with hepatocellular carcinoma after hepatectomy. *Ann Surg Oncol* 2009; 16(10):2805–2817.
18. Antoniello S, Auletta M, Magri P, Pardo F. Urinary excretion of free and acetylated polyamines in hepatocellular carcinoma. *Int J Biol Markers* 1998; 13(2):92–97.
19. Wu H, Xue R, Dong L, et al. Metabolomic profiling of human urine in hepatocellular carcinoma patients using gas chromatography/mass spectrometry. *Anal Chim Acta* 2009; 648(1):98–104.
20. Shariff MI, Ladep NG, Cox IJ, et al. Characterization of urinary biomarkers of hepatocellular carcinoma using magnetic resonance spectroscopy in a Nigerian population. *J Proteome Res* 2010; 9(2):1096–1103.
21. Jeng LB, Lo WY, Hsu WY, et al. Analysis of urinary nucleosides as helper tumor markers in hepatocellular carcinoma diagnosis. *Rapid Commun Mass Spectrom* 2009; 23(11):1543–1549.
22. Wishart DS, Tzur D, Knox C, et al. HMDB: the Human Metabolome Database. *Nucleic Acids Res* 2007; 35(Database issue):D521–D526.

26 Targeted gene therapy for hepatocellular carcinoma: a reality?

Christopher Binny[1], Marco Della Peruta[2], Amit C. Nathwani[1,2,3]

[1]Department of Haematology, UCL Cancer Institute, London, UK
[2]The Institute of Hepatology London, The Foundation for Liver Research, London, UK
[3]NHS Blood and Transplant, UK

LEARNING POINTS

- Targeted gene therapy is the delivery of therapeutic genes to a narrowly selected population of cells, in this case hepatocellular carcinoma (HCC) cells. Targeted delivery is necessary to avoid off-target cytotoxicity, and can be achieved using targeted liposomes and modified viruses
- Once inside the host cell, gene expression may be regulated through reliance on tumour-specific promoters (e.g. alpha-fetoprotein (AFP), survivin promoter) or by targeting messenger RNA (mRNA) of the therapeutic gene for destruction by micro-RNAs (miRNAs) normally absent in tumours.
- In gene therapy for cancer, therapeutic genes are typically intended to induce cell death through cytotoxicity (suicide genes such as herpes simplex virus (HSV) gene thymadine kinase (HSV-TK)), stimulate an antitumour immune response or inhibit the function of necessary oncogenic pathways
- Targeted gene therapies for HCC have shown safety and limited efficacy in phase I clinical trials, and more sophisticated techniques are making extremely promising progress through pre-clinical development.

Introduction

Hepatocellular carcinoma (HCC) accounts for more than 80% of liver cancers and is the fourth most common cause of cancer-related deaths. The incidence and mortality of HCC have increased globally in the last decade largely due to the dissemination of hepatitis B and C virus infection. Many patients are still not diagnosed until advanced stages of the tumour and have a very poor prognosis with a 5-year survival of around 7% [1]. Thus, there is an urgent need for novel therapies. Gene transfer has the potential to create ever-expanding therapeutic opportunities through the introduction of functional genes into a target cell that restore, modify or enhance cellular functions. Although gene therapy was originally conceptualised as a treatment for inherited genetic disorders, most of the effort so far has focused on cancer largely because of the often poor efficacy of conventional treatment and the dire prognosis overall for many malignancies. The first gene therapy product to be licensed (Gendicine) is an adenoviral vector engineered to express wildtype-p53 for the treatment of head and neck squamous cell carcinoma [2]. Gene therapy for HCC is under investigation with strategies focused on the inhibition of oncogenes, blockade of angiogenesis, immunotherapy and virotherapy. Results to date have been impressive in animal models. As our understanding of cellular and molecular biology of HCC increases, opportunities for attacking the tumour selectively will emerge through disruption of essential unique pathways. Examples of these approaches include the introduction or restoration of genes to inhibit the growth of the tumour; knockdown of genes necessary for tumour survival using shRNA and similar techniques; and expression of cytotoxic genes or drug precursor-activating enzymes under control of a tumour-specific mechanism. Therefore, with improvement in gene transfer technology and a better understanding of the cellular and molecular pathways involved in the development and progression of HCC, it should be possible to develop safe and effective strategies that target tumours at multiple sites with little or no toxicity to normal hepatocytes.

Clinical Dilemmas in Primary Liver Cancer, First Edition. Edited by Roger Williams and Simon D. Taylor-Robinson.

Targeted delivery of therapeutic genes

The success of gene therapy depends on the development of vehicles, known as vectors that can efficiently introduce therapeutic genes into the target somatic cells, a process often referred to as transduction. A number of gene transfer vehicles have been developed that can broadly be divided into two categories – non-viral and viral vectors.

Non-viral vectors include naked DNA and DNA encapsulated within cationic lipids known as liposomes. These vectors offer the advantages of relative ease of production and reduced toxicity. Additionally, it is possible to conjugate a molecular target to the liposomes, thus improving the prospects of targeting specific cells. For instance, use of a phage display library identified Hepatoma Cell Binding Protein 1 (HCBP1, also referred to as HBP), a homing peptide specific to a panel of HCC cell lines [3]. Cationic liposomes with pegylated HCBP1 embedded in their surface showed specific binding and entry to HCC cells, leading to expression of a reporter gene in the targeted cells [4]. While this preliminary work only showed efficacy in vitro, previous work with targeted liposomes using a different HCC-targeting peptide, SP94, demonstrated successful targeting of liposome contents to HCC cells in a mouse model [5]. Similar work in other cancer models have demonstrated the successful targeting of liposomes using monoclonal antibodies against tumour markers such as CD19 [6].

Viruses have the ability to gain access to specific cells and exploit the host's cellular machinery to facilitate their replication. Recombinant viral vectors are designed to harness the viral infection pathway. However, these vectors have been modified so that they are unable to replicate in the target cell. In general, viral vectors are more efficient at delivering their payload to target cells than non-viral approaches and have, therefore, been the focus of the majority of cancer gene therapy approaches. The number of different viruses under development as gene therapy vectors is steadily increasing, but can be divided into two general categories: integrating and non-integrating. At present, retroviral vectors based on oncoretro-, foamy- or lenti-virus are the only gene transfer systems that can mediate efficient integration of the transgene into recipient cells. In contrast, the genome of vectors based on herpes, adeno-associated or adeno-virus vectors is maintained mainly as episomes. These do not usually integrate into the host genome and are consequently lost over time. Therefore, expression from non-integrating vectors is often transient, especially in tissues and organs with a high cellular turnover. This may be ideal for a number of cancer strategies using a 'hit and run' approach. Just as wild-type viruses are able to exploit tissue- and cell-type-specific cell surface antigens to effect selective entry into their target cells, an understanding of cell surface antigens has allowed the targeting of tissues and, in some cases, cancer cells specifically. An example of a gene therapy vector tailored to specifically enter HCC cells is a mutated form of herpesvirus saimiri. The heparin sulphate-binding region of the protein responsible for this virus's adsorption to healthy liver cells was modified to bind to somatostatin receptors, which have been shown to be over-expressed on HCC cells [7]. This had the consequence of detargeting the virus from healthy hepatocytes, while maintaining its infectivity of HCC cells. At the time of writing this work is very preliminary, but demonstrates the potential for the modification of viral gene therapy vectors to specifically target HCC cells. However, it must be noted that interactions between viruses and their target cells are often complex and incompletely characterised. Consequently, the modification of a virus' known binding domains can have unpredictable effects, rendering the design of tumour-specific viruses unexpectedly difficult.

Targeted expression of therapeutic genes

Many viral vectors are able to efficiently transduce the liver of rodents, a property that is being exploited in developing gene transfer treatments for several diseases originating in the liver [8,9]. The challenge for gene therapy for HCC is to retain this efficient gene transfer to the tumour while preventing expression of the therapeutic gene in healthy liver, thus minimising off-target effects. Two main approaches can be used for this purpose: (1) transcriptional control through the use of promoters that restrict expression of therapeutic genes to the tumour and (2) post-transcriptional control, for instance the restriction of translation of the mRNA to HCC cells in preference to normal hepatocytes.

The AFP protein promoter has been most frequently used to limit transcription of a therapeutic gene in HCC. The basis for this is that the development of HCC is often (~50–80%) associated with up-regulation of AFP, a physiological counterpart of adult serum albumin. The human foetus has the highest amount of AFP found in humans. These AFP levels gradually decrease after birth. Elevation of AFP in adults occurs during hepatocyte regeneration, hepato-carcinogenesis and following development of embryonic carcinomas. This differential expression profile of AFP provides an opportunity for transcriptional targeting of therapeutic gene expression to HCC. An example is the use of a replication-defective adenovirus modified to express the pro-apoptotic protein tBid under the control of an AFP promoter in a xenograft murine model of HCC [10]. This vector was shown to efficiently deliver the modified viral genome to all liver cells, after which expression of the therapeutic gene was restricted to the AFP-expressing HCC cells. As hoped, an antitumour effect was observed without associated damage to the healthy (AFP-negative) liver. Similar work showed very promising results using a novel synthetic HCC-specific promoter based on the AFP promoter, directing expression of pro-apoptotic BikDD to create tumour-specific toxicity after delivery of therapeutic DNA within liposomes [11].

This approach can be applied to other tumour-specific promoter sequences. Recently, the tumour-specific survivin promoter has been exploited to demonstrate potent, tumour-specific expression of a therapeutic gene in an in vivo model of HCC [12]. Furthermore, analysis of microarray data from HCC samples led to the identification and subsequent validation of a further eight HCC-specific promoters [13], which may prove to be of great utility in selective expression of therapeutic genes for gene therapy of HCC.

A similar approach may be used to control the replication of lytic viruses and to create selectively oncolytic viruses. For example, an otherwise replication-competent adenovirus was put under the control of an AFP promoter sequence [14]. This modified virus showed selective replication in and lysis of AFP-positive HCC tumour cells in a mouse model with significant antitumour activity as a result, especially in combination with the chemotherapy 5-FU and paclitaxel.

Post-transcriptional control can be effected in a variety of different ways, the most elegant of which involves the use of miRNAs. They belong to a family of endogenous, short and non-coding RNAs that serve as post-transcriptional regulators of gene activity. When expressed, miRNAs are able to bind to target sequences within mRNAs, leading to their degradation and, therefore, silencing gene expression [15]. They have an important role in the control of numerous biological processes, such as development, differentiation, proliferation and apoptosis. It is not surprising, therefore, that miRNAs have been implicated in cancer, including HCC. Screening of miRNAs in samples of HCC and healthy liver tissue has identified a number of miRNAs differentially expressed in HCC [16,17]. One such miRNA currently receiving such attention is miR-122, being expressed at high levels in healthy liver tissue but absent from approximately 80% of examined HCCs [18–20]. This difference is exploited by designing gene therapy transcripts that include one or more target sites for miR-122. In healthy tissue, miR-122 will silence the transcript before translation of the therapeutic gene can occur by binding to its target sites, while in HCC cells miR-122 is absent or reduced and so translation of the therapeutic gene is able to continue to completion. This approach has already been exploited to show efficient and specific expression of Luciferase in HCC cells from a modified adeno-associated virus (AAV) vector [21].

Selection of therapeutic genes

Given the prospects of selective delivery of therapeutic genes to HCC cells, a range of approaches may be used to eradicate the tumour.

Amongst these is the targeted delivery of the HSV-TK, combined with systemic administration of the pro-drug Ganciclovir. HSV-TK catalyses the phosphorylation of the otherwise harmless pro-drug ganciclovir to form a chain-terminating dGTP analogue. The presence of this chain-terminating analogue prevents the targeted cell from replicating its DNA, leading to cell cycle arrest and death by apoptosis.

This approach has a potent bystander effect. Whilst the HSV-TK itself is retained within the targeted cell, the resulting dGTP analogue is able to exit the cell and cause chain-termination events in other dividing cells nearby. Such 'suicide gene' therapy may be a significant boon in the treatment of HCC. The densely packed and poorly vascularised nature of many tumours makes them a challenging environment for many gene delivery systems. With this bystander effect, the therapeutic DNA need not be expressed in every tumour cell: those cells that escape the initial gene transfer may still be killed by the nucleoside analogue diffusing from their neighbours.

The efficacy of HSV-TK:ganciclovir therapy has been demonstrated in a range of delivery systems and animal models [22] and has recently been used in a phase I clinical trial, expressed from an adenovirus vector [23].

A similar pro-drug/enzyme-based approach to suicide therapy has been explored using the enzyme linamarase to catalyse the local production of hydrogen cyanide from the otherwise harmless pro-drug linamarin. A modified adenovirus was used to deliver the linamarase gene to a xenograft model of HCC in mice, and the substrate delivered orally [24]. Significant inhibition of tumour growth was observed without toxic effects to the animals. As with the TK/ganciclovir system, a strong bystander effect was observed, obviating the need to infect every cell in the tumour.

Viral gene therapy approaches to targeted delivery of RNAi have shown efficacy in animal models of HCC after targeting oncogenic pathways involving p28GANK [25], survivin [26,27], VEGF [28] and URG11 [29]. Analysis of HCC samples has allowed the identification of many more oncogenes commonly associated with HCC, including *AFP*, *RAS*, *c-FOS*, *c-JUN*, *RHO*, *TGF-a*, *HGF*, *CerbB2*, *HER-2/neu*, *NEU*, *NGL*, *MDM2*, *MMP*, *IGF*-II and Aurora Kinase [20,30]. As our understanding of the genetic basis of HCC development expands along with our ability to classify HCC cases by their molecular profiles [31], it seems likely that the arsenal of available therapeutic gene therapy strategies will grow to reflect the range of identified molecular targets.

The potential of using differential miRNA expression in HCC as a biomarker to control selective expression of therapeutic genes has been described above. In addition to being exploited as a mechanism for ensuring tumour-specificity of a vector, miRNAs may themselves be used as therapeutic agents. One such example is miR-26a, an miRNA involved in establishing cell cycle arrest and known to be commonly down-regulated in human and mouse tumours, including HCC. Expression of this miRNA from an AAV vector in a mouse model of HCC resulted in inhibition of cancer cell proliferation and induction of tumour-specific apoptosis, with no off-target toxicity [32]. Similar results have been reported following the therapeutic restoration of expression of miRNA 223 [20], miRNA 122, which also reduced metastasis and angiogenesis [20,33] and miRNA 101, which also sensitised cells to killing by conventional chemotherapy [20,34].

Those miRNAs that have been identified as commonly up-regulated in HCC may be viewed similarly to common oncogenes in HCC. Silencing of these targets may result in the disruption of pathways necessary to tumour survival and development. For example, silencing of HCC-specific miR-21 and miR-221 each led to reduced viability and tumourogenicity of HCC cells [35,36].

Immune responses against tumour-specific antigens have been observed in the past, but these responses are often too weak to prevent the continuing development of tumours, thus allowing disease progression to continue [37,38]. One possible approach for the treatment of cancer is to stimulate the immune system into overcoming this tolerance, allowing it to mount an attack on the tumour. Tumour-specific expression of a membrane-anchored form of the powerfully antigenic protein Staphylococcus enterotoxin A (SEA) was demonstrated in a HCC xenograft model produced in immunocompetent mice [39]. This achieved the induction of tumour-specific cytotoxic T lymphocytes, leading to significant reduction in tumour growth and prolonged survival of treated mice.

An alternative approach to stimulating an immune response against tumour cells has been demonstrated, in which a recombinant adenovirus was used to express IL-12 at the tumour site [40]. The resulting up-regulation of cytolytic activities of T and NK cells had a moderate effect on the HCC xenograft model, and contributed to a larger antitumour effect when combined with a vector expressing the suicide gene HSV-TK.

Recent clinical trials of targeted gene therapy

Several approaches to targeted gene therapy have shown some success in animal models, summarised in Table 26.1, but the vast majority of these approaches are still in the pre-clinical stages. However, a handful of targeted gene therapies for HCC have entered clinical trials and are showing some promise.

A first-generation adenoviral vector encoding the suicide gene HSV-TK was administered to ten late-stage HCC patients by intratumoural injection in a phase I study [23]. Expression of the therapeutic gene was confirmed at all dose levels, with tolerable side effects (fever, sore site of injection, flu-like symptoms) without any associated hepatotoxicity. At the highest dose given to two patients, signs of intratumoural necrosis were observed and, in one of them, a sustained stabilisation of the tumour size was achieved, with the patient surviving for 26 months.

An adenovirus vector expressing TK has also been demonstrated to improve both recurrence-free survival (9.1–43.5%) and overall survival (19.9–63.6%) in HCC

TABLE 26.1 Notable animal trials of targeted gene therapy for HCC

Vector	Transgene	Model	Result	Notes	Reference
Adenovirus	IL-12 OR HSV-TK	BNL cells in immunodeficient model	Combination of vectors significantly improved mouse survival		[40]
Targeted liposome (SP94)	(None)	Mahlavu cells in immunodeficient mice	Efficient targeting to HCC cells and drug delivery	Targeting peptide discovery based on panel of HCC lines	[5]
Adenovirus	Staphylococcus enterotoxin A (under AFP promoter)	Hepa1-6 cells in immunocompetent mice	Tumour-specific toxicity, Improved survival	Induction of tumour-specific T lymphocytes	[39]
Adenovirus	tBid (under AFP promoter)	Hep3B in immunodeficient mice	Tumour-specific cell killing, improved survival		[10]
Adenovirus	BikDD (under AFP promoter)	HepG2-Luc or HuH7-Luc in immunodeficient mice; ML-1 cells in immunocompetent mice	Tumour-specific cell killing, improved survival		[11]
Adenovirus	TRAIL, firefly Luciferase (Under survivin promoter)	McA-RH7777 in immunocompetent rats	Tumour-specific gene expression.	Tumour load and survival not reported for this study	[12]
Adenovirus	None; virus replication under control of AFP promoter	HepG2 cells in immunodeficient mice	Tumour-specific cytotoxicity, significant reduction in tumour size	Synergistic cell killing effects in vitro with 5-FU, doxorubicin and paclitaxel in Hep3B cells	[14]
Adenovirus	Linamarase (under CMV promoter)	HepG2 cells in immunodeficient mice	Efficient cell killing, extensive bystander effect.	Killing observed only when pro-drug present. No tumour targeting: delivered by intratumoural injection	[24]
Adenovirus	siRNA targeting p28GANK	SMMC-7721 in immunodeficient mice	Strong inhibition of tumour growth, tumour-specific induction of apoptosis		[25]
siRNA (before tumour implantation)	siRNA targeting VEGF	Hepa129 in CH3 mice	Reduced tumour growth, reduced microvessel density	Cells transfected with siRNA before implantation	[28]
Adenovirus	siRNA targeting URG11	HepG2 in immunodeficient mice	Suppression of tumour growth (cell cycle arrest and apoptosis)	Intratumoural injection	[29]
AAV	miR-26a	tet-o-*MYC*; LAP-tTA mice (inducible HCC model)	Suppression of tumourigenesis, tumour-specific apoptosis	No targeting: transgene expressed systemically	[32]
Lentivirus (before tumour implantation)	mIR-122	Mahlavu in immunodeficient mice	Suppression of tumourigenesis and metastasis	Cells transformed with lentivirus before implantation	[33]

patients undergoing liver transplants [41]. In this study, HCC patients with tumours over 5 cm in diameter but no metastases received transplanted livers followed by immunosuppression therapy, with or without injections of a non-replicating Ad.HSV-TK vector around the transplant site. Sustained expression of TK was observed and a significant improvement in patient outcome was achieved, especially in patients whose tumours did not show signs of vascular invasion.

A recombinant adenovirus expressing p53 (rAd-p53; trademarked as Gendicine) has been demonstrated to have efficacy against HCC in conjunction with fractionated stereotactic radiotherapy [42]. This virally delivered tumour suppressor gene increased the cells' propensity to apoptotic death, thus enhancing their sensitivity to radiotherapy, to which HCC is normally remarkably resistant. As an example of using gene therapy to sensitise tumours to existing therapies, this study inspires a degree of optimism for the similarly designed interventions currently at earlier stages in the research pipeline.

Outlook

The clinical application of targeted gene therapy techniques to hepatocellular carcinoma is still in its very early stages. However, substantial progress in the efficiency of gene transfer technology has recently resulted in impressive clinical success in infants with immunodeficiency, adults with Leber's congenital amaurosis, patients with advanced melanoma as well as in patients treated in our haemophilia B trial. While targeted gene therapy for hepatocellular carcinoma is not yet a reality, improvements in vector design and an increasing understanding of the pathogenesis of this disorder will likely lead to the future success of this approach in the clinic.

References

1. Llovet JM, Burroughs A, Bruix J. Hepatocellular carcinoma. *Lancet* 2003; 362(9399):1907–1917.
2. Peng Z. Current status of gendicine in China: recombinant human Ad-p53 agent for treatment of cancers. *Hum Gene Ther* 2005; 16(9):1016–1027.
3. Zhang B, Zhang Y, Wang J, et al. Screening and identification of a targeting peptide to hepatocarcinoma from a phage display peptide library. *Mol Med* 2007; 13(5–6):246–254.
4. Tu Y, Kim JS. Selective gene transfer to hepatocellular carcinoma using homing peptide-grafted cationic liposomes. *J Microbiol Biotechnol* 2010; 20(4):821–827.
5. Lo A, Lin CT, Wu HC. Hepatocellular carcinoma cell-specific peptide ligand for targeted drug delivery. *Mol Cancer Ther* 2008; 7(3):579–589.
6. Allen TM, Mumbengegwi DR, Charrois GJ. Anti-CD19-targeted liposomal doxorubicin improves the therapeutic efficacy in murine B-cell lymphoma and ameliorates the toxicity of liposomes with varying drug release rates. *Clin Cancer Res* 2005; 11(9):3567–3573.
7. Turrell SJ, Whitehouse A. Mutation of herpesvirus Saimiri ORF51 glycoprotein specifically targets infectivity to hepatocellular carcinoma cell lines. *J Biomed Biotechnol* 2011; 2011:785158.
8. Davidoff AM, Gray JT, Ng CY, et al. Comparison of the ability of adeno-associated viral vectors pseudotyped with serotype 2, 5, and 8 capsid proteins to mediate efficient transduction of the liver in murine and nonhuman primate models. *Mol Ther* 2005; 11(6):875–888.
9. Nathwani AC, Rosales C, McIntosh J, et al. Long-term Safety and Efficacy Following Systemic Administration of a Self-complementary AAV Vector Encoding Human FIX Pseudotyped With Serotype 5 and 8 Capsid Proteins. *Mol Ther* 2011; 19:876–885.
10. Ma SH, Chen GG, Yip J, et al. Therapeutic effect of alpha-fetoprotein promoter-mediated tBid and chemotherapeutic agents on orthotopic liver tumor in mice. *Gene Ther* 2010; 17(7):905–912.
11. Li LY, Dai HY, Yeh FL, et al. Targeted hepatocellular carcinoma proapoptotic BikDD gene therapy. *Oncogene* 2011; 30(15):1773–1783.
12. Ahn BC, Ronald JA, Kim YI, et al. Potent, tumor-specific gene expression in an orthotopic hepatoma rat model using a Survivin-targeted, amplifiable adenoviral vector. *Gene Ther* 2011; 18(6):606–612.
13. Foka P, Pourchet A, Hernandez-Alcoceba R, et al. Novel tumour-specific promoters for transcriptional targeting of hepatocellular carcinoma by herpes simplex virus vectors. *J Gene Med* 2010; 12(12):956–967.
14. Mao CY, Hua HJ, Chen P, et al. Combined use of chemotherapeutics and oncolytic adenovirus in treatment of AFP-expressing hepatocellular carcinoma. *Hepatobiliary Pancreat Dis Int* 2009; 8(3):282–287.
15. Chekulaeva M, Filipowicz W. Mechanisms of miRNA-mediated post-transcriptional regulation in animal cells. *Curr Opin Cell Biol* 2009; 21(3):452–460.
16. Ji J, Wang XW. New kids on the block: diagnostic and prognostic microRNAs in hepatocellular carcinoma. *Cancer Biol Ther* 2009; 8(18):1686–1693.

17. Bala S, Marcos M, Szabo G. Emerging role of microRNAs in liver diseases. *World J Gastroenterol* 2009; 15(45):5633–5640.
18. Coulouarn C, Factor VM, Andersen JB, et al. Loss of miR-122 expression in liver cancer correlates with suppression of the hepatic phenotype and gain of metastatic properties. *Oncogene* 2009; 28(40):3526–3536.
19. Kutay H, Bai S, Datta J, et al. Downregulation of miR-122 in the rodent and human hepatocellular carcinomas. *J Cell Biochem* 2006; 99(3):671–678.
20. Zhang G, Wang Q, Xu R. Therapeutics based on microRNA: a new approach for liver cancer. *Curr Genomics* 2010; 11(5):311–325.
21. Qiao C, Yuan Z, Li J, et al. Liver-specific microRNA-122 target sequences incorporated in AAV vectors efficiently inhibits transgene expression in the liver. *Gene Ther* 2011; 18(4):403–410.
22. Pulkkanen KJ, Parkkinen JJ, Laukkanen JM, et al. HSV-tk gene therapy for human renal cell carcinoma in nude mice. *Cancer Gene Ther* 2001; 8(7):529–536.
23. Sangro B, Mazzolini G, Ruiz M, et al. A phase I clinical trial of thymidine kinase-based gene therapy in advanced hepatocellular carcinoma. *Cancer Gene Ther* 2010; 17(12):837–843.
24. Li J, Li H, Zhu L, et al. The adenovirus-mediated linamarase/linamarin suicide system: a potential strategy for the treatment of hepatocellular carcinoma. *Cancer Lett* 2010; 289(2):217–227.
25. Li H, Fu X, Chen Y, et al. Use of adenovirus-delivered siRNA to target oncoprotein p28GANK in hepatocellular carcinoma. *Gastroenterology* 2005; 128(7):2029–2041.
26. Zhang R, Ma L, Zheng M, et al. Survivin knockdown by short hairpin RNA abrogates the growth of human hepatocellular carcinoma xenografts in nude mice. *Cancer Gene Ther* 2010; 17(4):275–288.
27. Lu X, Zheng Q, Xiong J. Effect of siRNA targeting survivin gene on the biological behavior of hepatocellular carcinoma. *J Huazhong Univ Sci Technolog Med Sci* 2005; 25(1):48–50, 58.
28. Raskopf E, Vogt A, Sauerbruch T, et al. siRNA targeting VEGF inhibits hepatocellular carcinoma growth and tumor angiogenesis in vivo. *J Hepatol* 2008; 49(6):977–984.
29. Fan R, Li X, Du W, et al. Adenoviral-mediated RNA interference targeting URG11 inhibits growth of human hepatocellular carcinoma. *Int J Cancer* 2010.
30. Tanaka S, Arii S. Medical treatments: in association or alone, their role and their future perspectives: novel molecular-targeted therapy for hepatocellular carcinoma. *J Hepatobiliary Pancreat Sci* 2010; 17(4):413–419.
31. Hoshida Y, Toffanin S, Lachenmayer A, et al. Molecular classification and novel targets in hepatocellular carcinoma: recent advancements. *Semin Liver Dis* 2010; 30(1):35–51.
32. Kota J, Chivukula RR, O'Donnell KA, et al. Therapeutic microRNA delivery suppresses tumorigenesis in a murine liver cancer model. *Cell* 2009; 137(6):1005–1017.
33. Tsai WC, Hsu PW, Lai TC, et al. MicroRNA-122, a tumor suppressor microRNA that regulates intrahepatic metastasis of hepatocellular carcinoma. *Hepatology* 2009; 49(5):1571–1582.
34. Li S, Fu H, Wang Y, et al. MicroRNA-101 regulates expression of the v-fos FBJ murine osteosarcoma viral oncogene homolog (FOS) oncogene in human hepatocellular carcinoma. *Hepatology* 2009; 49(4):1194–1202.
35. Connolly E, Melegari M, Landgraf P, et al. Elevated expression of the miR-17-92 polycistron and miR-21 in hepadnavirus-associated hepatocellular carcinoma contributes to the malignant phenotype. *Am J Pathol* 2008; 173(3):856–864.
36. Gramantieri L, Fornari F, Ferracin M, et al. MicroRNA-221 targets Bmf in hepatocellular carcinoma and correlates with tumor multifocality. *Clin Cancer Res* 2009; 15(16):5073–5081.
37. Sahin U, Tureci O, Schmitt H, et al. Human neoplasms elicit multiple specific immune responses in the autologous host. *Proc Natl Acad Sci USA* 1995; 92(25):11810–11813.
38. Stockert E, Jager E, Chen YT, et al. A survey of the humoral immune response of cancer patients to a panel of human tumor antigens. *J Exp Med* 1998; 187(8):1349–1354.
39. Si S, Sun Y, Li Z, et al. Gene therapy by membrane-expressed superantigen for alpha-fetoprotein-producing hepatocellular carcinoma. *Gene Ther* 2006; 13(22):1603–1610.
40. Drozdzik M, Qian C, Xie X, et al. Combined gene therapy with suicide gene and interleukin-12 is more efficient than therapy with one gene alone in a murine model of hepatocellular carcinoma. *J Hepatol* 2000; 32(2):279–286.
41. Li N, Zhou J, Weng D, et al. Adjuvant adenovirus-mediated delivery of herpes simplex virus thymidine kinase administration improves outcome of liver transplantation in patients with advanced hepatocellular carcinoma. *Clin Cancer Res* 2007; 13(19):5847–5854.
42. Yang ZX, Wang D, Wang G, et al. Clinical study of recombinant adenovirus-p53 combined with fractionated stereotactic radiotherapy for hepatocellular carcinoma. *J Cancer Res Clin Oncol* 2010; 136(4):625–630.

27 Is immune modulation a possibility?

Tim F. Greten[1], Firouzeh Korangy[2]

[1]Gastrointestinal Cancer Section, National Cancer Institute, NIH, Bethesda, MD, USA
[2]National Cancer Institute, Center for Cancer Research, Medical Oncology Branch, Bethesda, MD, USA

LEARNING POINTS

- Understand the relevance of chronic inflammation for the development of hepatocellular carcinoma (HCC)
- Identify humoral and cellular markers in patients with HCC, which support or impair tumour-specific immune responses in HCC
- Understand how non-immune-based treatments affect immune responses in HCC patients
- Understand how immune responses affect patients' prognosis

Introduction

Systemic therapies for the treatment of HCC are limited and largely ineffective. While most conventional cytotoxic approaches have failed to provide a survival benefit for patients with HCC, recently molecular targeted therapies have shown for the first time an increased overall survival (OS) in treated patients. However, the survival benefit is limited to less than 3 months and accompanied by side effects in many patients treated [1]. Therefore, alternative treatment options are urgently needed.

Immune-based therapies represent an interesting alternative, which have gained a lot of attention. In 2010, the Food and Drug Administration (FDA) approved the first ever cancer vaccine for the treatment of hormone-resistant, metastatic prostate cancer. Patients treated received three vaccines consisting of autologous dendritic cells (DCs) pulsed with a prostate-specific antigen leading to an increase of 4.1 months in OS [2]. Using a different immune-based approach, Hodi and colleagues recently demonstrated a significant increase in OS in melanoma patients treated with anti-CTLA4-Ig (ipilimumab) [3]. Finally, the European Commission approved a bispecific, trifunctional antibody (catumaxomab), which targets T cells to EpCam positive tumour cells, for the intraperitoneal treatment of malignant ascites in patients with EpCAM-positive carcinomas [4]. These findings clearly mark the arrival of immune-based therapies in oncology.

HCC represents a potentially ideal tumour entity for an immune modulation treatment approach, which will be described in detail below:

1. In the vast majority of cases, HCC arises as a consequence of chronic viral hepatitis, suggesting that immune mechanisms are involved in disease development.
2. The patient's immune system affects the outcome of both non-immune-based and immune-based therapies. Therefore, specifically targeting one or a group of these mechanisms could have profound effects on tumour growth.
3. The outcome of conventional non-immune-based therapies seems to be influenced by the patients' immune responses. Modulating the response to non-immune-based therapies will enhance treatment efficacy.

Chronic viral hepatitis and HCC

This topic has been summarised by a number of authors including a recent study by Yang [5] and is only briefly summarised here. In Africa and southern Asia, hepatitis B

Clinical Dilemmas in Primary Liver Cancer, First Edition. Edited by Roger Williams and Simon D. Taylor-Robinson.

virus (HBV) infection is the major cause for HCC development, while in Japan and Western countries, the hepatitis C virus (HCV) is the predominant cause. According to the center of disease control, almost 4 million people are currently infected with HCV in the United States. Vaccination against HBV has already successfully led to a decrease in the number of new HCC cases in Thailand [6] and may, therefore, be recognised as the first successful cancer vaccine. Standard treatment for both chronic HBV and HCV infections include systemic interferon-α treatment, which is known to support antiviral immune responses [7].

The role of an 'immune signature' on the prognosis of patients with HCC.

A number of different aspects of the immune system have been analysed in patients with HCC and correlated with patients' outcome. These factors can be divided into germline immune signature, variations in the immune signature within the non-tumour liver and finally within the tumour, which will be summarised and discussed in the following.

Germline factors

HCC susceptibility is mediated by germline factors affecting the immune response and differences in T-cell receptor processing

A genome-wide variation analysis (copy number and single nucleotide polymorphism) in a population of unrelated Asian individuals with liver cirrhosis and HCC was performed to identify gene loci associated with the development of HCC. In this study, a strong association with copy number variations (CNV) at the T-cell receptor gamma and alpha loci ($p < 1 \times 10^{-15}$) was identified in HCC cases when contrasted with controls. This variation appeared to be somatic in origin, reflecting differences between T-cell receptor processing in lymphocytes from individuals with liver disease and healthy individuals that is not attributable to chronic hepatitis virus infection. Analysis of constitutional variation identified three susceptibility loci including the class II major histocompatibility complex (MHC), whose protein products present antigen to T-cell receptors and mediate immune surveillance. Statistical analysis of biological networks identified variation in the 'antigen presentation and processing' pathway as being significantly associated with HCC ($p = 1 \times 10^{-11}$)[8].

Spontaneous immune responses predict patients' outcome

Multiple studies have demonstrated a correlation between immune responses to tumours and outcome of disease (Table 27.1). We and others have shown the presence of tumour-specific T-cell responses in HCC patients [9,10], as well as different immune suppressor mechanism have been described in HCC. Initial studies suggested that tumour-infiltrating $CD4^+$ and $CD8^+$ T cells correlate with an improved survival after surgical resection of tumours [11]. Follow-up studies have demonstrated that an infiltration with T cells in not always beneficial for the patients' outcome and that a more detailed analysis is required.

Effector cells

T cells

In contrast to the increasing number of $CD4^+$ T cells, $CD8^+$, $CD3^-CD56^+$, $CD3^+CD56^+$ and gamma delta T cells are all under-represented in tumour-infiltrating lymphocytes (TILs). Tumour-infiltrating $CD4^+$ T cells tend to produce more interleukin (IL)-10 but less IFN-γ, whereas $CD8^+$ T cells are impaired in their capacity to produce IFN-γ and perforin [12]. These observations were corroborated in a second study, which demonstrated a global impairment in T-cell responses recognised by low IFN-γ production, cell proliferation and ATP production. Impaired T-cell responses correlated with tumour burden and poor outcome [13]. Further analysis could demonstrate that soluble factors derived from the serum of HCC patients induced this impairment of T cells. Significant elevations in serum levels of sCD25 are found in patients with HCC, which correlate with tumour burden and a worse survival. Since

TABLE 27.1 Different immune markers, which have been shown to correlate with patients' outcome

	Protein	Cell
Non-tumour tissue	M-SCF	Macrophages
Tumour	CCL-2	$CD3^+$ T cells
	TNF-α	NK cells
	IL-6	Th17 cells
	IDO	Monocytes
	PD-L1	Regulatory T cells
Peripheral blood	sCD25	Dendritic cells
	IL-10	Regulatory T cells

T cell reactivity was inversely proportional to serum levels of sCD25, the effect of sCD25 on effector T cells was analysed. Adding increasing doses of sCD25-suppressed effector T cells, which partly involves induction of apoptosis, while sCD25 depletion from HCC serum augmented T-cell responses.

NK cells

The frequency of peripheral and tumour-infiltrating $CD56^{dim}CD16^+$ NK subsets was shown to be reduced in HCC patients compared with healthy subjects or non-tumour regions in the livers from the same patients, respectively. Both peripheral and tumour-infiltrating NK cells exhibited poor capacity to produce IFN-γ and kill K562 targets in vitro [14]. One study provided preliminary data suggesting that the relative abundance of $CD3^+CD56^+$ cells correlated with patient survival [12]. Interestingly, $CD4^+$ Tregs and $CD14^+HLA\text{-}DR^{low}$ myeloid-derived suppressor cells (MDSCs), which both can be found at increased numbers in peripheral blood from HCC patients [15,16], have been shown to suppress NK cell function and are considered potential candidates responsible for impaired function of NK cells in HCC.

NKT cells

Natural killer T (NKT) cells are a heterogeneous group of T cells that share properties of both T cells and natural killer (NK) cells. Many of these cells recognise the non-polymorphic CD1d molecule, an antigen-presenting molecule that binds self- and foreign lipids and glycolipids. NKT cells represent only 0.2% of all peripheral blood T cells but are enriched in the liver. Increased numbers of Valpha24/Vbeta11 iNKT cells were detected in primary HCC specimen. In contrast similar frequencies of $CD4^+$, double negative and $CD8\alpha^+$ iNKT cell subsets were counted in the blood of patients and healthy donors. Interestingly, the proportion of $CD4^+$ iNKT cells increased gradually from blood to liver to tumour. Furthermore, $CD4^+$ iNKT cell clones generated from healthy donors were functionally distinct from their $CD4^-$ counterparts, exhibiting higher Th2 cytokine production and lower cytolytic activity. Thus, in the tumour micro-environment the iNKT cell repertoire is modified by the enrichment of $CD4^+$ iNKT cells, a subset able to generate Th2 cytokines that can inhibit the expansion of tumour Ag-specific $CD8^+$ T cells [17].

IL-17 producing T cells

Intratumoural $IL\text{-}17^+$ T cells can be found in HCC [18] and shown to correlate with poor survival. They represent both $CD4^+$ and $CD8^+$ T cells. In contrast to circulating $IL17^+$ T cells from HCC patients, tumour-infiltrating cells co-express IFN-γ and proliferate in response to IL-1β, IL-6 and IL-23, which can be secreted by tumour-activated monocytes [19], suggesting that the different tumour-infiltrating, -invading and -evading cells have direct effects on each other.

Antigen presenting cells

Dendritic cells

We have analysed circulating DCs in peripheral blood of HCC patients without in vitro maturation [15] and noticed a reduction in the frequency of $CD14^-CD19^-CD1c^+$ myeloid DCs. While no differences in the expression of co-stimulatory molecules (CD80, CD83 and C86) as well as MHC class II expression was detected, an impaired allo-stimulatory capacity and IL-12 secretion by myeloid DCs from HCC patients was seen. Others suggested that high alpha-fetoprotein (AFP) levels (>20 μg/mL) result in phenotypic changes of in vitro CD14 derived DCs [20]. Another study suggested that AFP impairs function of DCs by induction of apoptosis [21].

Monocytes

The role of monocytes in HCC has been extensively analysed by the group of Zheng and colleagues. PD-L1 expressing monocytes suppressed tumour-specific immune function. Furthermore, PD-L1 expression on tumour-infiltrating monocytes increased with disease progression. The intensity of the protein expression was associated with high mortality and reduced survival in the HCC patients [22].

Immune cells with suppressor function

Tregs

$CD4^+CD25^+Foxp3^+$ regulatory T cells that can be found at an increased frequency in peripheral blood and peri-tumoural region from patients with HCC [23,24] have been shown to suppress immune responses. Increased $CD4^+CD25^+FoxP3^+$ Treg also correlated with impaired effector function of $CD8^+$ T cells in patients with HBV-related HCC [25]. In one study, it was suggested that tumour-infiltrating Tregs are associated with an increased risk for vascular invasion [26], and a different study demonstrated that the presence of low intratumoural Tregs in combination with high intratumoural activated CD8$^+$ cytotoxic T cells (CTLs) was an independent prognostic factor for both improved disease free survival (DFS) and OS [27]. Recently a correlation between liver-infiltrating CD8$^+$FoxP3$^+$ infiltrating Tregs and tumour stage in HCC has been described (28]. On the basis of pre-clinical studies, we demonstrated that the removal of CD4+ Tregs from peripheral blood mononuclear cells derived from HCC patients unmasks AFP-specific T-cell responses in vitro. Consequently, we conducted a small clinical trial examining the effect of low-dose cyclophosphamide treatment (which has previously been shown to specifically target regulatory T cells in murine studies) on Tregs and tumour-specific T-cell responses in patients with HCC. In this proof of concept trial, we were not only able to demonstrate the safety of a low-dose cyclophosphamide treatment in advanced HCC patients, but our data also indicated removal of CD4$^+$ Tregs in HCC patients mounts AFP-specific T-cell responses in vivo [29]. Future studies will show if targeting Tregs in HCC patients will enhance immune responses to immune and also non-immune-based treatments.

MDSC

MDSCs represent a heterogenous population of cells that consist of myeloid progenitor cells and immature myeloid cells (IMCs). Murine MDSCs are characterised by the expression of Gr-1 and CD11b. CD11b$^+$Gr-1$^+$ MDSCs represent approximately 2–4% of all nucleated splenocytes, but can increase up to 50% in tumour-bearing mice [30,31]. These cells are a mixture of IMCs, immature granulocytes, mononcytes-macrophages, DCs and myeloid progenitor cells. In humans, different types of MDSCs have been described and characterised [32]. We observed an increase in the frequency of CD14$^+$HLA-DR$^{low/neg}$ cells in peripheral blood and the tumour micro-environment. These cells do not only fail to mature into functional DCs, but also suppress proliferation and cytokine secretion of CD8$^+$ T cells in an L-arginine-dependent manner. More importantly, we were able to demonstrate that depletion of these cells in vitro unmasked antigen-specific T-cell responses [16]. Further in vitro studies using freshly isolated human MDSCs demonstrated that CD14$^+$HLA-DR$^{low/neg}$ cells suppress T-cell responses not only directly but also indirectly. Co-culture experiments of MDSCs with autologous CD4$^+$ T cells induced a Foxp3$^+$ regulatory phenotype of T cells with suppressor function. Finally, MDSCs were capable to suppress the function of NK cells in vitro [33]. These findings make MDSCs a very interesting and important target for therapy aiming at the modulation of the immune system.

Immune suppressive cytokines

Different cytokines have been evaluated in the context of HCC including IL-6, IL-10, TGF-β and CSF. Increased levels of IL-10 have been described as a negative prognostic indicator for survival in patients with various types of cancer. IL-10 exerts tolerogenic and immunosuppressive effects on DCs and has been shown to impair function of NK cells. Serum levels of IL-10 were found to be higher in patients with HCC when compared with controls [34] and high IL-10 serum levels were associated with shorter OS in another study [35]. Macrophage colony-stimulating factor (M-CSF) has been assessed by immunohistochemistry in tissue micro-arrays consisting of paired tumour and peri-tumoural liver tissue derived from 105 patients with HCC who had undergone hepatectomy for HCC. In this study, it was demonstrated that neither intratumoural M-CSF nor macrophage density was associated with OS or DFS. However, peri-tumoural M-CSF and macrophage density was higher in patients with larger tumours and presence of intrahepatic metastasis and were independent prognostic factors for both OS and DFS in the analysed patient cohort [36]. Indoleamine 2,3-dioxygenase (IDO) is known to have an important role in immune tolerance [37]. In HCC over-expression of HCC can be found in selected cases (36%), which correlated with higher metastasis rates and poor prognosis [38].

Co-stimulatory molecules and MHC class I molecules

Immunohistochemical analysis of tumour biopsies obtained by surgical resection indicated a reduced expression of MHC class I, which correlated with tumour differentiation. Furthermore, B7-1 and B7-2 expression was reduced in primary tumours when directly compared with areas of liver tissue without tumour involvement [39]. The aberrant expression of programmed cell death ligands 1 and 2 (PD-Ls) on tumour cells dampens antitumour immunity, resulting in tumour immune evasion. Immunohistochemical analysis of tissue micro-arrays consisting of 240 randomly selected HCC patients, who had undergone curative surgery, demonstrated that higher tumour PD-L1 expression correlated with a significantly poorer prognosis [40]. These findings are of particular interest considering the fact that monoclonal antibodies targeting PD-1 are in early clinical trials [41].

Immune expression profiles

A number of investigators have done biased and unbiased immune gene expression analysis in HCC with the aim to identify specific signature genes suggestive for different clinical outcomes. In one study, the immune microenvironment within tumours was found to be heterogeneous, although globally more inert compared with the adjacent non-tumour liver tissue. An inflammatory signature within the primary tumour was associated with longer survival. Univariate analysis revealed that the expression of 11 immunological genes correlated positively with patients' outcome. TNF, IL-6 and CCL2 demonstrated the strongest correlation. Further analysis revealed that at least 8/11 of the molecules associated with survival were expressed by TILs [42]. Genome-wide expression profiling of tumour and tumour surrounding tissues from 307 patients with HCC failed to produce a gene expression profile of tumour tissue, which could be used to predict patients' survival in contrast to profiles of the surrounding non-tumour liver tissue. Here, a set of 186 genes was identified, which was predictive for patients' survival [43]. A different study demonstrated that a unique inflammation/immune response-related signature defined by the expression of 17 genes was a predictor for HCC venous metastasis [44].

Immune modulation induced by conventional 'non-immune-based' therapies

Recently, a number of interesting observations in patients with HCC suggest that immune modulation might become a potential therapeutic approach for the treatment of HCC in the near future. These findings show the presence of active antitumour immune responses and immune suppressor mechanisms as well as a direct effect of conventional therapies on immune responses in patients with HCC. Below we will discuss and summarise the recent data on the effect of local ablative therapies as well as targeted therapies using sorafenib on immune responses in patients with HCC.

Immune modulation induced by local destruction of the tumour

Local ablative therapies are widely used to treat patients with small tumours. Different types of devices are introduced into the intrahepatic tumour with the goal to cause a local destruction of the tumour. This can be achieved by different physical methods including application of heat, cold, chemically active substances etc. All these procedures cause massive tumour cell death followed by local inflammatory responses. Upon cell injury massive amounts of tumour antigens are being released along with endogenous adjuvants, which not only activate the innate immune response but can also have profound effects on the adaptive immune response as shown in multiple pre-clinical studies [45].

Radiofrequency thermal ablation (RFTA) has become the method of choice to ablate small tumours of the liver. Recently much focus has been put on its efficacy and safety in comparison to surgical resection [46]. RFTA treatment induces a localised and controlled disruption of the tumour by heating the tissue causing its coagulative necrosis, followed by an inflammatory response. The effect of this type of treatment on antitumour immune responses has become more and more the focus of attention of a number of new and interesting studies. Since it is impossible in patients to examine the local cellular response to RFTA, most studies have analysed cytokine levels as well as the composition and phenotype of different immune cells in the periphery of patients with HCC after RFTA. As one might have expected an increase of different pro-inflammatory cytokines including IL-1β and TNF-α was observed in blood from patients following RFTA. This increase was associated with an activation of circulating MDSCs upon RFTA [47], while a different study provided data suggesting that RFTA can release cytokines leading to a maturation of DCs [48].

In order to analyse the effect of RFTA on tumour-specific immune responses AFP-specific $CD4^+$ T-cell responses were followed in patients undergoing embolisation therapy. AFP-specific $CD4^+$ T-cell responses to three immunodominant epitopes in HCC patients were expanded during and after embolisation. The development of higher frequencies of AFP-specific $CD4^+$ T cells after treatment were significantly associated with the induction of >50% necrosis of the tumour and an improved clinical outcome again demonstrating the importance of generating an immune response from primarily non-immune-based treatments for patient's outcome [49]. An increase of patients responsive either to tumour antigens and a higher frequency of circulating tumour-specific T cells in response to RFTA was also observed in another study. However, no correlation between tumour-specific T-cell responses and disease relapse was observed [50]. In anther study, the frequency of

AFP-specific T cells was studied in HCC patients in response to transcatheter arterial embolisation (TAE). TAE also destroys a tumour by the induction of necrosis and/or apoptosis and causes inflammation with cytokine production. An increased frequency of AFP-specific T cells was observed in selected patients without any additional immune-based therapy after TAE [51]. Finally, very interesting results were reported recently on the phenotype, number and function of NK cells in response to RFTA in patients with HCC. In this study, 37 patients with HCC were treated with RFTA. Phenotype, number and function of NK cells were analysed 1 week before and 1 and 4 weeks after ablative therapy. Follow-up included 3 monthly contrast-enhanced ultrasound examinations and 6 monthly CT scans. Interestingly, in contrast to $CD3^+$, $CD4^+$, $CD8^+$ T cells and $CD19^+$ B cells, the absolute and relative frequency of $CD16^+CD56^+$ NK cells increased upon RFTA in HCC patients. Apart from an increase in expression of the activating receptors (NKG2D, CD16, NKp44 and NKp30) as well as a decrease in expression of the inhibitory receptor NKG2A on NK cells, an enhanced NK mediated cell-cytotoxicity and IFN-γ production was documented in HCC patients 4 weeks after RFTA. Further patient follow-up demonstrated that enhanced NK cell function after RFTA treatment was associated with improved disease-free survival [52]. Moreover the authors report that RFTA also increased the capacity of antibody-dependent cell mediated cytotoxicity supporting the idea of a new treatment modality, in which RFTA might be combined with monoclonal antibody-based therapies. Finally, the authors present preliminary data suggesting that enhanced NK cell function after RFTA treatment is associated with improved disease-free survival.

The effect of targeted therapies using multityrosine kinase inhibitors in tumour-specific immune responses and suppressor mechanisms in HCC

On the basis of the results from the Sorafenib HCC Assessment Randomized Protocol (SHARP) trial study, sorafenib can now be considered to be the standard of care for patients with advanced HCC according to Barcelona Clinic Liver Cancer (BCLC) classification and CHILD-Pugh A cirrhosis [1]. Sorafenib is a small molecule that inhibits tumour-cell proliferation and tumour angiogenesis and increases the rate of apoptosis in a wide range of tumour models. Its mode of action has been shown to depend on the inhibition of the serine–threonine kinases Raf-1 and B-Raf and the receptor tyrosine kinase activity of different vascular endothelial and platelet-derived growth factor receptors. A number of studies have examined the effect of sorafenib on different cells of the immune system including DCs, T cells, NK cells and Tregs.

Sorafenib was shown to inhibit the function of DCs, characterised by reduced secretion of cytokines and expression of CD1a, MHC, and co-stimulatory molecules in response to TLR ligands as well as by their impaired ability to migrate and stimulate T-cell responses. Furthermore, sorafenib inhibited the induction of antigen-specific T-cell responses in mice in vivo [53]. Sorafenib was also shown to inhibit the proliferation of primary human T cells in vitro as well as CD25 and CD69 expression and IL-2 production [54]. Analysis of the effect of sorafenib on NK cells revealed an impaired response of NK cells (cytotoxicity and IFN-γ production) to tumour cells upon sorafenib treatment. This was due to impaired PI3K and ERK phosphorylation, which directly controls NK cell reactivity [55]. Only one report was able to demonstrate a potentially beneficial effect of sorafenib on immune responses in renal cell carcinoma patents. In this recently published study, it was shown that sorafenib treatment results in a decrease in tumour-infiltrating Tregs [56].

Conclusion

Although many previous and ongoing studies focus on immune-based therapies for treatment of HCC, it is important to acknowledge that tumours have developed multiple pathways to module immune responses and evade tumour-specific immune responses. Furthermore, there is an increasing body of evidence suggesting that even non-immune-based therapies have profound effects on the immune system. Future research needs to aim at understanding how immune-based and non-immunological therapies can be combined optimally to modulate immune responses in the most effective way, leading to effective antitumour therapy.

References

1. Llovet JM, Ricci S, Mazzaferro V, et al. Sorafenib in advanced hepatocellular carcinoma. *N Engl J Med* 2008; 359(4):378–390.
2. Kantoff PW, Higano CS, Shore ND, et al. Sipuleucel-T immunotherapy for castration-resistant prostate cancer. *N Engl J Med* 2010; 363(5):411–422.

3. Hodi FS, O'Day SJ, McDermott DF, et al. Improved survival with ipilimumab in patients with metastatic melanoma. *N Engl J Med* 2010; 363(8):711–723.
4. Heiss MM, Murawa P, Koralewski P, et al. The trifunctional antibody catumaxomab for the treatment of malignant ascites due to epithelial cancer: results of a prospective randomized phase II/III trial. *Int J Cancer* 2010; 127(9):2209–2221.
5. Yang JD, Roberts LR. Hepatocellular carcinoma: a global view. *Nat Rev Gastroenterol Hepatol* 2010; 7(8):448–458.
6. Chang MH, Chen CJ, Lai MS, et al. Universal hepatitis B vaccination in Taiwan and the incidence of hepatocellular carcinoma in children. Taiwan Childhood Hepatoma Study Group. *N Engl J Med* 1997; 336(26):1855–1859.
7. Rehermann B, Nascimbeni M. Immunology of hepatitis B virus and hepatitis C virus infection. *Nat Rev Immunol* 2005; 5(3):215–229.
8. Clifford RJ, Zhang J, Meerzaman DM, et al. Genetic variations at loci involved in the immune response are risk factors for hepatocellular carcinoma. *Hepatology* 2010; 52(6):2034–2043.
9. Greten TF, Manns MP, Korangy F. Immunotherapy of hepatocellular carcinoma. *J Hepatol* 2006; 45(6):868–878.
10. Behboudi S, Boswell S, Williams R. Cell-mediated immune responses to alpha-fetoprotein and other antigens in hepatocellular carcinoma. *Liver Int* 2010; 30(4):521–526.
11. Wada Y, Nakashima O, Kutami R, Yamamoto O, Kojiro M. Clinicopathological study on hepatocellular carcinoma with lymphocytic infiltration. *Hepatology* 1998; 27(2): 407–414.
12. Pang YL, Zhang HG, Peng JR, et al. The immunosuppressive tumor microenvironment in hepatocellular carcinoma. *Cancer Immunol Immunother* 2009; 58(6):877–886.
13. Cabrera R, Ararat M, Cao M, et al. Hepatocellular carcinoma immunopathogenesis: clinical evidence for global T cell defects and an immunomodulatory role for soluble CD25 (sCD25). *Dig Dis Sci* 2010; 55(2):484–495.
14. Cai L, Zhang Z, Zhou L, et al. Functional impairment in circulating and intrahepatic NK cells and relative mechanism in hepatocellular carcinoma patients. *Clin Immunol* 2008; 129:428–437.
15. Ormandy LA, Farber A, Cantz T, et al. Direct ex vivo analysis of dendritic cells in patients with hepatocellular carcinoma. *World J Gastroenterol* 2006; 12(20):3275–3282.
16. Hoechst B, Ormandy LA, Ballmaier M, et al. A new population of myeloid-derived suppressor cells in hepatocellular carcinoma patients induces CD4(+)CD25(+)Foxp3(+) T cells. *Gastroenterology* 2008; 135(1):234–243.
17. Bricard G, Cesson V, Devevre E, et al. Enrichment of human CD4+ V(alpha)24/Vbeta11 invariant NKT cells in intrahepatic malignant tumors. *J Immunol* 2009; 182(8):5140–5151.
18. Zhang JP, Yan J, Xu J, et al. Increased intratumoral IL-17-producing cells correlate with poor survival in hepatocellular carcinoma patients. *J Hepatol* 2009; 50(5):980–989.
19. Kuang DM, Peng C, Zhao Q, et al. Tumor-activated monocytes promote expansion of IL-17-producing CD8+ T cells in hepatocellular carcinoma patients. *J Immunol* 2010; 185(3):1544–1549.
20. Ritter M, Ali MY, Grimm CF, et al. Immunoregulation of dendritic and T cells by alpha-fetoprotein in patients with hepatocellular carcinoma. *J Hepatol* 2004; 41(6):999–1007.
21. Um SH, Mulhall C, Alisa A, Ives AR, et al. Alpha-fetoprotein impairs APC function and induces their apoptosis. *J Immunol* 2004; 173(3):1772–1778.
22. Kuang DM, Zhao Q, Peng C, et al. Activated monocytes in peritumoral stroma of hepatocellular carcinoma foster immune privilege and disease progression through PD-L1. *J Exp Med* 2009; 206(6):1327–1337.
23. Ormandy LA, Hillemann T, Wedemeyer H, Manns MP, Greten TF, Korangy F. Increased populations of regulatory T cells in peripheral blood of patients with hepatocellular carcinoma. *Cancer Res* 2005; 65(6):2457–2464.
24. Yang XH, Yamagiwa S, Ichida T, et al. Increase of CD4+ CD25+ regulatory T-cells in the liver of patients with hepatocellular carcinoma. *J Hepatol* 2006; 45(2):254–262.
25. Fu J, Xu D, Liu Z, et al. Increased regulatory T cells correlate with CD8 T-cell impairment and poor survival in hepatocellular carcinoma patients. *Gastroenterology* 2007; 132(7):2328–2339.
26. Unitt E, Marshall A, Gelson W, et al. Tumour lymphocytic infiltrate and recurrence of hepatocellular carcinoma following liver transplantation. *J Hepatol* 2006; 45(2): 246–253.
27. Gao Q, Qiu SJ, Fan J, et al. Intratumoral balance of regulatory and cytotoxic T cells is associated with prognosis of hepatocellular carcinoma after resection. *J Clin Oncol* 2007; 25(18):2586–2593.
28. Yang ZQ, Yang ZY, Zhang LD, et al. Increased liver-infiltrating CD8+FoxP3+ regulatory T cells are associated with tumor stage in hepatocellular carcinoma patients. *Hum Immunol* 2010; 71(12):1180–1186.
29. Greten TF, Ormandy LA, Fikuart A, et al. Low-dose cyclophosphamide treatment impairs regulatory T cells and unmasks AFP-specific CD4+ T-cell responses in patients with advanced HCC. *J Immunother* 2010; 33(2):211–218.
30. Zhao F, Obermann S, von Wasielewski R, et al. Increase in frequency of myeloid-derived suppressor cells in mice with spontaneous pancreatic carcinoma. *Immunology* 2009; 128(1):141–149.
31. Gallina G, Dolcetti L, Serafini P, et al. Tumors induce a subset of inflammatory monocytes with immunosuppressive activity on CD8+ T cells. *J Clin Invest* 2006; 116(10):2777–2790.

32. Greten TF, Manns MP, Korangy F. Myeloid derived suppressor cells in human diseases. *Int J Immunopharmacol* 2011; 11:802–806 .
33. Hoechst B, Voigtlaender T, Ormandy L, et al. Myeloid derived suppressor cells inhibit natural killer cells in patients with hepatocellular carcinoma via the NKp30 receptor. *Hepatology* 2009; 50(3):799–807.
34. Beckebaum S, Zhang X, Chen X, et al. Increased levels of interleukin-10 in serum from patients with hepatocellular carcinoma correlate with profound numerical deficiencies and immature phenotype of circulating dendritic cell subsets. *Clin Cancer Res* 2004; 10(21):7260–7269.
35. Hattori E, Okumoto K, Adachi T, et al. Possible contribution of circulating interleukin-10 (IL-10) to anti-tumor immunity and prognosis in patients with unresectable hepatocellular carcinoma. *Hepatol Res* 2003; 27(4):309–314.
36. Zhu XD, Zhang JB, Zhuang PY, et al. High expression of macrophage colony-stimulating factor in peritumoral liver tissue is associated with poor survival after curative resection of hepatocellular carcinoma. *J Clin Oncol* 2008; 26(16):2707–2716.
37. Lob S, Konigsrainer A, Rammensee HG, Opelz G, Terness P. Inhibitors of indoleamine-2,3-dioxygenase for cancer therapy: can we see the wood for the trees? *Nat Rev Cancer* 2009; 9(6):445–452.
38. Pan K, Wang H, Chen MS, et al. Expression and prognosis role of indoleamine 2,3-dioxygenase in hepatocellular carcinoma. *J Cancer Res Clin Oncol* 2008; 134(11):1247–1253.
39. Fujiwara K, Higashi T, Nouso K, et al. Decreased expression of B7 costimulatory molecules and major histocompatibility complex class-I in human hepatocellular carcinoma. *J Gastroenterol Hepatol* 2004; 19(10):1121–1127.
40. Gao Q, Wang XY, Qiu SJ, et al. Overexpression of PD-L1 significantly associates with tumor aggressiveness and postoperative recurrence in human hepatocellular carcinoma. *Clin Cancer Res* 2009; 15(3):971–979.
41. Brahmer JR, Drake CG, Wollner I, et al. Phase I study of single-agent anti-programmed death-1 (MDX-1106) in refractory solid tumors: safety, clinical activity, pharmacodynamics, and immunologic correlates. *J Clin Oncol* 2010; 28(19):3167–3175.
42. Chew V, Tow C, Teo M, et al. Inflammatory tumor microenvironment is associated with superior survival in hepatocellular carcinoma patients. *J Hepatol* 2009; 52:370–379.
43. Hoshida Y, Villanueva A, Kobayashi M, et al. Gene expression in fixed tissues and outcome in hepatocellular carcinoma. *N Engl J Med* 2008; 359(19):1995–2004.
44. Budhu A, Forgues M, Ye QH, et al. Prediction of venous metastases, recurrence, and prognosis in hepatocellular carcinoma based on a unique immune response signature of the liver microenvironment. *Cancer Cell* 2006; 10(2):99–111.
45. Greten TF, Korangy F. Radiofrequency ablation for the treatment of HCC – Maybe much more than simple tumor destruction? *J Hepatol* 2010; 53:775–776.
46. Callstrom MR, Charboneau JW. Technologies for ablation of hepatocellular carcinoma. *Gastroenterology* 2008; 134(7):1831–1835.
47. Ali MY, Grimm CF, Ritter M, et al. Activation of dendritic cells by local ablation of hepatocellular carcinoma. *J Hepatol* 2005; 43(5):817–822.
48. Zerbini A, Pilli M, Fagnoni F, et al. Increased immunostimulatory activity conferred to antigen-presenting cells by exposure to antigen extract from hepatocellular carcinoma after radiofrequency thermal ablation. *J Immunother* 2008; 31:271–282.
49. Ayaru L, Pereira SP, Alisa A, et al. Unmasking of alpha-fetoprotein-specific CD4(+) T cell responses in hepatocellular carcinoma patients undergoing embolization. *J Immunol* 2007; 178(3):1914–1922.
50. Zerbini A, Pilli M, Penna A, et al. Radiofrequency thermal ablation of hepatocellular carcinoma liver nodules can activate and enhance tumor-specific T-cell responses. *Cancer Res* 2006; 66(2):1139–1146.
51. Mizukoshi E, Nakamoto Y, Arai K, et al. Enhancement of tumor-specific T-cell responses by transcatheter arterial embolization with dendritic cell infusion for hepatocellular carcinoma. *Int J Cancer* 2010; 126(9):2164–2174.
52. Zerbini A, Pilli M, Laccabue D, et al. Radiofrequency thermal ablation for hepatocellular carcinoma stimulates autologous NK-cell response. *Gastroenterology* 2010; 138: 1931–1942.
53. Hipp MM, Hilf N, Walter S, et al. Sorafenib, but not sunitinib, affects function of dendritic cells and induction of primary immune responses. *Blood* 2008; 111(12):5610–5620.
54. Zhao W, Gu YH, Song R, Qu BQ, Xu Q. Sorafenib inhibits activation of human peripheral blood T cells by targeting LCK phosphorylation. *Leukemia* 2008; 22(6):1226–1233.
55. Krusch M, Salih J, Schlicke M, et al. The kinase inhibitors sunitinib and sorafenib differentially affect NK cell antitumor reactivity in vitro. *J Immunol* 2009; 183(12):8286–8294.
56. Desar IM, Jacobs JH, Hulsbergen-Vandekaa CA, et al. Sorafenib reduces the percentage of tumour infiltrating regulatory T cells in renal cell carcinoma patients. *Int J Cancer* 2010; 129:507–512.

28 Systemic therapy for hepatocellular carcinoma: future directions

Daniel H. Palmer[1], Matthew E. Cramp[2]

[1]University of Liverpool, Liverpool, UK
[2]Plymouth Hospitals NHS Trust, Plymouth, UK

LEARNING POINTS

- Sorafenib is the first of many drugs in development that have the potential to improve outcomes for hepatocellular carcinoma (HCC)
- Understanding of the molecular pathways involved in angiogenesis and cell proliferation and how to block them has led to many new drugs entering clinical trials
- The efficacy and safety of these new treatments remains to be established particularly in the context of advanced liver fibrosis and portal hypertension
- Blocking several cellular pathways using drugs in combination or with drugs that have multiple actions may enhance responses and reduce the risk of tumour resistance
- There is considerable potential in the use of new drugs in combination with conventional chemotherapy
- There is considerable potential in the use of new drugs in combination with locoregional treatments such as transarterial chemoembolisation (TACE)
- The optimum strategy of when to use these drugs in combinations remains unknown although trials are under way

Introduction

The demonstration in well-designed randomised placebo-controlled trials that sorafenib can prolong survival in patients with advanced HCC (see Chapter X) provides proof-of-principle that targeted therapies can be effective in this clinical setting [1]. However, the absolute benefit derived from sorafenib is relatively modest. Recent advances in understanding the molecular pathogenesis of HCC is being used to guide development of better therapies and the selection of treatment combinations.

In this chapter, we examine novel systemic agents used singly and in combination that are entering clinical trials in the setting of advanced HCC and look at strategies that can be adopted for using new agents to potentially enhance the outcomes of currently available locoregional therapies.

Molecular pathogenesis of HCC

The molecular pathogenesis of HCC is complex. It is a heterogenous tumour at the molecular level and typically harbours a variety of genetic and epigenetic alterations and chromosomal aberrations. Although the transition from cirrhosis to carcinoma is poorly understood, it is clearly a multistep process characterised by an accumulation of oncogenes activated by point mutations or amplifications, and a loss of tumour suppressor genes through mutations or epigenetic silencing. These abnormalities allow acquisition of the hallmarks of cancer described by Hanahan and Weinberg, including cell cycle dysregulation, evasion of apoptosis, cell immortalisation through telomerase activity and angiogenesis [2]. These processes are frequently driven through deregulation of key signalling pathways including growth factor receptors and their intracellular signalling apparatus (e.g. EGFR, IGF, the ras/MAP Kinase pathway, PI3Kinase/Akt/mTOR and HGF/c-met signalling); wnt/β-catenin signalling; the hedgehog pathway and aberrations in apoptotic pathways (intrinsic and extrinsic) (Figure 28.1). Increasing understanding of these mechanisms has identified a variety of potential therapeutic targets for HCC,

Clinical Dilemmas in Primary Liver Cancer, First Edition. Edited by Roger Williams and Simon D. Taylor-Robinson.

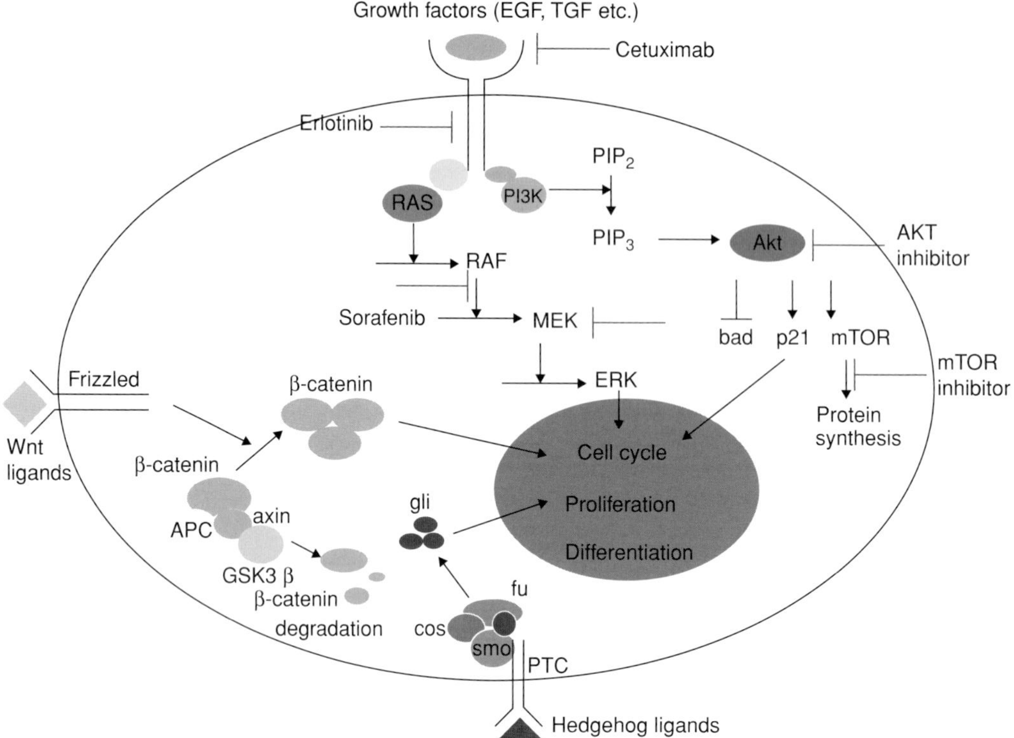

FIG 28.1 Molecular pathogenesis of hepatocellular carcinoma and potential therapeutic targets. The molecular pathogenesis of HCC is increasingly well characterised. In particular, the components of growth factor receptor signalling (EGF, IGF, etc.) present potential therapeutic targets. Similar molecular mechanisms contribute to endothelial cell proliferation that is a requisite for angiogenesis. Other key pathways that contribute to hepatocarcinogenesis such as wnt and hedgehog signalling are currently not readily amenable to drug therapy.

and many agents are currently in varying stages of clinical development.

Targeting angiogenesis

HCC is a highly vascular tumour and, indeed, this has been exploited therapeutically in the form of TACE. More recently, the molecular mechanisms mediating tumour angiogenesis have been elucidated and these have provided potential pharmacological targets. In particular, the fundamental role of angiogenic growth factor receptor signalling, most notably the importance of vascular endothelial growth factor (VEGF) signalling through VEGF receptors 2 and 3, has been recognised. These processes can be perturbed in a number of ways. Bevacizumab is a humanised murine monoclonal antibody against VEGF ligand and phase II trials have indicated some activity against HCC, although there have been concerns regarding the risk of significant gastrointestinal bleeding and recent studies has mandated prophylactic treatment of varices prior to treatment [3]. The downstream consequences of VEGF receptor signalling can also be inhibited by small molecules targeting receptor tyrosine kinase activity. Indeed, this mechanism is probably fundamental to the activity of sorafenib in HCC. A growing number of other molecules designed to perturb VEGF signalling are now in clinical trials in patients with HCC (Table 28.1). Sunitinib, an inhibitor of VEGF and platelet-derived growth factor (PDGF) receptors as well as c-kit and flt-3, has been tested in two phase II trials, using two different dosing schedules [4,5]. Both demonstrated evidence of activity sufficient to proceed to a randomised phase III trial comparing it with sorafenib, aiming to recruit in excess of 1000 patients. Unfortunately, this study closed prematurely for reasons of toxicity and serves as a reminder

TABLE 28.1 XXX

Agent(s)	Target(s)	Phase	Patient number	RR (%)	PFS at 4 mo	TTP (mo)	Overall survival (mo)
Sorafenib	Raf, VEGFR, PDGFR	II	137	2.2		4.2	9.5
Sorafenib vs. placebo	Raf, VEGFR, PDGFR	III	602	2.3 vs. 0.7	62% vs. 42%	5.5 vs. 2.8	10.7 vs. 7.9
Sorafenib vs. placebo	Raf, VEGFR, PDGFR	III	220	3 vs. 1		2.8 vs. 1.4	6.5 vs. 4.2
Bevacizumab brivanib	VEGF, VEGFR, FGFR	II II	46 55	13 8	65% @6 mo 18% @6 mo	2.7 (PFS)	12.4 10
Erlotinib	EGFR	II		9	32% @6 mo		13
Erlotinib	EGFR	II	40	0	43%		10.75
Sunitinib (50 mg 4 wk on, 2 wk off)	VEGFR, PDGFR, c-kit	II	37	2.7	35% @3 mo	5.3	8.0
Sunitinib (37.5mg 4wk on, 2wk off)	VEGFR, PDGFR, c-kit	II	34	2.9	50%	3.9 (PFS)	9.8
Sorafenib + doxorubicin vs. dox		Randomised phase II	96	4 vs. 2		6.4 vs. 2.8	13.7 vs. 6.5
Bevacizumab + GemOx		II		20	48% @6 mo		9.5
Bevacizumab + erlotinib		II	40	25 (1 CR)	62.5%	9 (PFS)	15.65

of the complexity of conducting studies in the context of HCC and underlying chronic liver disease. This toxicity was largely myelosuppression, which, interestingly, is not commonly observed with sorafenib. This difference may reflect the capacity of sunitinib to inhibit c-kit and flt-3, which are expressed on haematological precursors, as well as VEGF signalling. Other anti-angiogenic agents in trials for HCC include axitinib, vatalanib, cediranib, linifanib, brivanib and vargatef. Like sorafenib and sunitinib, these largely act through inhibition of VEGFR-2 but differ in their inhibition of other kinases, for example, brivanib and vargatef both also inhibit FGF receptor signalling. The monoclonal antibody ramicurimab/IMC-1121B also targets the VEGFR-2. Phase II data for these agents indicate median survival figures in the range 8–9 months, consistent with that achieved by sorafenib [6].

An understanding of the mechanisms of resistance to VEGF-targeted therapies may help improve therapeutic strategies. For example, there is some evidence that hepatocyte growth factor (HGF) signalling through its receptor, c-met, may play a role in mediating such resistance and, indeed, may contribute to the emergence of a more aggressive phenotype during anti-VEGF therapy [7]. This suggests a potential role for c-met inhibition as a second-line strategy, or in combination with anti-angiogenic therapy. The c-met inhibitor ARQ197 is currently under investigation in a randomised phase II trial for patients with HCC. Other agents, for example XL880 (foretinib) and XL184, that target both VEGFR and c-met are also entering clinical trials in HCC.

Pre-clinical data indicate that angiopoietin-2 (Ang-2), which signals through the Tie-2 receptor on vascular endothelium, works in cooperation with VEGF to promote tumour angiogenesis and a more aggressive tumour phenotype [8]. Inhibition of Ang-2 can reverse these effects in murine models of HCC such that dual inhibition of both Ang-2 and VEGF may induce a more potent anti-angiogenic effect [9]. Indeed, phase II trials of the anti-angiopoietin agent, AMG386, in combination with sorafenib are under way. Regorafenib, a fluorinated derivative of sorafenib, retains the ability to inhibit VEGFR, PDGFR and raf kinases, but differs from sorafenib in its ability to also inhibit the angiopoietin receptor Tie-2 and is also in phase II clinical development for HCC.

It is increasingly recognised that VEGF-targeted treatments act predominantly through 'vascular normalisation' rather than inhibiting new vessel formation. Thus, tumour angiogenesis results in the formation of immature, tortuous and highly permeable vessels, which leads to poor perfusion and high interstitial pressure within a tumour. This, in turn, may contribute to chemoresistance due to poor delivery of the chemotherapeutic agent. VEGF inhibition is thought to promote maturation of vessels and reduce tumour interstitial pressure and this may explain the successful combination of anti-VEGF therapies with conventional chemotherapy in other tumour types (see below). An alternative approach to the treatment of vascular tumours such as HCC is vascular disruption, which aims to directly collapse tumour circulation. This requires the identification of endothelial or perivascular targets that are specific to tumour rather than normal vessels. A number of tumour endothelial molecules have been identified, including the phospholipid phosphatidylserine (PS) [10]. PS is normally found on the inner leaflet of the endothelial cell membrane but is exposed on the outer leaflet of tumour endothelium. An anti-PS monoclonal antibody, bavituximab, is in clinical trials for HCC. PS expression on the surface of tumour endothelium is also increased by conventional chemotherapy, suggesting a rationale for combination studies

At present it is not known whether any one anti-angiogenic agent will be more potent against HCC. Whilst some agents have a greater affinity for VEGFR than sorafenib, sorafenib is the only agent that also potentially targets tumour cell proliferation (through raf inhibition). The relative importance of angiogenesis inhibition and raf inhibition in the efficacy of sorafenib is not known, since it is impossible to uncouple these effects in the clinic. These questions might be addressed by the studies comparing new agents against sorafenib as the standard of care that are now in progress.

Whilst it may be unlikely that agents with broadly similar mechanisms of action will result in clinically significant increments in survival compared to sorafenib, the availability of a number of active agents may still have utility. Thus, whilst one agent may not be significantly superior to another, there may be scope for sequential therapy when resistance emerges to first-line treatment. This is exemplified by phase II data suggesting that brivanib has clinical activity even when used as a second-line treatment in patients who have already received sorafenib [11]. Similarly a small study using bevacizumab following sorafenib failure reported a median survival of 9.5 months despite patients largely having poor performance status and often a Child-Pugh score of 7 [12]. Similar data have been observed using axitinib as a second-line agent in the setting of renal cancer, and a study of second-line axitinib following first-line anti-angiogenic therapy for advanced HCC is planned.

A choice of agents may also provide scope for 'personalised medicine' in the future with the choice of drug being made rationally on the basis of biomarkers predictive of benefit. Indeed, a critical challenge in the development of these therapies is the incorporation of translational endpoints into clinical trial design in order to identify the presence of the relevant target in the tumour and to correlate this with response so that patients most likely to benefit can be selected.

Antiproliferative therapies

Processes other than angiogenesis also contribute to the pathogenesis of HCC (Figure 28.1). For example, EGF and TGFα contribute to tumour cell proliferation and invasion through epidermal growth factor receptor (EGFR) signalling. Specific inhibitors of EGFR are growth inhibitory in HCC models in vitro and in vivo and early phase trials of anti-EGFR monoclonal antibody (cetuximab) and of small molecule EGFR tyrosine kinase inhibitor (erlotinib) suggest clinical activity [13,14] (Table 28.1). Downstream pathways of growth factor receptor signalling include the Map Kinase (Ras/Raf/Mek/Erk) and PI3Kinase/Akt/mTOR cascades. Indeed, sorafenib works, in part, through Raf inhibition. Downstream of Raf are Mek kinases that then phosphorylate and activate Erk kinases, promoting their translocation from cytoplasm to nucleus where they function as transcription factors regulating the expression of genes required for cell cycle regulation, cell survival and cell motility. This pathway can also be perturbed therapeutically through Mek inhibitors, such as AZD6244, which has entered trials for HCC. A phase II study recruited 19 patients but was discontinued after an interim analysis, since median time to progression was just 8 weeks and there were no radiological responses [15].

The PI3K pathway is commonly up-regulated in HCC either through constitutive activation of PI3K or loss of the tumour suppressor PTEN, leading to activation of mTOR, a key regulator of cell growth and proliferation. Inhibition of mTOR has shown promise in pre-clinical models, and clinical trials using the mTOR inhibitors rapamycin, everolimus and temsirolimus are under way with promising data emerging. For example, a phase I/II study of everolimus reported a median overall survival of 8.4 months, again in line with that achieved by sorafenib [16]. mTOR is also involved in production of angiogenic factors, including VEGF, and so its inhibition may also exert an anti-angiogenic effect and there is a rationale for its combination with VEGF-targeted therapies to enhance this effect. Akt inhibitors, such as MK2206, are also in clinical development for HCC. A phase II trial for patients failing a first-line anti-angiogenic agent is currently under way on the basis of pre-clinical data indicating that in cell lines, resistance to sorafenib is acquired through activation of the PI3K/Akt pathway and that sensitivity to sorafenib is restored by Akt inhibition, although these data may suggest that combination of Akt inhibitor with sorafenib may be a more effective strategy [17].

Insulin-like growth factor, IGF-II, is over-expressed in up to 30% of HCC and loss of IGF receptor-II, which normally binds and degrades IGF-II, is also commonly seen. Thus, IGF receptor signalling represents a rational target for HCC. Several monoclonal antibodies targeting the IGF-1 receptor (e.g. cixutumumab/IMC-A12) are in clinical trials either as a single agent or in combination [18].

There are a number of other pathways that are commonly perturbed in HCC, including wnt/β-catenin and hedgehog signalling cascades but, as yet, these have not lent themselves to pharmacological manipulation.

Combination therapy

The cross-talk within tumour cell and endothelial cell signalling suggests that inhibition of one single pathway is unlikely to result in durable tumour control. Better understanding of signalling processes is providing evidence for the rational combination of several agents and such combinations are now entering clinical trials. This may also underpin the activity of multitargeted kinase inhibitors such as sorafenib. Furthermore, combination of signal transduction inhibitors acting at different points in the same pathway offers the potential to maximise pathway inhibition to produce additive clinical benefit and to reduce potential development of resistance. Thus, EGFR activation results in secretion of angiogenic cytokines, including VEGF, such that EGFR inhibition may also mediate anti-angiogenic effects [19]. Indeed, pre-clinical models suggest that EGFR signalling is a pre-requisite for angiogenesis in HCC via up-regulation of VEGF. This process appears to be mediated through phosphorylation of AKT rather than ERK/MAPK and thus may be specifically susceptible to EGFR or mTOR inhibitors [19].

A phase II trial has investigated the combination of bevacizumab with erlotinib. Striking data have been reported, with an objective response rate of 25% (including one complete response), median progression free survival of 9 months and median survival 15.6 months [20] (Table 28.1). Clearly this combination warrants further investigation, although again some caution is required in terms of potential bevacizumab-associated GI bleeding in patients with cirrhosis. A biomarker study related to this trial reported that higher serum angiopoietin-2 and VEGFR-2 were associated with poorer outcome [21]. However, whether these may serve as prognostic or predictive markers cannot be elucidated from a single arm phase II trial. A randomised phase III trial investigating the addition of erlotinib to sorafenib is also ongoing.

mTOR is a downstream component of PI3K/AKT signalling, playing a critical role in regulating cell cycle progression, cell motility and angiogenesis. Combination of mTOR inhibitors with VEGFR antagonists has synergistic effects in pre-clinical models and trials of their combination with sorafenib are under way. Similarly, a phase II trial of everolimus with bevacizumab has demonstrated safety of this combination [22].

There is also cross-talk between IGF and VEGF receptor signalling, suggesting that combining drugs to target both may be beneficial. However, one such study combining an anti-IGF-1 receptor antibody with sorafenib was closed early due to problems with toxicity of the combination. This emphasises that tolerability, even with so-called targeted agents, can be an issue in the setting of HCC and may limit the use of some regimens despite a strong scientific rationale for their combination.

Novel therapies in combination with conventional chemotherapy

Response rates for conventional cytotoxic chemotherapy are low and significant durable remission is uncommon. The most widely used agent has been doxorubicin, and an early prospective randomised trial reported statistically significant increased survival compared with best supportive care [23]. However, this benefit was clinically insignificant and subsequent review of series containing over 700 patients suggests a typical response rate of only 10–15%, and convincing evidence that survival is improved has not been forthcoming. On this basis, HCC is generally regarded as being resistant to conventional chemotherapeutic drugs. However, pathways that are inhibited by novel targeted therapies, including raf/mek/erk, may contribute to this resistance and so combination of these agents with chemotherapy may overcome chemoresistance. Indeed, there is pre-clinical evidence of synergy between doxorubicin and raf inhibition. In a vascular endothelial model, resistance to doxorubicin is, at least in part, mediated via FGF-mediated raf-dependent survival signals, and can be overcome by inhibition of raf, providing rationale for combining doxorubicin with sorafenib or inhibitors of FGFR such as brivanib or vargatef [24]. Similarly, the combination of doxorubicin with the MEK inhibitor, AZD6244, was synergistic in a murine HCC model [25]. Furthermore, there is clear clinical evidence of benefit from the combination of anti-angiogenic agents with conventional chemotherapy in other tumour types. For example, in patients with metastatic colorectal cancer bevacizumab significantly prolongs survival when added to 5-FU, irinotecan or oxaliplatin based regimens [26]. Whilst the mechanism of action of bevacizumab is postulated to be anti-angiogenic, laboratory studies suggest that it may act through normalisation of tortuous, highly permeable tumour neovasculature, reducing intratumoural interstitial pressure, thereby increasing blood flow and improving chemotherapy delivery to the tumour.

A randomised phase II trial has investigated the combination of sorafenib and doxorubicin compared with doxorubicin alone. It was initiated at the same time as the SHARP trial and represented a reasonable combination to explore, since at that time doxorubicin was widely accepted as the control arm in HCC trials with a predictable and manageable toxicity profile in appropriately selected patients. The overall survival in the combination arm was more than double the control arm (13.7 months compared with 6.5 months, HR 0.45), but it must be remembered that the aim of a randomised phase II is simply to determine whether or not the combination should be taken into a phase III setting rather than to allow statistically robust comparisons between treatment arms [27]. To establish whether this benefit is attributable to synergy between the two agents or to sorafenib alone requires a further randomised trial of the combination using sorafenib as the control arm.

Another study has investigated the addition of bevacizumab to combination chemotherapy comprising gemcitabine and oxaliplatin (GemOx), demonstrating some activity with a response rate of 20% and median survival of 9.5 months [28]. The significance of these results within the context of a single arm phase II study is difficult to interpret but, whilst comparison across phase II studies is limited due to potential imbalances in prognostic factors in the two groups of patients, they do not appear to be significantly better than GemOx alone [29].

Conventional chemotherapy is often considered to be ineffective against HCC due to drug resistance. Chemoresistance can be intrinsic or acquired and is mediated through a variety of mechanisms. HCC cells are often intrinsically resistant to chemotherapy through the over-expression of drug transporter proteins including the multidrug resistance gene, MDR1, encoding p-glycoprotein. In vitro studies have demonstrated that over-expression of MDR1 leads to efflux of doxorubicin from the cell. A number of early phase clinical trials have investigated the role of p-glycoprotein inhibitors in combination with doxorubicin and other drugs without any clear indication of benefit to warrant their investigation in larger studies.

Cell replication pathways targeted by chemotherapy may be dysregulated in HCC. For example, topoisomerase 2a, an enzyme encoded by the TOP2A gene, is involved in DNA unwinding for replication and is the target for a number of chemotherapeutic agents. Mutations in the TOP2A gene are associated with doxorubicin resistance in HCC cell lines and its over-expression is reported to correlate with chemoresistance. In vitro studies have demonstrated that the topoisomerase 2 inhibitor, etoposide, can sensitise HCC cells to doxorubicin [30] and this may underpin the encouraging phase II data relating to etoposide in combination with the anthracycline epirubicin [31]. Nevertheless to confirm these data, phase III trials are required.

The proteosome is an intracellular enzyme complex responsible for degradation of ubiquitinated proteins and this process contributes to the regulation of transcription factors such as NFκB. NFκB coordinates many key cellular functions by regulating the expression of genes involved in cell survival and inflammation in response to a wide variety of stimuli and it has been implicated in acquired chemoresistance [32]. Bortezomib is a potent and selective proteosome inhibitor, which inhibits NFκB signalling.

Antitumour activity of bortezomib as a single agent and in combination with chemotherapeutic agents has been demonstrated in a pre-clinical models [32,33] and a phase I/II trial demonstrated good tolerance in HCC patients, with 7 of 15 evaluable patients achieving disease stability [34]. Since proteosome inhibition attenuates pathways implicated in anthracycline and other cytotoxic drug resistance, combination studies are of interest. However, results from a phase II study of doxorubicin plus bortezomib were disappointing with a response rate of 2.3% and median survival of 5.7 months [35].

Other novel therapeutic approaches

Immunotherapy

HCC possesses certain characteristics that render it a potential target for immunotherapy. There is an active recruitment of lymphocytes into the tumour and such tumour-infiltrating lymphocytes (TIL) can lyse autologous, but not allogeneic, tumour cells when manipulated ex vivo using appropriate stimulatory cytokines [36]. However, the very development of HCC in immunocompetent people indicates the presence of immunosuppressive mechanisms preventing effective maturation of TILs into useful effectors. A number of immunotherapeutic strategies aimed at overcoming this 'tolerance' to tumours are under investigation, including peptide vaccination and cellular therapies. A number of putative tumour-associated antigens have been identified in HCC including alpha-fetoprotein (AFP), glypican-3 (a molecule implicated in wnt and growth factor receptor signalling and commonly over-expressed in HCC) and telomerase (which, in common with many other tumours is over-expressed in HCC and is requisite for limitless cell replication), and peptide vaccines against these are in clinical trials [37,38]. GC33 is an antiglypican three monoclonal antibody that has demonstrated antitumour efficacy in HCC xenograft models via antibody-dependent cellular cytotoxicity rather than a direct effect on tumour cell proliferation and, perhaps through macrophage-dependent mechanisms [39]. A phase I trial in combination with sorafenib is under way.

Dendritic cells (DC) are professional antigen presenting cells that have the capacity to present tumour-associated antigens in the optimum co-stimulatory environment to elicit cytotoxic T-cell responses, and early phase clinical trials using autologous DC loaded ex vivo with tumour antigens prior to re-infusion have reported encouraging results with evidence of induction of immune and clinical responses [40].

Evasion of immune surveillance is, in part, mediated by immunosuppressive regulatory T cells (Treg). Recent work has shown that low-dose cyclophosphamide can selectively impair Treg and unmask cytotoxic T cells (CTL) responses to AFP, suggesting that this may form an important component of immunotherapy strategies [41]. However, significant challenges remain in the development of successful immunotherapy. These include the choice of target antigen, vaccination route and schedule and the disease context, with the highest chance of success being in earlier stage disease or in combination with locoregional therapies. Indeed, these challenges are exemplified by a recent phase II clinical trial combining telomerase peptide vaccination with low-dose cyclophosphamide in patients with advanced HCC, which failed to demonstrate any clear clinical benefit, with no detectable T-cell responses against the vaccine [38].

Death receptors and induction of apoptosis

Elucidation of the molecular processes that co-ordinate apoptotic cell death have facilitated an understanding of the mechanisms by which cytotoxic drugs kill cancer cells and the mechanisms by which cancers become resistant. Two pathways of apoptosis are well characterised: the 'intrinsic' pathway, which is mediated by permeabilisation of the mitochondrial membrane and release of cytochrome C through interactions of Bcl-2 family members; and the 'extrinsic' pathway, through engagement of cell surface 'death receptors' of the TNF receptor superfamily by their specific ligands including Fas ligand and TRAIL. Chemotherapeutic drugs typically induce apoptosis through activation of one or both of these pathways [42]. In normal physiology, these processes are counterbalanced by anti-apoptotic proteins, including Bcl-2, MCl-1 and members of the IAP (inhibitor of apoptosis) family, which may be over-expressed in cancers, contributing to chemoresistance [42].

TRAIL is a ligand of the death receptor family and its receptors (DR4 and DR5) have been targeted therapeutically using monoclonal antibodies, recombinant soluble ligand and gene therapy to deliver the TRAIL gene to tumour cells in early phase clinical trials. However, despite claims that TRAIL has tumour specificity there have been reports of liver toxicity.

The inhibitor of apoptosis, XIAP, is commonly over-expressed in HCC and may contribute to drug resistance.

AEG35156 is an antisense oligonucleotide that specifically targets XIAP mRNA to suppress its function. This compound is currently in early phase clinical trial in combination with sorafenib.

Mapatumumab is a fully human agonist antibody against DR4. Sorafenib targets MCl-1 over-expression of which may confer resistance to TRAIL, suggesting potential synergy between sorafenib and TRAIL-targeted therapy. A phase I trial has confirmed the safety of the combination (specifically in pts with hepatitis B or C) with dose-limiting toxicity seen and in 19 pts there were two objective radiological responses and four patients with stable disease lasting more than 3 months [43]. On this basis a phase II trial is planned.

PARP inhibition

Temozolomide is a DNA damaging drug and resistance to it is mediated by PARP-dependent DNA repair. Thus, PARP inhibition may prevent repair of temozolomide-induced DNA damage and enhance its cytotoxicity [44]. To test this concept, a phase II trial combining temozolomide with the PARP inhibitor, ABT 888 in HCC patients, is ongoing.

Src inhibition

Src is central to several oncogenic processes including MAP-Kinase signalling and it can contribute to chemoresistance. Cell line studies suggest a subgroup of HCCs with a 'hepatoblast' (rather than a hepatocyte) molecular profile, which may be sensitive to src inhibition [45]. Dasatinib is an inhibitor of src family kinases and a phase II trial is under way, although this study does not attempt to correlate response with molecular subtype of HCC.

Arginine depletion

Arginine is a non-essential amino acid synthesised through the urea cycle enzyme arginosuccinate synthase (ASS). Some cancers, including HCC, are deficient in ASS and are dependent on exogenous arginine for their growth. Arginine deiminase (ADI) is a bacterial enzyme that catalyses the conversion of arginine to citrulline and has an antitumour effect in pre-clinical HCC models. However, since ADI is non-mammalian it is strongly immunogenic, limiting its clinical utility. Pegylation of ADI reduces its immunogenicity, and phase II studies have confirmed its ability to reduce serum arginine levels in patients with a promising median survival of 11 months in a group of patients largely naive to prior systemic therapy [46].

Epigenetics

Histone deacetylation plays a key role in the transcriptional regulation of key genes involved in cell cycle progression, differentiation and apoptosis. Thus, histone deacetylase (HDAC) inhibitors have antitumour activity through histone modulation, which increases immunogenicity, inhibits angiogenesis and enhances chemotherapeutic effects. Vorinostat is the first Food and Drug Administration (FDA) approved HDAC inhibitor indicated for refractory cutaneous T-cell lymphoma [47]. A Phase I study of vorinostat in combination with sorafenib is under way.

Improving efficacy of systemic therapies through application in earlier stage disease

Recent years have seen major advances in treatment options for HCC to the extent that effective local control can now be achieved in many cases by the application of surgical resection, liver transplantation and ablative therapies such as radiofrequency ablation (RFA) and percutaneous ethanol injection (PEI). TACE can also induce extensive tumour necrosis and in appropriately selected cases is associated with improved overall survival. However, as tumour size increases, so does the frequency of vascular invasion and with it the risk of metastases increases, thereby limiting the impact of local control.

The limitations of locoregional therapies might be ameliorated by more effective systemic therapies. This could be applied in a neo-adjuvant setting (thereby 'downstaging' tumours and expanding the indication for local treatments) or the adjuvant setting (thereby decreasing post-operative/procedure recurrence and, if successful, expanding current size limits).

The questions that now arise are, having developed an effective agent and learnt lesson from the trials undertaken to date, how should active systemic therapies be integrated with currently available locoregional therapies.

Liver transplantation

Considerable controversy surrounds the value of local therapies, such a TACE, whilst patients are on the waiting list for liver transplantation [48]. The primary aim of such therapy is to maintain the patient within the limits of current criteria for transplantation for sufficient time for a graft to become available; currently the shortage of available grafts leads to 'drop out' and this is a significant factor impacting on the overall effectiveness of transplantation. A secondary aim may be to decrease the rate of tumour recurrence *after* transplantation. The question of whether or not sorafenib may be helpful in this situation arises. Whilst at first sight, it seems logical to seek a clinical trial to answer this question the primary aim of systemic treatment in this situation is, in effect, to prolong the 'time to progression'. Although strictly speaking this has only been shown for sorafenib in patients with advanced disease, there is no reason to believe that the result would be different in the case of earlier disease and hence the use of sorafenib for patients awaiting transplantation would seem reasonable simply based on currently available evidence. Although this does not address the second question of whether sorafenib could impact on recurrence if used as an adjuvant following transplant, with currently employed criteria recurrence is, in fact, already rare and any impact would likely be marginal. This may be different if transplant criteria were broadened but at present this is primarily limited by availability of donor organs.

Surgery and ablative therapies

Surgical resection and ablative treatments such as RFA and PEI are widely regarded as radical therapies that have the potential, in well-selected cases, to achieve complete local control and thereby improve overall survival. A systemic therapy might be applied in two settings. Firstly, in the neoadjuvant setting it might render tumour initially considered non-resectable, resectable. This has, on occasion, been achieved with doxorubicin and doxorubicin-based combinations [49]; it is unlikely to be achieved with drugs such as sorafenib where significant reduction in tumour size is uncommon. On the other hand, in the post-operative setting it could be hypothesised that effective agents might decrease the relapse rate. A recent randomised phase II study suggested that the heparinase inhibitor PI-88 might be effective in this role [50]. A similar study for sorafenib has been launched (STORM) trial in which patients achieving complete local control by surgery or ablative therapy are randomised to receive either sorafenib or placebo and has recently successfully completed accrual of more than 1000 patients. Design of such studies raises interesting questions regarding the nature of HCC recurrence. On the one hand, like other cancers, recurrence may be mediated by micrometastatic spread occurring prior to the ablative therapy and this typically becomes clinically apparent within the first 1–2 years of treatment. On the other hand, since patients still have underlying cirrhosis, so-called recurrence may reflect occurrence of de novo tumours and may occur later. Thus, the duration of adjuvant therapy may be difficult to determine and its ability to prevent progression of pre-malignant lesions to invasive carcinomas is unknown.

Transarterial chemoembolisation

There are several potential attractions to the addition of a systemic agent such as sorafenib to chemoembolisation. It might be expected that the systemic agent could impact on the two major factors that limit the effectiveness of such procedures, namely, residual disease (local and distant) and recurrent disease (both directly and by inhibiting re-vascularisation). Indeed, since TACE induces profound tumour hypoxia, there is activation of hypoxia-inducible signalling pathways and angiogenic factors such as VEGF, b-FGF and IGF-2 are frequently over-expressed following embolisation. Higher serum levels of these angiogenic factors are associated with metastasis and reduced survival, perhaps through the mediation of the re-vascularisation that is characteristic of TACE failure, or through stimulating the growth and vascularisation of micrometastases. This may help guide rationale selection of systemic agents to combine with TACE.

The optimal design for such a study is challenging. The major choice lies between addition of the systemic agent prior to TACE and continuing thereafter or only instituting the systemic therapy once all planned TACE procedures have been completed (Figure 28.2). A theoretical advantage of commencing sorafenib immediately is the potential for a synergistic interaction between sorafenib and doxorubicin since, as noted above, levels of doxorubicin are similar whether the drug is administered locally or systemically and the safety of this drug combination has already been demonstrated [27]. Furthermore, pre-treatment with sorafenib may stabilise the tumour microvasculature to enhance local chemotherapy delivery. Some caution with this schedule is required since the pharmacokinetics of sorafenib may be altered by the temporary impairment of liver function that typically follows TACE.

The endpoints of the trial are similarly challenging. There is no reason to believe that sorafenib efficacy would be any greater or less if given after TACE when recurrence has been documented hence studies should be powered on

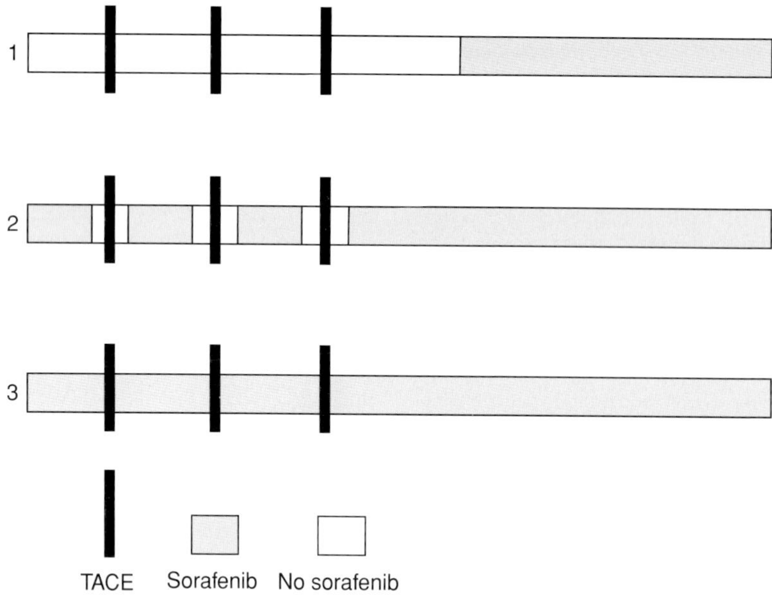

FIG 28.2 Strategies for combination of sorafenib with TACE. 1: Sequential treatment. Sorafenib is given as an adjuvant treatment once all planned TACE sessions are completed. This approach avoids any potential additional toxicity during the TACE procedures. However, it misses an opportunity for synergistic interactions and delays treatment of micrometastatic disease by several weeks. 2: Intermittent treatment. Sorafenib is commenced immediately to avoid the problem of delayed systemic therapy, but is suspended at the time of TACE to reduce the risk of complications. Again, the opportunity for synergy may be missed. 3: Continuous treatment. The anti-angiogenic agent will be present when the TACE procedure induces angiogenic cytokines and there is an opportunity for synergy between sorafenib and the chemotherapy component of TACE. However, the risk of complications may be greater.

the basis that its effect might be synergistic with TACE. On this basis, the UK NCRN has launched a randomised placebo-controlled trial in which patients will immediately receive sorafenib or placebo followed by TACE and with sorafenib/placebo continued until progression.

A Japanese randomised phase II study combining TACE with TSU-68 (an inhibitor of VEGF, PDGF and FGF receptor tyrosine kinases) in 101 patients reported an improvement in the primary endpoint of progression-free survival from 4 to 5.2 months with the addition of the anti-angiogenic agent (hazard ratio 0.699; $p = .054$) [51]. However, this benefit appears modest and larger studies are required to determine if there is any significant impact on overall survival. Another study conducted in Japan and Korea randomised patients to receive sorafenib or placebo after completion of, and recovery from, a course of TACE, with no improvement in survival [52]. A potential explanation for this failure may be the scheduling of treatment, with the median time from last TACE to commencing drug/placebo being 2 months, which may have missed the peak of angiogenic cytokines released as a result of embolisation. This question will be addressed by the UK study.

Conclusions

Increased understanding of the molecular pathogenesis and an ever-expanding number of drugs available to modify these processes is contributing to incremental improvements in survival for patients with HCC. However, the future beyond sorafenib remains unclear and carefully designed clinical trials addressing the impact of these new treatments on the tangible patient benefits of survival and quality of life are required. A number of such trials are currently ongoing and their results are eagerly awaited.

The HCC population presents unique challenges to cancer drug development and trial design with the interplay of the HCC itself with the underlying liver disease aetiology and liver disease severity. In general, HCC-specific phase

I trials are required to determine safety and tolerability in the context of chronic liver disease. Phase II trial design continues to present challenges in terms of identifying a key efficacy signal to justify proceeding to larger phase III studies. The traditional phase II outcome measure of radiological response rate is largely unhelpful and 'progression' endpoints such as progression-free survival and time-to-progression are variable depending on the baseline demographics of the patient group such that single-arm phase II trials are difficult to interpret. These problems may be addressed by increasing use of randomised phase II trials, but these are not substitutes for adequately powered randomised phase III trials with overall survival as the primary endpoint.

Finally, with increasing recognition of the molecular heterogeneity of HCC and the rapid rise in number of potential drugs, there is an urgent need to identify molecular predictors of benefit in order to select the most appropriate therapy for patients. Some studies have reported tantalising results. Indeed, the sorafenib phase II study suggested that phosphorylation of Erk detected immunohistochemically in tumour biopsies was associated with improved survival and speculated that, since this may reflect activation of the MAPKinase pathway, it may be predictive of benefit from raf inhibition [53]. However, since this was a single-arm phase II trial in which all patients received sorafenib, it is not possible to conclude whether Erk phosphorylation is a predictive biomarker or whether it is associated with better prognosis irrespective of treatment received. It is imperative, therefore, that such translational studies are embedded in randomised studies so that these questions may be resolved. In this way a better understanding of specific tumour biology can be used in the future to individualise treatment and reap the full benefits of the broad array of molecular agents under development.

References

1. Llovet JM, Ricci S, Mazzaferro V, et al. SHARP Investigators Study Group. Sorafenib in advanced hepatocellular carcinoma. *N Engl J Med* 2008; 359(4):378–390.
2. Hanahan D, Weinberg RA. Hallmarks of cancer: the next generation. *Cell* 2011; 144(5):646–674.
3. Siegel AB, Cohen EI, Ocean A, Lehrer D, et al. Phase II trial evaluating the clinical and biologic effects of bevacizumab in unresectable hepatocellular carcinoma. *J Clin Oncol* 2008; 26(18):2992–2998.
4. Zhu AX, Sahani DV, Duda DG, et al. Efficacy, safety, and potential biomarkers of sunitinib monotherapy in advanced hepatocellular carcinoma: a phase II study. *J Clin Oncol* 2009; 27(18):3027–3035.
5. Faivre S, Raymond E, Boucher E, et al. Safety and efficacy of sunitinib in patients with advanced: an open-label, multicentre, phase II study. *Lancet Oncol* 2009; 10(8):794–800.
6. Park JW, Finn RS, Kim JS, et al. Phase II, Open-label study of brivanib as first-line therapy in patients with advanced hepatocellular carcinoma. *Clin Cancer Res* 2011; 17(7):1973–1983.
7. Shojaei F, Lee JH, Simmons BH, et al. HGF/c-Met acts as an alternative angiogenic pathway in sunitinib-resistant tumors. *Cancer Res* 2010; 70(24):10090–100100.
8. Zhang ZL, Liu ZS, Sun Q. Expression of angiopoietins, Tie2 and vascular endothelial growth factor in angiogenesis and progression of hepatocellular carcinoma. *World J Gastroenterol* 2006; 12(26):4241–4245.
9. Hashizume H, Falcón BL, Kuroda T, et al. Complementary actions of inhibitors of angiopoietin-2 and VEGF on tumor angiogenesis and growth. *Cancer Res* 2010; 70(6):2213–2223.
10. Heath VL, Bicknell R. Anticancer strategies involving the vasculature. *Nat Rev Clin Oncol* 2009; 6(7):395–404.
11. Raoul JL, Finn RS, Kang YK, et al. An open-label phase II study of first- and second-line treatment with brivanib in patients with hepatocellular carcinoma (HCC). *J Clin Oncol* 2009; 27(suppl):15s (abstract 4577).
12. Pazo Cid RA, Esquerdo G, Puertolas T, et al. Bevacizumab (BVZ) as second-line treatment after sorafenib (SFB) progression in patients (pts) with advanced hepatocellular carcinoma (HCC). *J Clin Oncol* 2010; 28(suppl; abstract e14619).
13. Zhu AX, Stuart K, Blaszkowsky LS, et al. Phase 2 study of cetuximab in patients with advanced hepatocellular carcinoma. *Cancer* 2007; 110(3):581–589.
14. Thomas MB, Chadha R, Glover K, et al. Phase 2 study of erlotinib in patients with unresectable hepatocellular carcinoma. *Cancer* 2007; 110(5):1059–1067.
15. O'Neil BH, Williams-Goff LW, Kauh J, et al. A phase II study of AZD6244 in advanced or metastatic hepatocellular carcinoma. *J Clin Oncol* 2009; 27 (suppl; abstract e15574).
16. Blaszkowsky L, Abrams TA, Miksad RA, et al. Phase I/II study of everolimus in patients with advanced hepatocellular carcinoma (HCC). *J Clin Oncol* 2010 (suppl; abstract e14524).
17. Chen KF, Chen HL, Tai WT, et al. Activation of phosphatidylinositol 3-kinase/Akt signaling pathway mediates acquired resistance to sorafenib in hepatocellular carcinoma cells. *J Pharmacol Exp Ther* 2011; 337(1):155–161.
18. O'Donnell R, El-Khoueiry AB, Lenz H, Gandara DR. A phase I trial of escalating doses of the anti-IGF-1R monoclonal antibody (mAb) cixutumumab (IMC-A12) and sorafenib for

treatment of advanced hepatocellular carcinoma (HCC). *J Clin Oncol* 2010; 28(suppl):15s (abstract TPS212).
19. Ueda S, Basaki Y, Yoshie M, et al. PTEN/Akt signaling through epidermal growth factor receptor is prerequisite for angiogenesis by hepatocellular carcinoma cells that is susceptible to inhibition by gefitinib. *Cancer Res* 2006; 66(10):5346–5353.
20. Thomas MB, Morris JS, Chadha R, et al. Phase II trial of the combination of bevacizumab and erlotinib in patients who have advanced hepatocellular carcinoma. *J Clin Oncol* 2009; 27(6):843–850.
21. Kaseb AO, Morris J, Hassan M, et al. Molecular predictors of response to antiangiogenic therapy in HCC: data from bevacizumab and erlotinib phase II study. *J Clin Oncol* 2010; 28(suppl):15s (abstract 4046).
22. Treiber G. Treatment of advanced or metastatic hepatocellular cancer (HCC): interim analysis of a single-arm phase II study of bevacizumab and RAD001. *J Clin Oncol* 2010; 28(suppl):15s (abstract 4102).
23. Lai CL, Wu PC, Chan GC, Lok AS, Lin HJ. Doxorubicin versus no antitumor therapy in inoperable hepatocellular carcinoma. A prospective randomized trial. *Cancer* 1988; 62(3):479–483.
24. Alavi A, Hood JD, Frausto R, Stupack DG, Cheresh DA. Role of Raf in vascular protection from distinct apoptotic stimuli. *Science* 2003; 301(5629):94–96.
25. Huynh H, Chow PK, Soo KC. AZD6244 and doxorubicin induce growth suppression and apoptosis in mouse models of hepatocellular carcinoma. *Mol Cancer Ther* 2007; 6(9):2468–2476.
26. Hurwitz H, Fehrenbacher L, Novotny W, et al. Bevacizumab plus irinotecan, fluorouracil, and leucovorin for metastatic colorectal cancer. *N Engl J Med* 2004; 350(23):2335–2342.
27. Abou-Alfa GK, Johnson P, Knox JJ, et al. Doxorubicin plus sorafenib vs doxorubicin alone in patients with advanced hepatocellular carcinoma: a randomized trial. *JAMA* 2010; 304(19):2154–2160.
28. Zhu AX, Blaszkowsky LS, Ryan DP, et al. Phase II study of gemcitabine and oxaliplatin in combination with bevacizumab in patients with advanced hepatocellular carcinoma. *J Clin Oncol* 2006; 24(12):1898–1903.
29. Louafi S, Boige V, Ducreux M, et al. Gemcitabine plus oxaliplatin (GEMOX) in patients with advanced hepatocellular carcinoma (HCC): results of a phase II study. *Cancer* 2007; 109(7):1384–1390.
30. Wong N, Yeo W, Wong WL, et al. TOP2A overexpression in hepatocellular carcinoma correlates with early age onset, shorter patients survival and chemoresistance. *Int J Cancer* 2009; 124(3):644–652.
31. Bobbio-Pallavicini E, Porta C, Moroni M, et al. Epirubicin and etoposide combination chemotherapy to treat hepatocellular carcinoma patients: a phase II study. *Eur J Cancer* 1997; 33(11):1784–1788.
32. Hideshima T, Richardson P, Chauhan D, et al. The proteasome inhibitor PS-341 inhibits growth, induces apoptosis, and overcomes drug resistance in human multiple myeloma cells. *Cancer Res* 2001; 61(7):3071–3076.
33. Cusack JC Jr, Liu R, Houston M, et al. Enhanced chemosensitivity to CPT-11 with proteasome inhibitor PS-341: implications for systemic nuclear factor-kappaB inhibition. *Cancer Res* 2001; 61(9):3535–3540.
34. Hegewisch-Becker S, Sterneck M, Schubert U, et al. Phase I/II trial of bortezomib in patients with unresectable hepatocellular carcinoma (HCC). *Journal of Clinical Oncology, 2004 ASCO Annual Meeting Proceedings (Post-Meeting Edition). Vol 22, No 14S (July 15 Supplement),* 2004:4089.
35. Berlin JD, Powell ME, Su Y, et al. Bortezomib (B) and doxorubicin (dox) in patients (pts) with hepatocellular cancer (HCC): A phase II trial of the Eastern Cooperative Oncology Group (ECOG 6202) with laboratory correlates. *Clin Oncol* 2008; 26 (May 20 suppl; abstract 4592).
36. Butterfield LH. Immunotherapeutic strategies for hepatocellular carcinoma. *Gastroenterology* 2004; 127(5 suppl 1):S232–S241.
37. Butterfield LH, Ribas A, Meng WS, et al. T-cell responses to HLA-A∗0201 immunodominant peptides derived from alpha-fetoprotein in patients with hepatocellular cancer. *Clin Cancer Res* 2003; 9(16 Pt 1):5902–5908.
38. Greten TF, Forner A, Korangy F, et al. A phase II open label trial evaluating safety and efficacy of a telomerase peptide vaccination in patients with advanced hepatocellular carcinoma. *BMC Cancer* 2010; 10:209.
39. Takai H, Kato A, Kinoshita Y, et al. Histopathological analyses of the antitumor activity of anti-glypican-3 antibody (GC33) in human liver cancer xenograft models: the contribution of macrophages. *Cancer Biol Ther* 2009; 8(10):930–938.
40. Palmer DH, Midgley RS, Mirza N, et al. A phase II study of adoptive immunotherapy using dendritic cells pulsed with tumor lysate in patients with hepatocellular carcinoma. *Hepatology* 2009; 49(1):124–132.
41. Greten TF, Ormandy LA, Fikuart A, et al. Low-dose cyclophosphamide treatment impairs regulatory T cells and unmasks AFP-specific CD4+ T-cell responses in patients with advanced HCC. *J Immunother* 2010; 33(2):211–218.
42. Petak I, Houghton JA, Kopper L. Molecular targeting of cell death signal transduction pathways in cancer. *Curr Signal Transduct Ther* 2006; 1:113–131.
43. Sun W, Nelson D, Alberts SR, et al. Phase Ib study of mapatumumab in combination with sorafenib in patients with advanced hepatocellular carcinoma (HCC) and chronic viral hepatitis. *J Clin Oncol* 2011; 29 (suppl 4; abstract 261).

44. Palma JP, Rodriguez LE, Bontcheva-Diaz VD, et al. The PARP inhibitor, ABT-888 potentiates temozolomide: correlation with drug levels and reduction in PARP activity in vivo. *Anticancer Res* 2008; 28(5A):2625–2635.
45. Finn RS, Aleshin A, Rivera D, et al. Effect of dasatinib, an orally active small molecule inhibitor of both *src* and *abl* kinases, on growth of hepatic progenitor subtype human hepatocellular carcinoma cells in vitro. *ASCO Gastrointestinal Cancers Symposium*, 2009 (abstract 169).
46. Glazer ES, Piccirillo M, Albino V, et al. Phase II study of pegylated arginine deiminase for nonresectable and metastatic hepatocellular carcinoma. *J Clin Oncol* 2010; 28(13):2220–2226.
47. Duvic M, Talpur R, Ni X, et al. Phase 2 trial of oral vorinostat (suberoylanilide hydroxamic acid, SAHA) for refractory cutaneous T-cell lymphoma (CTCL). *Blood* 2007; 109(1):31–39.
48. Palmer DH, Johnson PJ. Pre-operative locoregional therapy and liver transplantation for hepatocellular carcinoma: time for a randomized controlled trial. *Am J Transplant* 2005; 5(4 Pt 1):641–642.
49. Leung TWT, Patt YZ, Lau WY, et al. Complete pathological remission is possible with systemic combination chemotherapy for inoperable hepatocellular carcinoma. *Clin Cancer Res.* 1999; 5:1676–1681.
50. Liu CJ, Lee PH, Lin DY, et al. Heparanase inhibitor PI-88 as adjuvant therapy for hepatocellular carcinoma after curative resection: a randomized phase II trial for safety and optimal dosage. *J Hepatol* 2009; 50(5):958–968.
51. Arai Y, Inaba Y, Yamamoto T, et al. A randomized phase II study of TSU-68 in patients (pts) with hepatocellular carcinoma (HCC) treated by transarterial chemoembolization (TACE). *J Clin Oncol* 2010; 28(suppl):15s (abstract 4030).
52. Okita K, Imanaka K, Chida N, et al. Phase III study of sorafenib in patients in Japan and Korea with advanced hepatocellular carcinoma (HCC) treated after transarterial chemoembolization (TACE). *ASCO 2010 Gastrointestinal Cancers Symposium.* LBA 128.
53. Abou-Alfa GK, Schwartz L, Ricci S, et al. Phase II study of sorafenib in patients with advanced hepatocellular carcinoma. *J Clin Oncol* 2006; 24:4293–4300.

Index

Note: Page numbers with italicised *f*'s and *t*'s refer to figures and tables, respectively.

Clinical Dilemmas in Primary Liver Cancer, First Edition. Edited by Roger Williams and Simon D. Taylor-Robinson.